DATE DUE

FEB 16 1995	
FEB 22 1995	
MAR - 7 1995	
MAR 18 1995	
MAR 3 1 1995	
OCT 17 1996	
JUL 24 1997	
APR 15 1999	
OCT - 8 1999	
JAN - 5 2000	
FEB - 1 2000	
FEB 2 2 2000	
APR 2 2 2000	
OCT 2 0 2001	
FEB 1 2 2002	
MAR 2 7 2002	

BRODART   Cat. No. 23-221

FORENSIC ANALYSIS OF THE SKULL

Craniofacial Analysis, Reconstruction, and Identification

FORENSIC ANALYSIS OF THE SKULL
Craniofacial Analysis, Reconstruction, and Identification

Editors

Mehmet Yaşar İşcan
Department of Anthropology
Florida Atlantic University
Boca Raton, Florida

Richard P. Helmer
Experimentelle Rechtsmedizin
Institut für Rechtsmedizin der Universität Bonn
Bonn, Germany

(W) **WILEY-LISS**
A JOHN WILEY & SONS, INC., PUBLICATION
New York • Chichester • Brisbane • Toronto • Singapore

Address all Inquiries to the Publisher
Wiley-Liss, Inc., 605 Third Avenue, New York, NY 10158-0012

Copyright © 1993 Wiley-Liss, Inc.

Printed in the United States of America.

Library of Congress Cataloging-in-Publication Data

Forensic analysis of the skull : craniofacial analysis,
   reconstruction, and identification / edited by Mehmet Yaşar İşcan
   and Richard P. Helmer.
      p. cm.
   Includes bibliographical references and index.
   ISBN 0-471-56078-2
    1. Forensic osteology. 2. Skull—Examination. I. İşcan, M.
Yaşar. II. Helmer, Richard P.
RA1059.F67   1993
611'.91—dc20   93-6838
                                        CIP

The text of this book is printed on acid-free paper.

Dedicated to
Ordinarius Professor Şevket Aziz Kansu (1903–1983)
The Founder of Turkish Biological Anthropology

Contents

Contributors

Tatiana S. Balueva (Doctorate, 1980) is a Senior Researcher at the Institute of Ethnography and Anthropology, Moscow. Specializing in facial reconstruction, her publications (in Russian) include: "Anthropological types in the ancient population in the USSR" (with Veselovskaya E, Lebedinskaya G, and Pestryakov A), in AA Zubov (ed.): *Anthropological Reconstructions,* 1988; "Neolithic cemeteries of northern Baraba, West Siberia" (with Polosmak NV and Chikisheva TA), in *Novosibirsk,* 1989; "Techniques of investigation of interconnections between morphological features of the face and their bony support" (with Lebedinskaya GV), *Antropologicheskaya rekonstrukciya,* 1991; and "Facial reconstruction from the skull by the combined graphic method with application of special pictures" (with Davyidova GM, Lebedinskaya GV, and Stepin VS), *Antropologicheskaya rekonstrukciya,* 1991.

Fred Brix (Ph.D., Medizinische Fakultät, 1987) is currently Privatdozent at Radiologische Abteilung of the Städtisches Krankenhaus in Kiel. Specializing in radiology, his publications include: "Vorstellung eines Styrodurschneide- und Fräsgerätes für Strahlentherapie," *Strahlentherapie,* 1981; "Verfahren und Vorrichtung für den Modellbau in Rahmen der orthopädischen und traumatologischen Operationsplanung" (with Hebbinghaus D and Meuer W), *Röntgenpraxis,* 1985; "Three typical clinical applications of a new irradiation technique" (with Christianse FR, Hancken C, and Quinn A), Radiotherapy and Oncology, 1988; and "Individuelle Schädelmodellherstellung auf der Grundlage computer-tomographischer Informationen" (with Lambrecht J), *Thieme-Verlag: Fortschritte der Kiefer- und Gesichts-Chirurgie,* 1988. He was awarded the 1987 Wilhelm C. Röntgenpreis Award and is a member of the Deutsche Röntgengesellschaft.

Cai Dongsheng is the Chief Forensic Medical Expert at the Tieling City Public Security Bureau. Specializing in forensic anthropology and identification, his publications include: "Study on photographic angle of skull-image superimposition," "Study on photographic distance in skull-image superimposition," and "Study on photographic method in skull-image superimposition" (all with Lan Y), *Criminal Technology (suppl.),* Beijing, 1982; and *Research Report of Skull-Image Superimposition on 3 Chinese Han Females,* Reference Room of 213 Institute, Tieling City. He was awarded the Second Class National Invention Prize for new technology in skull identification in December 1988 with Lan Y. He is a member of the Chinese Inventor Association.

P. Chandra Sekharan (Ph.D., University of Madras, 1986) is currently Director of the Forensic Sciences Department in Madras, India. He specializes in forensic skull identification and individualization. Some of his publications include: "Forensic science as is what is" (with Damodaran C), *Forensic Sci. Soc. India,* 1987; "A treatise on bank crime, prevention and detection," *Forensic Sci. Soc. India,* 1988; and "Frontiers of forensics," *Forensic Sci. Soc. India,* 1989. He was awarded the 1988 J.L. Eustace Memorial Award (Adelaide), and the 1992 Bharatiya Udyog Jyoti Award (New Delhi). He has served as the President of the Forensic Society of India, and is

ix

a member of the Forensic Science Society of the United Kingdom, and a Patron of the International Association of Forensic Odontologists.

Massimo Colonna is a Professor at the Institute of Legal Medicine of the University of Bari, Italy. His publications include: "Considerations sur cinq cas d'identification par superposition télevisée entre photo du visage et crâne" (with Pesce Delfino V and Introna F), *Pro. XII Cong. Int. Acad. Forensic Med.*, 1982; "Computer-aided skull-face superimposition by analytical procedures" (with Introna F, Potente F, Vacca V, and Pesce Delfino V), *Acta Medicinae Legalis et Socialis*, 1984; "Computer aided skull-face superimposition" (with Pesce Delfino V, Introna F, Potente M, and Vacca E), *Am. J. Forensic Med. Pathol.*, 1986; and "Identificazione personale," in P Martini (ed.): *Medicina Legale in Odontoiatria*, 1988. He is a member of the International Academy of Legal Medicine and Social Medicine, the Société Méditerrané de Medicine Legale, and the Società Italiana di Medicina Legale e Delle Assicurazioni.

Gloria Jean y'Edynak (Ph.D., Harvard University, 1974), formerly a Curator at the Armed Forces Medical Museum, is now an Instructor in the University College at the University of Maryland. Her publications include: "Yugoslav Mesolithic dental reduction," *Am. J. Phys. Anthropol.*, 1989; "Dental pathology: A factor in post-Pleistocene Yugoslav dental reduction," in JR Lukacs (ed.): *Culture, Ecology and Dental Anthropology*, 1992; and "Microevolution and biological adaptability in the transition from food-collecting to food-producing in the Iron Gates of Yugoslavia" (with S. Fleisch), *J. Hum. Evol.*, 1983. She is a member of the Dental Anthropology Association and the American Association of Physical Anthropologists.

Boris D. Fedosyutkin (Dr.Med.Sc., Russian Institute of Forensic Medicine, 1970) is currently a Senior Researcher at the Scientific Research Laboratory of the Criminalistics Center of the Russian Ministry of Internal Affairs, Moscow. An expert in personal identification, his publications include: *Identification from Skeletonized Remains* (with Dvorkin AI), 1977; *Facial Reconstruction from the Skull in Criminalistics* (with Korovjansky

OP, Usacheva LL, Kuzin VM, Savushkin AV, and Hohlov AE), 1990; *Crime Scene Determination of the Time of Death* (with Loktev VE), 1992; and "The first application of ultrasound for studies of the thickness of soft tissues of the face" (with Lebedinskaya G, Stepin V, Surnina T, and Tscherbin L), *Soviet Ethnography* (in Russian), 1979. He is a member of the Scientific Association of Forensic Medicine of Russia.

Robert McClellan George (Ph.D., University of Washington, Seattle, 1973) is presently a Professor of Anatomy at the Universidad Central del Caribe in Puerto Rico. Specializing in facial reconstruction, his publications include: "The limb musculature of the Tupaiidea," *Primates*, 1977; and "The lateral crainographic method of facial reconstruction," *J. Forensic Sci.*, 1987. He is a member of the American Academy of Forensic Sciences, the International Association for Identification, and the Association of Forensic Artists.

Holle Greil (Dr. sc. nat.) is currently at the Institut für Anthropologie of Humboldt Universität, Berlin. Her publications include: "Der Korperbau im Erwachsenenalter—repräsentative anthropologische Querschnittsstudir," *Promot. B.*, 1989; and "Mehrdimensionale Variabilität von Korperbaumassen im Erwachsenenalter," *R. Med.*, 1988.

Helmut Gremmel (Prof. Dr. med., Kiel, 1966) is currently Professor Emeritus Ehemaliger Ordinarius at the Universitätsklinik Kiel. Specializing in radiology, his many publications include: "Offene Verletzungen und Fremdkörper des Herzens und der herznahen Gefäße" (with Löhr HK, Kaiser K, and Vieten H), *Handbuch der med. Radiologie*, 1979; "Stumpftraumatische Schäden des Herzens und der großen herznahen Gefäße" (with Löhr HK, Kaiser K, and Vieten H), *Handbuch der med. Radiologie*, 1979; and "Strahlenschäden" (with Vieten H), *Das ärtzliche Gutachten im Versicherungswesen*, 1969. He is a member of the Deutsche Röntgengesellschaft and Norddeutsche Röntgengesellschaft.

Oskar Grüner became a full Professor in 1964 at the University of Giessen and is now Professor Emeritus (and former director) at the Institut für Rechtsmedizin der Christian-Albrechts-Universität Kiel. His publications include: "Bestimmung des Körperwassergehaltes mit Hilfe von Alkohol," *Klin. Wechr.*, 1957; "Ein photographisches Verfahren zur Schädelidentifizierung" (with Reinhard R), *Dtsch. Z. ges. gerichtl. Med.*, 1959; "Identification d'un crâne par superimposition à l'aide du mixage éléctronique des images" (with Helmer P), *Acta Med. Leg. Soc.*, 1980; and "Die rechtsmedizinische Identifizierung Bedeutung und Beweiswert," Z. Rechtsmed., 1957. In 1983 he received the Widmark Award from the International Committee on Alcohol, Drugs, and Traffic Safety. He is a member of the International Academy of Legal and Social Medicine, Deutsche Gesellschaft für Rechtsmedizin, and Deutsche Gesellschaft für Unfallchirurgie.

Hans-Joachim Hammer (Dr. med. habil., University of Leipzig, 1987) is a Senior Physician at the Institut für Gerichtliche Medizin, University of Leipzig. Specializing in forensic anthropology and hair, fingerprint, and ear analysis, his publications include: "Die metrischen und deskriptiven morphologischen Merkmale des Menschen—ein Studie über ihre Verteilung in einer DDR Population und ihre Bedeutung für die forensische Praxis," *Promot. B.*, 1986; "Zur Anwendbarkeit morphologischer Gesichtsmerkmale bei der Identifikation" (with Hunger H and Leopold D), *Kriminalistik forens. Wiss.*, 1981; *Identifikation* (edited with Leopold D), 1978; and "The identification of earprints secured at the scene of the crime," *Fingerprint Whorld*, 1986. He is a member of the Fingerprint Society.

Richard P. Helmer is presently a Professor in the Department of Experimental Forensic Medicine at the Institut für Rechtsmedizin, Bonn. His publications include: "Identifizierung" (with Grüner O), in B Mueller (ed.): *Gerichtliche Medizin,* 1975; "Schädelidentifizierung durch superprojection nach dem Verfahren der elektronischen Bildmischung, modifiziert zum Trickbild" (with Grüner O), *Differenz-Verfahren Z. Rechtmed.*, 1977; "On the conclusiveness of skull identification via the video superimposition technique" (with Schimmler J and Rieger J), *Can. Soc. Forensic Sci. J.*, 1989.

Mehmet Yaşar İşcan (Ph.D., Cornell University, 1976) is currently Professor and Chairman of the Department of Anthropology at Florida Atlantic University, Boca Raton, and a board certified Diplomate of the American Board of Forensic Anthropology. Specializing in skeletal biology and forensic anthropology, he has published numerous books and articles including: *The Human Skeleton in Forensic Medicine* (with Krogman WM), 1986; *Age Markers in the Human Skeleton* (editor), 1989; *Reconstruction of Life From the Skeleton* (edited with Kennedy KAR), 1989; and "Rise of forensic anthropology," *Yrbk. Phys. Anthropol.*, 1988. He was the recipient of the Aleš Hrdlička Fellowship (1968) and named Sigma Xi Distinguished Researcher of 1993. He has been awarded grants from the Japanese National Research Institute of Police Science, the Smithsonian Institution, and the United Nations. He is the founder and past president of the Dental Anthropology Association, a fellow of the American Academy of Forensic Sciences, and is a member of the American Anthropological Association and the American Association of Physical Anthropologists.

J. Thomas Lambrecht is currently Professor and Chairman of the Department of Oral Surgery at the University of Basel, Switzerland. Specializing in oral and maxillofacial plastic surgery, his many publications include: "Planning orthognathic surgery with three-dimensional models," *Int. J. Adult Orthodontics & Orthognathic Surgery,* 1989; "Morphological changes of isolated osteoclasts in cell culture" (with Ewers R, Kerscher A, and Jentzsch R), *Mar. Res. Soc. Symp. Proc.*, 1989; "Three-dimensional operation simulation in functional skeletal surgery" (with Brix F), *J. Japan Soc. Cranio-Maxillo-Facial Surgery,* 1990; and "Individual skull model fabrication for craniofacial surgery" (with Brix F), *Cleft Palate J.*, 1990. He received the best annual award of the German Association of Oral Surgery (1987) and the University Research Award of the German Federal Chamber of Dentistry. He is a member of the International Association for Oral and Maxillofacial Surgeons, the European Association for Cranio-Maxillo-Facial

Surgery, and the German Association for Plastic and Reconstructive Surgery.

Lan Yuwen is Director and Senior Engineer for the Tieling Public Security Bureau. He specializes in the study of skull-image superimposition, and his publications include: "Study on photographic angle of skull-image superimposition," "Study on photographic distance in skull-image superimposition," and Study on photographic method in skull-image superimposition" (all with Cai D), *Criminal Technology (suppl.),* 1982; and *Research Report of Skull-Image Superimposition on 3 Chinese Han Females,* Reference Room of 213 Institute, Tieling City. He was awarded the Second Class National Invention Prize for new technology in skull identification in December 1988 with Cai D.

Galina V. Lebedinskaya (Doctorate, 1970) heads the Laboratory of Anthropological Reconstruction at the Institute of Ethnography and Anthropology of the Russian Academy of Sciences, Moscow. Specializing in facial reconstruction, her numerous publications (in Russian) include: "On the problem of reproduction of the actual shape of the eyes in reconstructions of the face of the skull," *Short Communications of the Ethnographic Institute of USSR Academy of Sciences, Moscow,* 1957; "Correlations between the upper part of the facial skull and the tissues covering it," in *Anthropological Reconstructions and Problems in Palaeoethnography* (edited with GV Rabinovich), 1973; "Plastic reconstruction of the face on the skull and its developmental trends," *Soviet Ethnography,* 1976; and "The first experience of application of ultrasound for the studies of the thickness of soft tissues of the face" (with Stepin VS, Surnina TS, Fedosyutkin BA, and Tscherbin LA), *Soviet Ethnography,* 1979.

Dieter Leopold (Dr. med. habil., University of Leipzig, 1969) is presently working as Director of the Institut für Gerichtliche Medizin at the Medizinische Akademie Erfurt, where he is also a Professor. His areas of specialization include identification of the living and the dead, head and vertebral injury, and medical aspects of death and alcohol. His many books and articles include:

Identifikation (with Hunger K), 1978; "Identifikation durch Scädeluntersuchungen unter besonderer Berücksichtigung der Superprojektion," *Habil. Schr.,* 1968; "Die Superprojecktion—eine Möglichkeit zur Identifikation," *Kriminalistik u. forens. Wiss.,* 1971; and "Erfahrungen bei Katastrophenuntersuchungen in der DDR unter besonderer Berücksichtigung der Superprojektion," *Acta Med. Leg.,* 1973. He is a member of the Royal Society of Medicine, Society of Forensic Medicine, Society of Neuro-Surgery and Neuro-Traumatology, and the Association of German Anthropology.

Teresa Lettini (Ph.D., 1992) is currently a Researcher at the Digamma Research Consortium in Bari, Italy, and specializes in image processing and morphometry, anthropology, and forensic pathology. Her publications include: "A case of identification by skull-face computer aided superimposition" (with Colonna M, Potente F, Vacca E, and Pesce Delfino V), *12th International Congress of Anthropological and Ethnological Sciences,* 1988; "Valutazione computerizzata della sovrapposizione cranio-foto del viso: Utilizzazione de un nuovo parametro" (with Potente F, Vacca E, and Pesce Delfino V), *Rassegna Medico-Forense,* 1987; and "Analytical description of cranial profiles by means of Kth order polynomial equations, and application of *Plesianthropus transvaalensis* (STS5)" (with Pesce Delfino V, Vacca E and Potente F), *Anthropologie,* 1987.

Susan R. Loth (Ph.D. candidate, University of the Witwatersrand) is Adjunct Professor of Anthropology at Florida Atlantic University. Specializing in human skeletal biology, her numerous publications include: "Age estimation from the rib by phase analysis: White males" (with İşcan MY and Wright RK), *J. Forensic Sci.,* 1984; "Racial variation at the sternal extremity of the rib and its effect on age determination" (with İşcan MY and Wright RK), *J. Forensic Sci.,* 1987; "A comparative analysis of the ribs of Terry Collection blacks," *Adli Tip Dergisi (Istanbul),* 1990; and "Morphological indicators of skeletal aging: Implications for paleodemography and paleo-gerontology" (with İşcan MY) in DE Crews and RM Garruto (eds.): *Biological Anthropology and Aging,* 1993. She was awarded the Lambda Alpha National Scholarship Award and Certificate of Distinguished Achievement, and grants from Sigma Xi, the Smithsonian Institution, and Florida Atlantic University, and has been inducted into The Honor Society of Phi Kappa Phi. She served as editor of the *Dental Anthropology Newsletter* and is currently on the editorial board. She is a member of the American Association of Physical Anthropologists and the Dental Anthropology Association.

F. Möhr is a design artist on the staff of the Opera in Hamburg, Germany.

Jonas V. Nainys (Dr.Med.Sc., Kaunas University Medical Faculty, 1945) headed the Department of Anatomy and Forensic Medicine at the Kaunas Medical Institute in Lithuania until his death on September 18, 1989. Credited with founding the field of forensic medicine in Lithuania, his more than 200 publications included: "Ergebnisse und Aussichten der forensisch-osteologischen Forschungen zur Personenidentifizierung" (with Swajagin WJ), *Kriminalistik u. forens. Wiss.,* 1984; and "Postmortale Veränderungen in den Nervenzellen und Transmitteraktivität des begetativen Nervensystems des Herzens" (with Ashelis V and Stropus R), *Kriminalistik u. forens. Wiss.,* 1980. He was Chairman of the Lithuanian Scientific Medico-Legal and Criminalistic Association.

Vladimír Novotný (Ph.D., Masaryk University, 1982) formerly of the Czechoslovak Academy of Sciences, is currently a Professor in the Department of Anthropology at Masaryk University, Brno, Czech Republic. Specializing in morphology, his publications include: "Sex determination of the pelvic bone: A systems approach," *Anthropologie,* 1986; "Systems approach in morphology," in *General Questions of Evolution,* Czech. Academy of Sciences, 1983; "Sex differences of pelvis and sex determination in paleoanthropology," *Anthropologie,* 1983; and "Systems aspects of the sexual dimorphism in human lower limb" (with Vancata V), in *Evolution and Morphogenesis,* 1985. He is a member of

the European Anthropological Association, Czech Anthropological Association, and the Craniofacial Identification Group.

Vittorio Pesce Delfino is associated with the Consorzio di Ricerca Digamma. Specializing in analytical morphometry, his many publications include: "Remarks on analytic morphometry in biology: Procedure and software illustration" (with Ricco R), *Acta Stereologica,* 1983; "Identification by computer aided skull face superimposition" (with Colonna M, Introna F, Potente F, and Vacca E), *11th International Congress of Anthropological and Ethnological Sciences,* 1983; "Computer-aided skull/face superimposition (with Colonna M, Vacca E, Potente F, and Introna F), *Am. J. Forensic Med. Pathol.,* 1986; and "Analytical description of cranial profiles by means of Kth order polynomial equations, and application on *Plesianthropus transvaalensis* (STS5)" (with Vacca E, Lettini T, and Potente F), *Anthropologie,* 1987.

D. Petersen is a dentist in Flensburgh, Germany. His publications include: "Die plastische Gesichts-weichteilrekonstruction als Möglichkeit zur Identifizierung unbekannter Schädel" (with Röhricht S), *(I) Med. Dis.,* 1989.

F. Potente (Università degli Studi di Bari, 1984) is presently a Researcher at the Consorzio di Ricerca "Digamma." Her publications include: "Computer aided skull-face superimposition" (with Pesce Delfino V, Colonna M, Vacca E, and Introna F Jr), *Am. J. Forensic Med. and Pathol.,* 1986; "Shape Evaluation in Medical Image Analysis" (with Pesce Delfino V, Lettini T, Vacca E, Ragone P, and Ricco R), *European Microscopy and Analysis,* 1990; and "Analytical Morphometry of the Neanderthal Cranium from Monte Circeo (Circeo 1)" (with Pesce Delfino V, Vacca E, Lettini T, and Ragone, P), in *The Circeo 1 Neanderthal Skull, Studies and Documentation,* 1991. She is a member of the European Anthropological Association, the Unione Antropologi Italiani, and the Società Italiana di Biologia Sperimentale.

Jürgen Rieger is a dentist in Berlin. His publications include: "On the conclusiveness of skull identification via the video superimposition technique" (with Helmer R and Schimmler J), *Can. Soc. Forens. Sci. J.*, 1989; and "Value of skull identification as evidence using a superimposed videoimage technic with reference to individual craniometric differences in the human skull" (with Helmer R and Schimmler J), *Zeitschrift für Rechtsmedizin* (in German), 1989.

Stefan Röhricht is a dentist in Kiel, Germany. His publications include: "Die plastische Gesichtsweichteilrekonstruction als Möglichkeit zur Identifizierung unbekannter Schädel" (with Petersen D), *Med. Dis.*, 1989.

Jörg Burkhard Schimmler (Ph.D., 1974) is presently at the Rechenzentrum of the Christian-Albrechts-Universität Kiel. Specializing in applied statistics, his publications include: "On the conclusiveness of skull identification via the video superimposition technique" (with Helmer R and Rieger J), *Can. Soc. Forens. Sci. J.*, 1989; and "Value of skull identification as evidence using a superimposed videoimage technic [sic] with reference to individual craniometric differences in the human skull" (with Helmer R and Rieger J), *Zeitschrift für Rechtsmedizin* (in German), 1989.

Sueshige Seta (Ph.D., University of Tokyo, 1972) is Director of Research at the National Research Institute of Police Science in Tokyo. He specializes in comparative anatomy and has also worked in the areas of cell pathology, electron microscopic analysis, and forensic DNA typing. His publications include: "Forensic hair investigation" (with Sato H and Miyake B), *Forensic Sci. Progress*, 1986; "Classification system of frontal sinus patterns by radiography, its application to identification of unknown skeletal remains" (with Yoshino M, Miyasaka S, and Sato H.), *Forensic Sci. Int.*, 1987; *Personal Identification of the Human Skull: Superimposition and Radiographic Techniques* (with Yoshino M), 1989; and "Microscopical study on estimation of time since death in skeletal remains" (with Yoshino M, Kimijima T, Miyasaka S, and Sato H), *Forensic Sci. Int.*, 1991. He is a member of Japanese Association of Anatomists, Clinical Electron Microscopy Society of Japan, and the Medico-Legal Society of Japan.

E. Vacca (Ph.D., Università degli Studi di Bari, 1991) is a Researcher at the Consorzio di Ricerca "Digamma" at the Università di Bari. His publications include: "Computer aided skull-face superimposition" (with Pesce Delfino V, Colonna M, Potente F, and Introna F), *Am. J. Forensic Med. and Pathol.*, 1986; "Shape Evaluation in Medical Image Analysis" (with Pesce Delfino V, Potente F, Lettini T, Ragone P, and Ricco R), *European Microscopy and Analysis,* 1990; "Analytical morphies on mid-sagittal craniograms glabella-opisthocranion of *Homo erectus* and *Homo sapiens neanderthalensis*" (with Pesce Delfino V), *Boll. Soc. It. Biol. Sper.*, 1991; and "Analytical Morphometry of the Neanderthal Cranium from Monte Circeo (Circeo 1)" (with Pesce Delfino V, Potente F, Lettini T, and Ragone, P), in *The Circeo 1 Neanderthal Skull, Studies and Documentation,* 1991. He is a member of the European Anthropological Association, the Unione Antropologi Italiani, and the Società Italiana di Biologia Sperimentale.

Elizabeth V. Veselovskaya (Doctorate, 1990) is a Junior Researcher at the Institute of Ethnography and Anthropology at the Russian Academy of Sciences, Moscow. Specializing in facial reconstruction, her publications (in Russian) include: "Age-dependence of changes in the facial soft tissues in Bashkirs," in VV Koroteyeva (ed.): *Ethnography, Anthropology and Related Disciplines: Interrelations Between Objects and Methods,* 1989; "Anthropological types of ancient populations in the USSR" (with Lebedinskaya GV, Balueva TS, and Pestryakov AP), in AA Zubov (ed.): *Anthropological Reconstructions,* 1988; "New anthropological features in plastic reconstruction" (with Balueva TS), *Sovetskaya yetnografiya,* 1989; "Variability of soft tissue thickness of the face of Bashkirs in comparison with other groups" (with Lebedinskaya GV), *Antropologiya Bashkirskogo Naroda,* 1990; and "Peculiarities of intergroup variability of features of facial soft tissue thickness," *Antropologicheskaya rekonstrukciya,* 1991.

Mineo Yoshino (Ph.D., Saitama Medical School, 1992) is currently a Senior Researcher at the National Research Institute of Police Science in Tokyo. He specializes in legal medicine and has also worked in forensic osteology and cell pathology. His publications include: "Classification system of frontal sinus patterns by radiography, its application to identification of unknown skeletal remains" (with Miyasaka S and Sato H), *Forensic Sci. Int.,* 1987; *Personal Identification of the Human Skull: Superimposition and Radiographic Techniques* (with Seta S), 1989; "Ultrastructural and cytochemical changes of rabbit brains in hypoxic state" (with Kimijima T, Miyasaka S, Sato H, Miyake B, and Seta S), *Proc. Int. Symp. Adv. in Legal Med.,* 1990; and "Microscopical study on estimation of time since death in skeletal remains" (with Kimijima T, Miyasaka S, and Sato H), *Forensic Sci. Int.,* 1991. He is a member of the Japanese Association of Anatomists, Clinical Electron Microscopy Society of Japan, and the Medico-Legal Society of Japan.

Preface

For over a century, attempts have been made to translate the bony skull into a likeness of its owner, yet the greatest strides in this quest have resulted from technological advances in only the last few decades. Therefore, the purpose of this book is to bring together reports on the latest progress in identifying individuals from their skulls and photographic evidence.

This international effort offers a critical review of the scientific literature and an assessment of methodological advances and problems. The topics are put in perspective with the inclusion of factors arising from human evolution and growth, the importance of such basic determinations as age, sex, and race from the skull, and facial constitution. This book introduces diverse technical and methodological developments in the area of skull-photo superimposition and facial reconstruction from the skull, as well as the first attempt to establish standards for photographic comparisons.

The idea for this volume originated when the editors met at the annual meeting of the International Association of Forensic Sciences held in Vancouver, British Columbia, Canada, in 1987. They discussed organization of a special workshop on these recent advances. Under Helmer's direction, "Advances in Skull Identification via Video Superimposition," was held on August 3-5, 1988 in Kiel, Germany. Invited speakers came from Australia, Canada, the People's Republic of China, Czechoslovakia, France, India, Italy, Japan, Russia, the United Kingdom, and the United States. To arrange the most comprehensive treatment of the subject, several additional respected members of the profession were later invited to contribute to this book.

The authors are most grateful to Susan R. Loth for her editorial work. She struggled through every chapter, skillfully "translating" foreign expressions that had been rendered literally into English. We are very appreciative of the assistance of Natileene Cassel for taking care of details needed for figures and non-English characters. She also organized the Contributors section. We thank Bill Watkins, Kay Gutierrez, and Jude Turner for their photographic expertise, and Steve Kika and Sherri L. Hartman for the art work. We also appreciate the patience of Dr. Bill Curtis of Wiley-Liss, especially with all the delays, and thank Mr. Rick Mumma of the production department at Wiley-Liss for his helpfulness and attention to detail. Finally, this project would not have been possible without the hard work and cooperation of the contributors.

The symposium and the preparation of this book were partially supported by the Deutsche Forschungsgemeinschaft, Germany, and Florida Atlantic University, USA.

Mehmet Yaşar İşcan
Richard P. Helmer

Chapter 1
Craniofacial Image Analysis and Reconstruction

Mehmet Yaşar İşcan

Department of Anthropology, Florida Atlantic University, Boca Raton, Florida 33431

One of the goals of forensic science is to reconstruct the scene of a crime, including the identities of all involved. Every bit of evidence must be analyzed to recreate the events surrounding a death or robbery. This requires the well-coordinated participation of many types of forensic scientists, each contributing their own particular expertise to add another piece of the puzzle.

There are basically two kinds of evidence: biological and peripheral. Biological evidence consists of both the solid and liquid components of the body itself (e.g., isolated teeth and bones, blood, saliva, etc.). Peripheral evidence encompasses anything in physical proximity to the remains or having a causal or circumstantial connection to the case. This constitutes the context of the crime scene and may include personal belongings of both the victim and the criminal. Such items as personal photographs, videotapes, and antemortem X-rays are of particular interest when identification is the aim.

A key focus of any investigation is the identification of criminals and their victims. This is the realm of forensic anthropology. One of the most difficult but important tasks these scientists undertake is to recapture the living appearance of an individual from skeletonized remains or to connect a photograph with a person or another photograph. This process often begins with an analysis of a skeleton to determine its most basic characteristics—age, sex, race, stature, etc. The next step is to uncover skeletal peculiarities that may further distinguish this individual from others and to attempt to recreate a likeness. These activities center on bio-logical evidence. In cases where there are no other clues, an attempt to reconstruct the face from the skull is the only option if a general description of the victim does not elicit a possible match from authorities or the public.

The next phase including superimposition or photo matching—requires the interaction of biological and peripheral evidence. This may include a picture of a missing person or clothing that may indicate size and confirm sex. If there is a picture, the forensic anthropologist may try to superimpose it on the skull. Finally, in some cases there might be no biological evidence—only peripheral items like photographs of a missing person or a surveillance videotape of a bank robber. In this case the expert can only analyze this piece of evidence against pictures of a known individual.

Within the scientific tradition of biological anthropology, skeletal biologists study the human skeleton, including cranial and facial morphology. Forensic anthropology is a subdiscipline that covers all aspects of the analysis of human skeletal remains in a legal context. This of course extends to encompass facial reconstruction, superimposition, and photographic comparison. The field is well established and was pioneered by scholarly contributions from around the world (Krogman and İşcan, 1986). The history of its development has been summarized in a number of publications.

Of the identification techniques mentioned above, facial reconstruction is the most popular and enduring. Krogman and İşcan (1986) trace the origin of this method to His's work in 1895. Facial reconstruction was originally attempted to give fleshed form to early hominids and to validate remains of historic figures, as well as for forensic applications. Gerasimov (1964, 1971) was probably the first to try paleo-anthropological reconstruction to gauge the physiognomic appearance of ancient people. His tradition continued through his students, such as Lebedinskaya and others (e.g., Lebedinskaya, 1957; Balueva et al., 1988), whose attention turned to the many ethnic groups of the former USSR. Gerasimov's influence can also be seen in the work of Rişcuţia (1966), Yordanov (1981), and Ullrich (1966) in Eastern Europe. Although they later used their skills in assisting law enforcement agencies, it was Krogman who popularized its application to the forensic field (Krogman and McCue, 1946; Krogman et al., 1948). In his 1962 book, Krogman presented his method in detail, showing step by step how to reconstruct a face on a skull (Krogman and İşcan, 1986). The method was later modified in the enlarged and expanded version by Krogman and İşcan (1986). In a relatively short time, this method became a standard technique, routinely used by many practitioners (Snow et al., 1970; Suzuki, 1973; Farrar, 1977; Gatliff, 1984). While reconstruction may give a more "lifelike" three-dimensional appearance, some forensic anthropologists also advocated the creation of two-dimensional drawings from the skull (Cherry and Angel, 1977; İşcan and Charney, 1981; Krogman and İşcan, 1986). The advantages of drawings are that the procedure is simpler and less expensive and that the skull is kept uncovered and available for other types of analysis.

Superimposition can also lead to identification by comparing a skull with the photograph of a missing person. In this approach, one image is usually superimposed over another. Krogman and İşcan (1986) note that as early as 1883, Welcker made the first attempt to compare a skull with the portrait of a historical figure. One of the earliest superimpositions was done by Pearson (1926), who matched the skull of George Buchanan with his portrait. In this work, Pearson offered a detailed list of steps to follow. The first forensic application of skull-to-photo com-

parison was carried out by Glaister and Brash (1937) for the Buck Ruxton case. The case involved two skulls presumably from the bodies of Isabella Ruxton and housemaid Mary Rogerson. These were compared with ¾, full, and profile portraits of Mrs. Ruxton.

This successfully proven case gained considerable attention and was followed by many other attempts (Malinowski and Porawski, 1970; Yoshino et al., 1981; McKenna et al., 1984; Taylor et al., 1984). The earlier studies were mostly modifications of the procedure used by Glaister and Brash (1937); that is, photographs of the portrait and skull were enlarged and compared in transparencies with features on the skull. The superimposition procedure changed from a simple overlaying of negatives to drawing the contours of the face in the picture and superimposing this on the skull, as was done in the Ruxton case (Prinsloo, 1953; Sen, 1962; Gupta, 1969; Chandra Sekharan, 1971; Janssens et al., 1978). The most technical approach was pursued by Grüner and Reinhard (1959) using a transparent optical stand and is detailed by Grüner in Chapter 3, this volume.

Although considerable attention was concentrated on the technical development of superimposition, there were other problems and improvements needed, such as gauging the enlargement of the photograph and positioning the skull to match the picture. Approaches ranged from estimation of the size of background objects in the photograph to use of the interpupillary to bizygomatic breadth and facial tissue thickness (Chandra Sekharan, 1973; Reddy, 1973; Maat, 1989; Chee and Cheng, 1989; Yoshino and Seta, 1989). Mechanical mounting devices have greatly improved skull positioning (Grüner and Reinhard, 1959; Ishibashi, 1986; Chandra Sekharan, 1988; McKenna, 1988; Brocklebank and Holmgren, 1989; Seta and Yoshino, 1990; Kumari and Chandra Sekharan, 1992).

Once video cameras and accessories such as mixing and editing units became readily available, the traditional approach to superimposition was supplanted by electronic methods. With these modern tools, one image can simply be superimposed over another taken by a second camera. This procedure eliminates many of the problems associated with earlier methods. Instantaneous, precise sizing is accomplished by simply turning a knob. This saves many hours in the darkroom making photographic enlargements. Mixers create many types of overlay comparisons (fading, side-to-side, and top-to-bottom sweeps). Another advantage of a video-based system is that the procedure and results are easy to demonstrate and explain in court because each step is recorded and can be illustrated when needed. If, for example, one is particularly concerned with the relationship of the dentition and jaws on the skull to the mouth on the picture, the cameras can be focused on those areas in both the skull and photograph. Video superimposition quickly became the method of choice for many practitioners (Koelmeyer, 1982; Hagemeier, 1983; Pesce Delfino et al., 1986; Krogman and İşcan, 1986; Helmer, 1987; Chai et al., 1989). One of the earliest attempts at video superimposition was carried out by Helmer and Grüner (1977). An authoritative book on the subject was written by Helmer (1984).

The technologic advantages offered by personal computers have led many investigators to attempt to overcome the challenge of superimposition through the development of different ways of comparing skulls and photographs. Most of these new studies rely on digitization to objectively quantify the characteristics that make faces different. Thus human subjectivity and the physical limits on our ability to detect minute differences can be nearly eliminated by entrusting the evaluation and comparison to a computer. Examples of this approach include Pesce Delfino et al. (Chapter 11, this volume) and a number of other recent publications (e.g., Majumdar and Sinha, 1989; Nickerson et al., 1991; Evenhouse et al., 1992).

The need for another kind of analysis, identification of an individual from a photograph or video image, is arising more often, presumably because of the plethora of surveillance cameras to deter crime. Since this is a relatively new phenomenon, there has not been much method-ological development or case studies published in this area. Standards must be set for both the assessment of morphologic variation and photoanthropometric analysis based on a solid understanding of facial anatomy and how it can be quantified from photographs.

As indicated above, the purpose of this book is to provide a state-of-the-art treatment of craniofacial identification and reconstruction. The editor realized the need for a publication on this subject and decided that research presented at Helmer's 1988 symposium in Kiel, Germany, would be an excellent basis for a book. To make this work the most complete compilation on the subject to date, the editor also added chapters from other experts.

This book is divided into five parts. Part 1 deals with the evolution and growth of the human craniofacial complex, and historical development in skull–face identification. Chapter 2 by y'Edynak and İşcan sets the stage in terms of evolutionary and growth-related changes in the cranium, particularly the masticatory apparatus. The major changes in the skull are described from the enlargement of the brain case to cranial flexure that reorganized the relationship of the head and face. The chapter addresses the causes and effects of temporal changes in the craniofacial structure and masticatory apparatus as well as tooth size in terms of environmental and genetic factors. There is a summary of growth-related changes in the head and face. It is noted that growth in this part of the body is complete in the first decade of life, but remodeling continues to alter appearance throughout life.

Grüner provides historical perspective in Chapter 3 with a summary of the development of skull–photo superimposition from its early years until today. He credits individuals such as Schaaffhausen (1875), Welcker (1883), and His (1895) for their early technical contributions to skull–portrait matching and discusses technical problems associated with superimposition. The author reintroduces his superprojection technique (Grüner and Reinhard, 1959), preferring the term "superprojection" to separate it from video-based superimposition. A list of step-by-step instructions for positioning the skull and photograph is included. The chapter ends by emphasizing the individuality of the human head.

Part 2 deals with facial morphology and constitution and the vital role they play in the developing field of photo-to-photo comparison. Chapter 4, by Leopold, Hammer, and Greil, presents a somatometric analysis of the head and face. The authors first describe the range of facial appearance and associate it with somatological types. Their purpose is to develop a systematic and objective analysis of the face using anthropometric data. Using stepwise discriminant function analysis, they found that sexing accuracy was 61% for male and 78% for female pyknomorphs. These figures were somewhat lower in leptomorphs. The chapter discusses facial morphology and overall body constitution based on numerous anthropometric dimensions of the head and body. The authors also conducted a factor analysis in which these dimensions were coordinated with robusticity and plasticity.

In Chapter 5, İşcan describes the methods he has developed for photographic comparison. This technology is needed to determine if a photograph or video image matches a known individual. The author offers three approaches, of which morphological comparison should be the most effective. He includes a table listing basic features of the face that should also act as a guide to a systematic examination. The photo-anthropometric approach applies standard anthropometric methods to photographic measurements. This is particularly useful for eliminating individuals rather than proving identity. Finally, İşcan ends with a discussion of the difficulties of photo-to-photo superimposition.

Part 3 is designed to provide basic information for skull identification and individualization in terms of age, sex, and race. Novotný, İşcan, and Loth (Chapter 6) review several current techniques to determine these characteristics from the skull, and make it clear that identification and reconstruction cannot proceed if these attributes are not correctly ascertained. Age assessment in children is easy using dental development and epiphyseal closure, but differ-

entiating the sexes is very difficult until adolescence. The opposite is true in adults—race and sex are often clearly demonstrable in the skull, while only the roughest guess of age is possible from this part of the skeleton. Sutural closure and dental attrition should only be used if the skull is the only part recovered. These authors stress the importance of postcranial age estimation methods for adults, like that of the rib-phase technique, which has proven accurate and reliable in forensic cases. This chapter presents a number of ways that sex can be determined both morphologically and metrically. Although the pelvis is the best site for sexing, the skull is a close second. Despite the proliferation of discriminant function formulae from the skull and elsewhere, the authors recommend a morphologic approach. The discussion of race includes a clear statement of the significance of and specific need for this often controversial term in the forensic arena. This section focuses on differentiating the three major groups—Caucasoid, Mongoloid, and Negroid. As with sexing, the authors present statistical formulae using cranial dimensions, but conclude that morphologic evaluation is the most effective.

Although it is commonly assumed that the human cranium is unique, the question has not been systematically analyzed. In Chapter 7, Schimmler, Helmer, and Rieger use their earlier work as a starting point to tackle this issue (Helmer et al., 1989a,b). Using eight cranial measurements, they statistically demonstrate that craniometric individuality is as distinctive as fingerprints. They note that lateral views exhibit more uniqueness than frontal ones, but a combination of the two increases the likelihood of successful discrimination. The success rate drops when the statistical model is applied to (two-dimensional) photographs. This determination is also affected by mensural errors.

Chapter 8 (by Lambrecht, Brix, and Gremmel) features the development of a reverse reconstruction technique. They use computed tomographic (CT) data and a video visualization system on a living subject's head and feed that information to a three-dimensional carving machine that recreates the skull from a styrofoam block. The system is based on Gillespie and Isherwood's (1986) three-dimensional anatomic modeling procedure and a carving machine developed by Brix et al. (1985). Once the CT series is obtained, the skull is carved from a styrofoamlike substance. The authors claim that the system would be especially beneficial when a skull is incomplete, damaged, or needs restoration.

Part 4 covers new technical developments in skull–photo superimposition. Chandra Sekharan (Chapter 9) sets forth his revised technique for orienting the skull on a motor-driven stand. He demonstrates how to estimate the orientation angle in a picture, calculate its equivalent in the skull, and precisely place it in the same position.

In Chapter 10, Lan and Cai introduce a new technique to determine objective length, the angle of superimposition, and head size from the photograph. Using 19 angles from 100 Chinese males, the authors explain how they obtain the photographic angle from the tilt (pitch) and rotation (deflection) of the head. They calculate a deflection index formed from the distances from glabella to the right and the left ectoconchions. The pitch index is formed by comparing the distances from nasospinale to glabella and gnathion. Both of these indices decrease as the photographic angle increases. Next, the authors calculate natural head size using photographs in an experiment on 120 Chinese females. They found that the estimation of natural head size (based on bi-ectoconchionic distance) becomes less accurate as the deflection angle increases, especially if it is greater than 40°. The chapter continues with the determination of ideal camera–subject distance. Tests on 10 skulls using various distances from 0.7 m to 3 m revealed that a 1-m objective length is optimal. They also note that some areas on the face—primarily where the face is perpendicular to the camera–subject axis—remain unchanged, no matter what length is chosen. The authors conclude with the introduction of their own superimposition apparatus, consisting of an optical system, skull-positioning

device, and a mechanism for viewing the superimposition.

Chapter 11, by Pesce Delfino, Vacca, Potente, Lettini, and Colonna, delineates their highly technical shape-analysis system, called Shape Analytic Morphometry (SAM), and details improvements since it was first introduced in 1980 (Colonna et al., 1980, 1984). The authors begin by explaining that shape-analytic morphometry allows reliable superimposition, as well as evaluating congruency between the skull and photographs. Necessary equipment for SAM includes a video camera, optical device, digital monitor attached to a computer, an analog monitor, video image printer, and VCR. The video camera is used to take the images of both skull and picture through the optical device, which is placed in front of the camera. The image is processed by the computer, sent to the analog monitor to avoid distortion, and then sent to the digitized monitor for viewing. Once the superimposition is accomplished, congruency is analyzed numerically using three different approaches. The polynomial procedure is used to smooth the curve of the profile and reduce anomalies on the photograph. Fourier harmonics assess the superimposition by calculating the sine–cosine coefficients and determining the amplitude and phase values of each harmonic contributor. The third (Janus) procedure is designed to judge the symmetry between the profiles of the skull and photographs. The authors test their method on a number of skulls and photographs and conclude that SAM incorporates both size and shape differences between the two objects. Furthermore, although the three procedures are independent, they can be combined to arrive at a final single evaluator. They indicate that at its present stage of development, the method may be more effective in excluding, rather than proving, a match. Similar conclusions were also reached by İşcan (1988) and Seta and Yoshino in the next chapter.

Seta and Yoshino developed an apparatus for setting up cameras and objects to be analyzed and describe it in Chapter 12. During my visit to the Japanese National Research Institute of Police Science, I observed this system and can report that it is very precise and efficient. It consists of a well-lit chamber containing a skull-positioning device flanked by separate video cameras for the skull and picture, a mixer, VCR, and monitor. With the mixing unit, images can be shown and compared in a number of ways (e.g., fade-out and wiping). The results are recorded with the VCR. The authors discuss several of their cases and agree that skull–photo superimposition may be reliable under exacting conditions. However, as noted earlier, they state that it is more effective in ruling out a match rather than in establishing one.

Chapter 13, by Cai and Lan, reports an elaborate test of skull–photo superimposition. In their study, the authors took radiographs of 224 Chinese males and females on whom numerous facial landmarks were identified and marked in lead prior to X-raying. They developed four groups of standards, including landmarks, examination lines, soft tissue thickness, and contours, and applied them to 1,000 female photographs. The contour curve and examination lines yielded the best result. The authors recommend that this method be tested across a wider age range and different racial groups.

Part 5 concentrates on facial reconstruction from the skull. Tissue depth calculation, radiographic analysis of facial dimensions and bony features, and palpation of the facial tissues are discussed in Chapter 14, using samples from many ethnic groups in the former USSR. Lebedinskaya, Balueva, and Veselovskaya present a partial summary of Veselovskaya's (1989) doctoral dissertation. Their use of an ultrasound system to measure tissue thickness was pioneered by Lebedinskaya et al. in 1979. In their radiographic analysis of the face, these authors stress that the reconstruction of the nose is the most difficult part and they present their own procedure. They consider their palpatory examination of the face and underlying skull features more effective than the radiographic approach, which has numerous technical problems. Their findings are accompanied by regression analyses.

In this regard, it should be noted that since tissue thickness is population-specific, all racial and geographic groups should be assessed, be-cause the results from one may not apply to another. Therefore, I think it is important to refer to other radiographic studies of tissue thickness. Altemus (1963) researched American whites and blacks of both sexes (ages 12 to 16), and Heglar and Parks (1980) studied white boys and girls (age range of 10–18 years). There are a number of studies of adult facial tissue thickness (e.g., Helmer, 1984; Hodson et al., 1985). Before the popularity of the ultrasonic technique, a needle with measuring scale was probed into standard locations on the face. This was done extensively over the years, but most recently by Rhine and Campbell (1980) and Rhine et al. (1982) on American whites and blacks of both sexes. Suzuki (1948) and Ogawa (1960) conducted pioneering work on facial tissue thickness in the Japanese.

Chapter 15 was written by Fedosyutkin and Nainys (who died on September 18, 1989, about a year after the presentation of his paper at the symposium in Kiel). This chapter begins with a summary of facial reconstruction attempts in Eastern Europe and Russia, but is basically a detailed description of the relationship of bony features of the skull to soft tissue features of the face. Their use of illustrations of each feature makes it easier to follow.

George (Chapter 16) introduces a set of standard guidelines for facial reconstruction. He explains and compares facial reconstruction techniques, e.g., two-dimensional versus three-dimensional procedures. Basic Caucasoid features that seem to play an important role in facial recognition are outlined, along with some of the most frequently used landmarks for facial analysis. He also covers the more subjective phase of reconstruction with step-by-step artistic canons for such areas as facial heights, proportional relationships between the nose, lips, and chin, and features in the orbital region and facial triangle formed by the canthi and the mid-upper lip. George advises that these canons should be followed carefully and care must be taken not to substitute artistic "ideals." The chapter ends with the admonition that forensic facial reconstruction is at best a "scientific art" and it is not possible to achieve 100% accuracy with our current state of technology.

The last chapter, by Helmer, Röhricht, Petersen, and Möhr, is a double-blind test of facial reconstructions made by two of the authors. They each reconstructed the same 12 skulls. When compared to each other, a "close resemblance" was produced in 33% of the cases and "slight resemblance" was seen in only 17%. When the reconstructions were compared to photographs of the actual individuals, an average of 38% bore a "close resemblance," while 42% evinced only "slight resemblance." When hair color, length, and style were made available, the reconstructions became even more recognizable.

The papers presented here leave no doubt that there is considerable international interest in developing and improving techniques that would make identification easier and more reliable. This book contains the experience and results of scientific investigations from scholars around the world. In all cases they have enunciated the problems affecting the reliability of their methods in craniofacial identification.

Finally, it must be concluded that the skull does not provide all of the clues needed to indicate many aspects of soft tissue formations. Therefore, despite recent advances, it is still valid to state that a person is recognized by "many little *details*, [and] so many subtle *nuances*" that even a relative likeness is considered an achievement (Krogman and İşcan, 1986).

REFERENCES

Altemus A (1963) Comparative integumental relationships. Angle Orthod 33:217–221.

Balueva TS, Veselovskaya EV, and Lebedinskaya GV (1988) Antropologecheskie Tiipu Drevnego Naseleniaj na Territoree (Anthropological Types of the Ancient Population of the USSR). Moscow: Nauka (in Russian).

Brix F, Hebbinghaus D, and Meyer W (1985) Verfahren und Vorrichtung für den Modellbau im Rahmen der orthopädischen und traumatologischen Operationsplanung. Röntgenpraxis 38:290–292.

Brocklebank LM, and Holmgren CJ (1989) Development of equipment for the standardization of skull photographs in personal identifications by photographic superimposition. J Forensic Sci 34(5):1214–1221.

Chai DS, Lan YW, Tao C, Gui RJ, Mu YC, Feng JH, Wang WD, and Zhu JA (1989) A study on the standard for forensic anthropologic identification of skull-image superimposition. J Forensic Sci 34(6):1343–1356.

Chandra Sekharan P (1971) A revised superimposition technique for identification of the individual from the skull and photograph. J Criminal Law Criminol Police Sci 62:107–113.

Chandra Sekharan P (1973) A scientific method for positioning of the skull for photography in superimposition studies. J Pol Sci Admin 1:232–240.

Chandra Sekharan P (1988) Positioning skull for video superimposition. Indian J Forensic Sci 2:166–172.

Chee LF, and Cheng CT (1989) Skull and photographic superimposition: A new approach using a second party's interpupil distance to extrapolate the magnification factor. J Forensic Sci 34(3):708–713.

Cherry DG, and Angel JL (1977) Personality reconstruction from unidentified remains. FBI Law Enforcement Bull 46:12–15.

Colonna M, Pesce Delfino V, and Introna F Jr (1980) Identificazione mediante sovrapposizione craniofoto del viso a mezzo di circuito televisivo: Applicazione sperimentale di una nuova metodica. Boll Soc Ital Biol Sper 56:2271–2278.

Colonna M, Introna F Jr, Potente F, Vacca E, and Pesce Delfino V (1984) Computer-aided skull–face superimposition by analytical procedures. Acta Medicinae Legalis et Socialis 34:139–149.

Evenhouse R, Rasmussen M, and Sadler L (1992) Computer-aided forensic facial reconstruction. J Biocommun 19(2):22–28.

Farrar F (1977) From skull to visage: A forensic technique for facial restoration. Police Chief 44:78–86.

Gatliff BP (1984) Facial sculpture on the skull for identification. Am J Forensic Med Pathol 5:327–332.

Gerasimov MM (1964) Ljudi Kamennogo Veka (The People of the Stone Age). Moscow: Nauka (in Russian).

Gerasimov MM (1971) The Face Finder. Philadelphia: Lippincott.

Gillespie JE, and Isherwood I (1986) Three-dimensional anatomical images from computed tomographic scans. Br J Radiol 59:289–292.

Glaister J, and Brash JC (1937) The Medico-legal Aspects of the Buck Ruxton Case. Edinburgh: E and S Livingston.

Grüner O, and Reinhard R (1959) Ein photographisches Verfahren zur Schädelidentifizierung. Dtsch Z Gerichtl Med 47:247–256.

Gupta SR (1969) The superimposition technique in the identification of unknown skulls. J Indian Acad Forensic Sci 8:33–38.

Hagemeier H (1983) Identification of a skull by electronic superimposition of images. Int Criminal Police Rev 38:286–290.

Heglar R, and Parks CR (1980) Juvenile facial restoration: Pediatric and cephalometric expectations. Am Acad Forensic Sci Prog, p 62 (abstr).

Helmer RP (1984) Schädelidentifizierung durch Elektronische Bildmischung. Heidelberg: Kriminalistik Verlag.

Helmer RP (1987) Identification of the cadaver remains of Josef Mengele. J Forensic Sci 32:1622–1644.

Helmer RP, and Grüner O (1977) Vereinfachte Schädelidentifizierung nach dem Superprojektionsverfahren mit Hilfe einer Video-Anlage. Z Rechtsmed 80:183–187.

Helmer RP, Schimmler JB, and Rieger J (1989a) On the conclusiveness of skull identification via the video superimposition technique. Can Soc Forensic Sci J 22(2):177–194.

Helmer R, Schimmler JB, and Rieger J (1989b) Zum Beweiswert der Schädelidentifizierung mit Hilfe der Video-Bildmischtechnik unter Berucksichtigung der kraniometrischen Individualitat menschlicher Schädel. Z Rechtsmed 102(7):451–459.

His W (1895) Johann Sebastian Bach. Forshungen uber dessen Grabstätte, Gebeine und Antlitz. Bericht an den Rath der Stadt Leipzig. Leipzig: FCW Vogel.

Hodson G, Liebermann S, and Wright P (1985) In vivo measurements of facial tissue thickness in American Caucasoid children. J Forensic Sci 30(4):1100–1112.

İşcan MY (1988) Rise of forensic anthropology. Yrbk Phys Anthropol 31:203–230.

İşcan MY, and Charney M (1981) Two-dimensional vs. three-dimensional facial reconstruction. Am Acad Forensic Sci Prog, p 47 (abstr).

Ishibashi H (1986) Identification of a person by the superimposition method. Japanese J Legal Med 40:445.

Janssens PA, Hänsch CF, and Voorhamme LL (1978) Identity determination by superimposition with anthropological cranium adjustment. Ossa 5:109–122.

Koelmeyer TD (1982) Videocamera superimposition and facial reconstruction as an aid to identification. Am J Forensic Med Pathol 3:45–48.

Krogman WM, and İşcan MY (1986) The Human Skeleton in Forensic Medicine. Springfield, Ill: Charles C Thomas.

Krogman WM, and McCue MJ (1946) The reconstruction of the living head from the skull. FBI Law Enforcement Bull 15(7):11–18.

Krogman WM, McGregor J, and Frost B (1948) A problem in human skeletal remains. FBI Law Enforcement Bull 17(6):7–12.

Kumari TR, and Chandra Sekharan P (1992) Remote control skull positioning device for superimposition studies. Forensic Sci Int 54(2):127–133.

Lebedinskaya GV (1957) On the problem of reproduction of the actual shape of the eyes in reconstructions of the face on the skull. Short communications of the Ethnographic Institute of USSR Acad Sci, No 27, Moscow (in Russian).

Lebedinskaya GV, Stepin VS, Surnina TS, Fedosyutkin BA, and Tscherbin LA (1979) The first experience of application of ultrasound for the studies of the thickness of soft facial tissues. Sov Ethnogr 4:121–131 (in Russian).

Maat GJ (1989) The positioning and magnification of faces and skulls for photographic superimposition. Forensic Sci Int 41(3):225–235.

Malinowski A, and Porawski, R (1970) L'utilité de l'expertise anthropométrique pour les essais d'identification des crânes humaines par la méthodes de la superprojection photographique. Zaccharia 45(1):77–97.

McKenna JJ (1988) A method of orientation of skull and camera for use in forensic photographic investigation. J Forensic Sci 33(3):751–755.

McKenna JJI, Jablonski NG, and Fearnhead RW (1984) A method of matching skulls with photographic portraits using landmarks and measurements of the dentition. J Forensic Sci 29:787–797.

Majumdar T, and Sinha P (1989) Photographs of the human face and broken projective symmetry. J Forensic Sci Soc 29:387–395.

Nickerson BA, Fitzhorn PA, Koch SK, and Charney M (1991) A methodology for near-optimal computational superimposition of two-dimensional digital facial photographs and three-dimensional cranial surface meshes. J Forensic Sci 36(2):480–500.

Ogawa H (1960) Anatomical study on the Japanese head by the X-ray cephalometry. Shika Gakuho 60:17 (in Japanese).

Pearson K (1926) On the skull and portraits of George Buchanan. Biometrica 18:233–256.

Pesce Delfino V, Colonna M, Vacca E, Potente F, and Introna F (1986) Computer-aided skull/face superimposition. Am J Forensic Med Pathol 7:201–212.

Prinsloo I (1953) The identification of skeletal remains. J Forensic Mcd 1:11–17.

Reddy KSN (1973) Identification of dismembered parts: The medicolegal aspects of the Nagaraju case. Forensic Sci 2:351.

Rhine JS, and Campbell HR (1980) Thickness of facial tissues in the American Negro. J Forensic Sci 25:847–858.

Rhine JS, Moore CE II, and Weston JT (eds) (1982) Facial Reproduction: Tables of Facial Tissue Thickness of American Caucasoids in Forensic Anthropology. Maxwell Museum Technical Ser 1. Albuquerque: University of New Mexico.

Rişcuţia C (1966) Recontituirea plastica a fetei unei femei cultura bolan faza vidra de la Boian-Varasti, dupa metoda lui M. M. Gherasimov. Studii Cercetari Anthropol 3:3–5.

Schaaffhausen H (1875) Über die Totenmaske Shakespeares. JB Dtsch Shakespeares Ges 10:26–49.

Sen NK (1962) Identification by superimposed photographs. Int Criminal Police Rev 162:284–286.

Seta S, and Yoshino M (1990) Hakkotsu-Shitai no Kantei (Identification of Human Skeletal Remains). Tokyo: Reibunsha Publishing (in Japanese).

Snow CC, Gatliff BP, and McWilliams KR (1970) Reconstruction of facial features from the skull: An evaluation of its usefulness in forensic anthropology. Am J Phys Anthropol 33:221–227.

Suzuki K (1948) On the thickness of the soft parts of the Japanese face. J Anthropol Soc Nippon 60:7–11.

Suzuki T (1973) Reconstitution of a skull. Int Criminal Police Rev 264:76–80.

Taylor JV, DiBennardo R, Lianres GH, Goldman AD, and DeFrost PR (1984) Metropolitan Forensic Anthropology Team (MFAT) studies in identification: 1. Race and sex assessment by discriminant function analysis of the postcranial skeleton. J Forensic Sci 29:787–797.

Ullrich H (1966) Kritische Bemerkungen zur plastischen Rekonstruktionsmethode nach Gerassimow aufgrund persönlicher Erfahrungen Ethnogr-Archäol-Z (Berlin) 7:111–123.

Veselovskaya EV (1989) Zonal'noe Raspredelenie Tolshinu Myagkish Tkanei Litsa (Zonal Distribution of the Soft Tissue of the Face). Doctoral dissertation, Moscow State University.

Welcker H (1883) Schiller's Schädel und Todtenmaske, nebst Mittheilungen über Schädel und Todtenmaske Kant's. Braunschweig: Fr Viehweg and Sohn.

Yordanov Y (1987) Portraits From Antiquity. Atlanta: Oglethorpe University Art Gallery.

Yoshino M, and Seta S (1989) Personal identification of the human skull: Superimposition and radiographic technique. Forensic Sci Rev 1:23–42.

Yoshino M, Sato H, Ichikwa K, and Seta S (1981) An investigation on the anatomical consistency in personal identification with the superimpose method. Rep Nat Inst Police Sci 34:42–46.

Chapter 2
Craniofacial Evolution and Growth

Gloria Jean y'Edynak and Mehmet Yaşar İşcan

Department of Anthropology, University of Maryland, University College,
College Park, Maryland 20742-1660 (G.J.y'E.); Department of Anthropology,
Florida Atlantic University, Boca Raton, Florida 33431-0991 (M.Y.İ.)

Our basic knowledge of variation in the human face is far from complete. We are becoming increasingly knowledgeable about the differential analysis of soft tissue configurations by population, sex, and age. Yet it is difficult to deal with facial expressions produced independently of the underlying bony tissue. It also seems that with some practice one can mimic the expressions of others, as do actors and impersonators. Another area of concentration has been the morphological assessment of the human cranium and facial skeleton. These studies focus on pinpointing variation, as, for example, in orbit shape, nasal aperture size, or nasal root configuration. The gonial region of the mandible shows differences, but its significance can be traced to a myriad of causes—diet, heredity, disease, or unusual musculoskeletal activity. Zygomatic arches are strong in some individuals, thin in others; they may be laterally flared to support a strong masseter muscle for the masticatory system.

A third field of research deals with the interrelationship of soft tissue with the facial skeleton. This assessment is critical because it ultimately leads to the approximation of which faces can realistically "fit" the skull in question. One would like to be certain, for example, exactly how the subnasal spine is related to the shape and size of the nose.

Most existing forensic studies seem to emphasize that human facial morphology and its underlying bony structures is primarily genetically based and predictable. This rather simplistic approach often leads to difficulties because many other independent factors can affect the phenotype. With this line of thinking, many craniofacial studies, especially those that relate to human identification, assume one's face is a "mask" missing from the skull. Reconstructions have been based on identifying the most dominant characteristics and proportions of that mask, even though it is often the small nuances and variations that separate the individual from others who share the same prevailing features that characterize a particular population.

Modern humans are the products of a long (and ongoing) evolutionary process. This process has acted on human physiognomy in many ways, and thus its outcome is very complex. Evolutionary changes can be seen in nearly every part of the human face. The nasal region is highly varied in both extinct and extant hominids. The range of forms of the mouth and teeth has no doubt been heavily influenced by dietary adaptations. The dentition can also be affected by nondietary (e.g., tool or cosmetic mutilation) use in certain cultures. Configurations of the orbits and forehead are inexorably linked to the size and distribution of supraorbital ridges. Thus, it is necessary to understand craniofacial evolution and growth in order to see the human face as plastic—anatomically and environmentally interactive. Only then can one see the error of treating the face as a "mask" to fit a static bony framework.

THE PREHISTORIC CONNECTION

When Raymond Dart of the University of the Witwaterstrand announced the discovery of the first australopithecine fossil in 1925, the professional world did not believe this represented a human ancestor. The "Taung baby" did not support the conception that a large cranial capacity would always distinguish the human line. The Taung baby possesses a very small cranial capacity, estimated not to exceed 400 cc in the adult. In addition, the fossil has a large, toothy, protruding face (Fig. 1).

Preceding this evolutionary reduction in maxillofacial structure, erect posture and bipedalism became the habitual mode of locomotion in *Australopithecus*. The professional world had to totally reorder its thinking regarding the sequence of changes in anatomical structure in hominid evolution. The general sequence of evolutionary changes in anatomical structure now seems to be clear: First came foot, pelvic, spinal, and lower leg anatomical changes as adaptations to opportunistic, behavioral bipedalism. Second, reduction in tooth size and the maxillofacial complex developed as an adaptation to feeding strategies. Third, brain size and cranial capacity increased, especially in lines leading to our own species.

Masticatory Function in *Australopithecus*

The dentition in *Australopithecus* seems to have had a primarily masticatory function. Anterior teeth were very small (smaller than in humans) and were not used extensively for biting. Canines were small, leading us to infer that shearing and tearing were not important masticatory functions. Premolars were molarized and molars were extraordinarily large, exceeding modern human size by about 100% (Fig. 2).

A functional interpretation of australopithecine teeth is that they were used for grinding vegetables or seeds. *Australopithecus* may have used sticks or bones as tools or in aggressive displays, but it appears they did not use tools to replace or supplement masticatory function. There is no evidence of meat in the diet of *Australopithecus*, although we cannot exclude that possibility.

Dental Function and Craniofacial Form

One of the forms that arose from the first hominids—the australopithecines—is the genus *Homo*. Traced to about 2 million years ago, it is characterized by a decrease in facial and back tooth size and accompanied an increase in the anterior dentition and brain size. This arrangement appears more "balanced," or proportioned, and is more similar to the modern human dental arcade. Early *Homo*'s teeth were approximately 25–50% smaller than *Australopithecus*, and 50 to 75% larger than our own (*H. sapiens sapiens*). Complete anatomical bipedalism had been achieved by early *Homo* and stature exceeded 5 feet.

There is evidence that early *Homo* manufactured stone tools, which would have allowed manual cutting and grinding to replace some of the more strenuous mastication, thus perhaps explaining this early dental reduction. At Olduvai Gorge, Tanzania, there is evidence that early *Homo* made tools out of stone, manufactured from raw materials that were transported from a considerable distance. We infer that the stones were deliberately collected because of their naturally occurring fractures or battered appearance. In addition, they were modified by chipping flakes off the core. The resultant tool is called a chopper and was used for cutting or piercing.

It is not so clear how much was scavenged or hunted and what was the proportion of meat to vegetable in the diet (Potts, 1988). However, early *Homo* seems to be associated with (1) the use of tools to process food (vegetable and meat), (2) an omnivorous diet, (3) a "balanced" dental arcade, and (4) a reduction of tooth size from *Australopithecus*.

The first evidence of fire and roasting meat occurs with *Homo erectus*. Processing meat and bones with tools, and roasting them, is associated with a 25–50% reduction in tooth size relative to *Australopithecus*. Although *Homo erectus* teeth are approximately 50–75% larger than our own, the anterior dentition is not disproportionately larger than the posterior, or vice versa. Tooth size in *Homo erectus* appears "balanced" or proportioned along the dental arcade, as in our own (see Fig. 2). Relative to *Australopithecus*, the facial skeleton is reduced

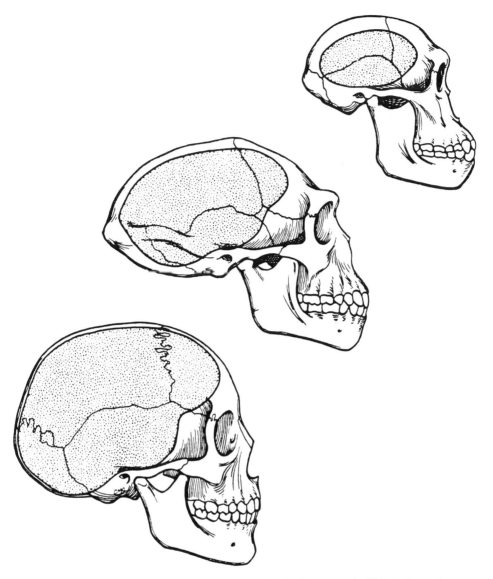

Fig. 1. Profile drawings of *Australopithecus* (**top**), *H. erectus* (**middle**), *H. sapiens* (**bottom**). In *Homo*, facial size and posterior tooth size are reduced, anterior tooth size enlarged, and brain size increased.

in both facial height and prognathism. The face has moved under the larger cranial vault as the probable result of increased cranial base flexure (Biegert, 1963) (Fig. 1).

By the Middle Paleolithic, approximately 250,000–40,000 years ago, anterior teeth were exposed to intensive loads, and selected for larger size. Such appears to be the case for the Classic Neanderthals in western Europe, who developed the largest incisors of any hominid group. In addition, the entire infraorbital portion of the Classic Neanderthal face became

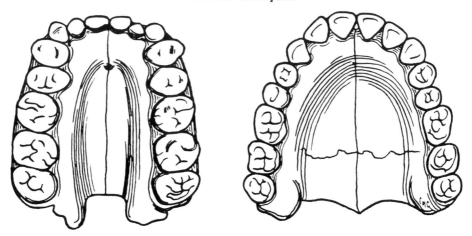

Fig. 2. Dental arch of *Australopithecus* (**left**) and *Homo sapiens* (**right**).

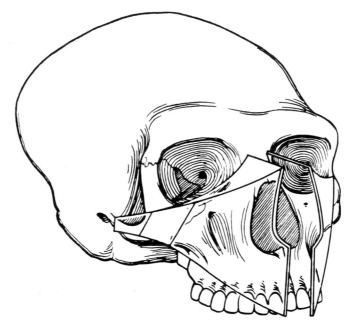

Fig. 3. The infraorbital plates of the Classic Neanderthal face. Modified from Rak (1986, Fig. 2).

oriented in a parasagittal plane to provide biomechanical support for the anterior dental load (Rak, 1986) (Fig. 3).

The heavy occlusal loads on the anterior dentition seemed to determine the midfacial prognathism and steepness of the nasoalveolar slope.

It has been claimed that Neanderthal facial morphology was advantageous in resisting vertical bite forces (Smith, 1988). Trinkhaus (1987) states that the maintenance of total facial prognathism among Neanderthals is best seen as a secondary consequence of their large anterior dentition. In addition, he observed a "zygomatic retreat," reflecting a posterior positioning of the masticatory muscles. The point here is that biomechanical factors or occlusal loads on the anterior dentition in Neanderthals apparently affected their facial morphology, but biomechanical experiments are needed to test this hypothesis. Extensive loads on the anterior dentition are suggested by the extreme wear of the incisors relative to molars in this group.

It is not clear, however, how the anterior dentition was used. Archaeologically, we observe a consistency in the patterns of stone tools used by Neanderthals over a 100,000-year period. The incisors may be viewed as part of the tool kit of these people. The interpretation that Neanderthal incisors were used as tools (Brace, 1979) is supported by observations of extreme tooth wear and evolutionary increase in tooth size between *Homo erectus* and *Homo sapiens neanderthalensis*! It is believed that large incisors were genetically selected for in Neanderthals in response to functional demand over many generations. According to Molnar (1972), living human groups have been observed to use the anterior dentition in many ways, including (1) use of the incisors as knives and the jaw as a third hand, (2) splitting willow shafts or yucca leaves for use in the manufacture of baskets, (3) tearing and cutting fresh seal meat, (4) opening frozen steel gasoline drums, (5) holding a bone drill between the teeth, (6) tightening a sled harness by clinching the end between the teeth and leaning backward, (6) finishing the edge of a stone projectile point or adze by pressure flaking with the teeth, (7) holding strips of bark while fashioning bark sandals, (8) using teeth as a vise to hold a spear in preparation, (9) stripping bark off a branch or sapling to make spear shafts and digging sticks, and (10) holding sinew while hafting a projectile or ax onto a wooden shaft. It is possible that the Classic Neanderthals, who lived in Europe during cold weather, may have used their anterior dentition in similar ways.

CONCEPTS IN CRANIOFACIAL EVOLUTION

Genetic and Biomechanical Components of Face

Head shape has strong heritability in measurements of breadth, facial and nose heights, jaw breadth, and head circumference (Clark, 1956; Osborn and DeGeorge, 1959). Heritability is a measure of the proportion of the variation in a trait that is genetically determined. It is not a direct measure of the genetic component of the trait itself. These estimates, based on twin studies (soft tissue measurements), range between 0.54 and 0.76 in white children. Clark's cephalic module (head height + head length + head breadth) has a heritability of 0.80. Howells (1973), in his study of cranial variation in recent world populations, has shown that major metrical differences are found in cranial base breadth, facial height and breadth, facial projections, nasal shape, vault height, and sagittal profile. Even though the genetic contribution to the variance in these variables is high, we see change precisely in these variables in many populations after the Ice Age. Most likely, the subtle and consistent changes in head shape in many populations parallel changes in diet, physical texture of food, and stresses of mastication.

Endo (1966) describes the facial skeleton in physical terms as a structure adapted to withstand the stresses of mastication. The face receives most of the stresses, while the vault, with the exception of the glabella and superciliary arches, receives little. The vault is protection for the brain, and the facial skeleton provides protection for sensory organs and resistance to the forces of mastication. He describes the facial skeleton as a "rigid frame model" that resists bending movement produced by the muscles of mastication (Fig. 4).

The strength of the facial skeleton is mainly determined by the resistibility to this bending moment. The thickness and breadth of every part of this structure may be regarded as a kind of beam or column roughly parallel to the magnitude of the internal forces acting on it. The facial skeleton is an example of the principle of

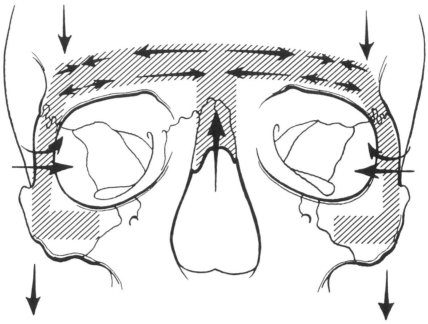

Fig. 4. Endo's (1966) "rigid frame model" of the face.

lightest structure that can resist bending movement. "In other words, the mechanical factors relative to the masticatory action could modify the form and structure of the facial skeleton to a considerable extent" (Endo, 1966:100).

Influence of Masticatory Muscles

Masticatory muscles seem to affect adult facial shape through the growth process. Following masseterectomy, the mandible is partially resorbed, including the ramus (see Moore and Lavelle, 1974, for a review). Weijs and Hillen (1986) found that the cross-sectional area of the temporalis and masseter muscles correlates positively with cranial and facial widths. This suggests that the masseter and temporalis locally stimulate bone deposition at their attachments at the jaw angle, zygomatic arch, and squamous portion of the temporal bone. The masseter and medial and lateral pterygoid muscles affect mandibular length. The cross-sectional area of the lateral pterygoid correlates positively with lower facial height and negatively with cranial base

length. Weijs and Hillen (1986) believe that the observed correlations between jaw muscle sizes and skull dimensions can be traced to local mechanical influences on growth sites. "[I]n man too the jaw muscles affect facial growth and partly determine the final facial dimensions" (Weijs and Hillen, 1986:423).

Secular Trends in Masticatory Apparatus

Waugh (1937) observed more than 50 years ago that the Eskimo jaw and face became reduced in one generation with the switch to a soft-textured diet. The native Eskimo ate hard-textured, sun- and air-dried marine and terrestrial mammal meat, as well as birds and fish. In the winter, the meat froze solid and required even more vigorous chewing. The native Eskimo jaw is large and strong, with a very developed angle of the ramus and wide bigonial breadth. The dental arch is large and the body of the jaws and alveolus are very thick and strong. Women exercised jaws in softening the raw, dry hides to make muk-luks, clothing, harnesses, and boots, and thus had larger jaws than males. There is no decay or malocclusion on the native diet. The children, however, preferred "white man's food" when they came into contact with prospectors, miners, traders, and missionaries. The worst dental conditions seem to occur among Eskimos at missionary stations in Labrador, where the children of rugged-jawed parents preferred sweet, soft food that demanded little chewing. These children had noticeably smaller and less strongly formed jaws. Their teeth became irregular, crowded, carious, and abscessed. There was early loss of deciduous teeth and malocclusion of permanent teeth.

Genetic and Environmental Components of Tooth Size

Since the appearance of modern *H. s. sapiens* about 40,000 years ago, the dentition has grown progressively smaller. There are many conflicting explanations for dental reduction in modern humans. They include natural selection (y'Edynak, 1978, 1989a; Frayer, 1978, 1984; y'Edynak and Fleisch, 1983; Calcagno and Gibson, 1988), accumulation of random mutations (probable mutation effect) (Brace, 1963; McKee, 1984), and nutritional or secular factors (Garn and Burdi, 1971; Garn et al., 1979; Larsen, 1983; Smith, 1988; y'Edynak, 1989b). Whatever the mechanism(s), it is believed that changes in human culture, most likely food-processing/cooking technology, provided the external condition or sociocultural matrix in which one or more evolutionary or secular mechanisms affected tooth size development (Brace, 1962, 1967, 1978; Brace and Mahler, 1971; Frayer, 1978, 1984). Whatever mechanisms may have operated, it is necessary to understand the nature of biological plasticity inherent in the development of tooth size. The current theories of dental reduction are summarized by y'Edynak (1989a).

Tooth length and breadth appear to be under separate genetic control, and they respond to environmental factors differently. At least 74% of their tooth size variance indicates a different genetic or developmental basis (Garn et al., 1967; Lombardi, 1976; Potter and Nance, 1976; Potter et al., 1976). Tooth length is more affected by attrition and breadth by developmental, local environmental factors (Sofaer et al., 1971). Common environmental factors accounted for more of the variance in breadth than length in half-sib data (Potter et al., 1968; Townsend and Brown, 1978).

Animal and human studies suggest that prenatal, gestational, nutritional, and secular/environmental factors affect tooth size in the developing individual and over subsequent generations. In rat studies, protein and vitamin A deficiency, fluoride supplementation, and low calcium/phosphorus ratio during pregnancy and lactation result in offspring with reduced molars or cusp size and/or delayed eruption of the third molar (Paynter and Grainger, 1956; Holloway et al., 1961; Tenczar and Bader, 1966). Shaw and Griffiths (1963) add that positive alteration of the postweaning diet to include adequate protein for the offspring did not correct the dental abnormalities. In white children, maternal health status during gestation affects tooth size in the offspring. Maternal diabetes, hypothyroidism, and high birth length and weight increase both deciduous and permanent crown size. Maternal hypertension, protein–caloric malnutrition, reduced birth weight, and crown–heel length decrease dental dimensions (Garn et al., 1979, 1980). Garn and associates (1965) stated that "a hazardous prenatal existence is not easily overcome, and the teeth, and imperfect twin concordance in the teeth, may preserve such evidence, not just in developmental timing and size, but even in cusp pattern and crown morphology."

Finally, such developmental plasticity can explain secular trends seen in modern and archaeological populations. In the United States and England, children have larger teeth than their parents (Hanna et al., 1963; Goose, 1971). In archaeological native American populations that appeared to have suffered stress, tooth size decreased between adults and juveniles (Perzigian, 1976; Guagliardo, 1982).

RECENT MICROEVOLUTIONARY REDUCTION IN CRANIOFACIAL STRUCTURE

Reduction in Mandibulofacial Robusticity

In cranial vault size, Upper Paleolithic humans were larger than populations after the Ice Age in the Holocene about 7,000 years ago (Henneberg, 1988). They were muscular and medium to tall in stature, with large, robust, long heads and broad, low orbits. The face was hung low and projected at glabella. The jaws were large and robust, the dental arch was wide and shallow, and the teeth were worn and well aligned.

Hunt (1959) explained these trends as, in part, related to less growth in the aboriginal upper sutures of the face, and to increased growth at the median palatine suture, which produces the broad dental arch. The following trends are observed from the Upper Paleolithic through Mesolithic (the cultural period of small-scale fishing, hunting, and collecting that succeeded the Ice Age): Upper facial projections reduced, including projections of the brow region and nasal spine; the skull shortened and became lower; and sexual dimorphism decreased because greater craniofacial reduction occurred in males (Frayer, 1984). Frayer (1978, 1984) observed that anterior tooth size reduced sharply during the middle Upper Paleolithic period. Males showed more reduction not only in craniofacial structure and teeth but also in body size. According to Frayer (1978, 1984) and Brace (1962, 1967, 1978), increasing technocultural sophistication lessened the need for robust craniofacial structure and skeleton. During the Upper Paleolithic, a new stone technology based on the production of blades from a prepared core appeared. In addition, other materials for tool use were discovered, such as antler, bone, ivory, and the innovation of handles and composite tools. There were advances in preparing and cooking foods, such as the introduction of a semisubterranean ventilation system for hearths, and the introduction of baking meat and other foods, as in a clam bake or luau. Such long cooking techniques made meat succulent and tender, which in turn demanded less biomechanical power from the jaw and less buttressing of the facial skeleton.

From the Mesolithic (7,500–5,500 B.C.) through the early Neolithic or farming period in Yugoslavia (5,500–4,500 B.C.), for example, it is clear that both size and biomechanical robusticity of the jaw reduced (y'Edynak, 1978, 1989a, 1992; y'Edynak and Fleisch, 1983). This marked reduction of the masticatory apparatus occurred during the transition from hunting and gathering to domestication. This reduction in functional measurements, tori, and the power function of the mandible is not surprising in view of the fact that the Neolithic group ate domesticated animal meat (which is more tender than wild), domesticated grains, and had pottery for boiling, cooking, or baking. During this time, ovens appeared for baking, replacing the Mesolithic open air, dirt hearth.

Brachycephalization

In 1977 Carlson and van Gerven proposed the "masticatory-functional hypothesis" to account for craniofacial changes among Nubians since 12,000 B.P. Their samples included Mesolithic (ca. 11,000 B.C.), transitional hunting/gathering, agricultural (3,400–1,000 B.C.), and fully agricultural/historic (350 B.C.–1,100 A.D.) groups. These authors state that

systematic reduction in functional demand . . . on the masticatory complex from the Mesolithic led, . . . to an alteration of growth of the maxillomandibular complex such that the face became progressively less robust, and more inferoposteriorly located relative to the cranial vault. The increase in the height of the vault, relative to its length, produced a more globular appearance. The reduction in dental size was tertiary to these changes. Dental reduction was a compensatory response to altered facial size and position.

They analyzed 16 anterior–posterior measurements of the cranium with multiple discriminant analysis. The first function described 85.3% of the variation among the groups (Table 1). This first function indicates that crania with large mandibles had a large masseter muscle insertion and a long cranial vault. These crania were mostly Mesolithic. Conversely, a short skull with a relatively high vault had a smaller mandible and a decreased size of the masseter muscle insertion. These crania tended to be from the later groups. Mandibular measurements, which had higher coefficients on the first function, discriminated between the Mesolithic and later groups in Nubia.

Measurements of the relative height of the cranial vault and face slightly increased over time (7% change). Measurements of masticatory robusticity showed the greatest reduction through time (15–30%), while those concerned with craniofacial length and mandibular height decreased slightly through time (0–8%). The progressive decrease in size and robusticity of the mandible and masticatory apparatus was the dominant feature in the transition from the Mesolithic period through the Christian horizon in Nubia. Carlson and van Gerven (1977) summarized their results as follows: (1) There was a decrease in robusticity of the entire craniofacial complex, especially in those features primarily associated with masticatory function; (2) there was a definite tendency for the mid- and lower face to become more inferoposteriorly situated relative to the anterior cranial vault; and (3) there was a relative increase in height and decrease in length of the cranial vault (Fig. 5).

Carlson's (1976) cephalometric study of the series supported the findings of anthropometry. The skull became shorter and more globular. The maxillomandibular region became posteriorly located. His study suggests, but does not directly measure, an increase in cranial base flexure, which may account for the inferior and posterior migration of the face.

In historic times, head shape continued toward brachycephalization (round-headedness) in Sweden, Great Britain, Germany, Switzerland, Italy, Russia, Egypt, India, Central Asia, and among native Americans, along with foreshortening of jaws (Weidenreich, 1945). In Poland, the mean cephalic index (cranial breadth/cranial length) increased from the 11th through the 20th centuries (Bielicki and Welon, 1966)(Table 2).

In less than 700 years (30 generations), the mean cephalic index increased by 10 units, almost three times the present standard deviation of this trait. Bielicki and Welon (1966) acknowledge the possibility of nongenetic, developmental response to environmental factors, and explore the possibility of natural selection. In two separate studies, one on Poles, the other on Ukrainians from northeastern Poland, data on army recruits between the ages of 21 and 25 were collected in the late 1920s in the Military Anthropological Survey of Poland. In both populations, the round-headed groups had slightly more living siblings than the long-headed groups. This indirect method, with all its assumptions, suggests that differential fertility may be favoring round-headed individuals.

y'Edynak (1974) studied craniometric variation in the Dinaric mountainous zone and karst region of central Yugoslavia between 900 B.C. and 1900 A.D. The samples included (1) Iron Age, Roman, and late Antique skulls dating between 900 B.C. and 600 A.D., (2) Slavic and Croatian skulls (8–11th centuries A.D.), (3) Late Medieval skulls (14–15th centuries A.D.), and (4) Recent material (18–19th centuries A.D.).

TABLE 1. Discriminant Function Coefficients

Measurement[a]	Coefficient
Cranial length	+0.40
Masseter insertion length	+1.15
Symphyseal height	+0.53
Sigmoid notch height	+0.50

[a]These measurements are large in the Mesolithic group, but small in the Christian group. Modified from Carlson and van Gerven (1977, Table 3).

TABLE 2. Increase in Mean Cephalic Index in Poland[a]

Century	Mean Cephalic Index
20th	83–84
17th	81
11-12th	73.5–74.0

[a]Adapted from Bielicki and Welon (1966, Table 1).

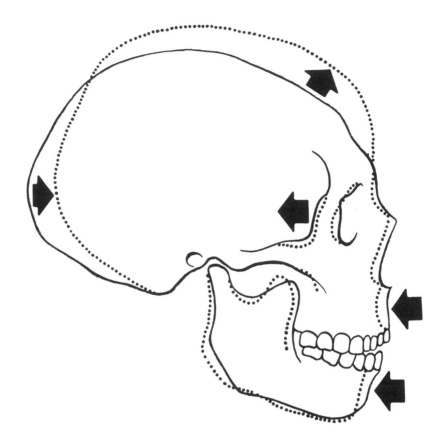

Fig. 5. Craniofacial reduction in Nubia.

Strong similarity in cranial size and shape was found among all these groups. They resembled each other more than other European populations. Through time, the Dinaric Yugoslav skull shortened in length and vault contour, reduced facial and occipital projection, and increased in vault height. In sum, the skull became shorter, higher, and less projecting in recent centuries (Table 3).

In the United States, Boas (1912) showed that head length, width, facial width, and stature changed in children of immigrants born in the United States, compared with those of the same immigrant parents born in Europe. The cephalic index decreased in Bohemians and Hebrews, but increased in Sicilians and Neopolitans, while facial width decreased in all groups.

[C]hanges in the values of the averages occur at all ages, these are found among individuals born almost immediately after the arrival of their mothers, and they increase with the length of time elapsed between the arrival of the mother and the birth of the child as long as we do not know the causes of the observed changes, we must speak of a plasticity (as opposed to permanence) of types, including selection, changes of prenatal or postnatal growth, or by changes in the hereditary constitution (Boas, 1912).

TABLE 3.　Cranial Changes in Yugoslavia (Males)[a]

Measurements	900 B.C.–600 A.D. X	N	8–11th A.D. X	N	14–15th A.D. X	N	18–19th A.D. X	N
Glabella occ. 1	186.7	35	189.7	28	183.7	30	180.3	23
Nasion occ. 1	183.9	33	186.9	28	180.8	30	178.4	23
Breg. lamb. ch.	115.6	33	120.3	28	116.9	9	113.7	23
Maximum br.	146.1	35	142	28	148.5	30	145.8	23
EAM-opisthion	42.6	24	42.9	25	41.3	30	41.2	21
EAM-lambda	105.7	25	108	26	104.2	30	104	21
Basion-nasion	105.5	33	106.9	28	102.4	30	102.9	23
EAM-vertex	122.6	32	125.5	25	124	30	124.3	21

[a]Adapted from y'Edynak (1974, Appendix C, Table B).

Maxillo-dental Maladjustment and Dental Reduction

Carlson and van Gerven (1977) state that dental reduction is the tertiary event in the sequence of changes transforming the long, projecting, early modern skull to the gracile, globular, less projecting current skull shape. Sofaer (1973) summarizes his research and that of others as follows:

Assuming that dental change has been largely secondary to skeletal change, the following conclusions can be drawn. Since the dental changes must have lagged behind the skeletal changes, the teeth must have always been, on average, genetically too large for the jaw in which they developed. Environmental deviations, expressed most by the latest tooth to develop in each class, would then have been overwhelmingly negative due to the restriction of space. Lack of harmony between tooth size and jaw size would therefore have been the result of inability of the individual to respond sufficiently by negative environmental deviations, and selection would have operated against genotypes that failed to produce negative deviations large enough to accommodate all the teeth comfortably in the restricted jaw.

This concept is illustrated by the following research on post-Pleistocene Yugoslav populations:

From the Mesolithic period (7500 BC to 5500 BC) through the early Neolithic period in Yugoslavia (5500 BC to 4500 BC) both size and mechanical robusticity of the jaw reduced. This marked reduction of the masticatory apparatus occurred during the major food-producing revolution, in which the domestication of animals and plants replaced hunting and gathering. All functional measurements of the mandible decreased between the Mesolithic and Neolithic periods in Yugoslavia [Table 4] In addition, mandibular tori, which were present in 42 percent of Mesolithic mandibles, did not occur in the Neolithic sample [Table 5] Apparently a softer diet allowed a biomechanical reduction in the phenotypic development of the mandible in the Neolithic group.

When reduction occurs in the mandible and maxilla, tooth size reduction lags behind. This maladjustment between dental and osseous tissue may occur in one or several generations within a population [D]entomandibular malocclusion appeared to have caused dental pathology, which in turn formed a focus of biologic stress on the posterior dentition (particularly in the mandibular arch). This stress acted as the selective agent for tooth reduction. By the Neolithic period posterior teeth comfortably fit the jaw, and biologic stress, as indicated by pathology, shifted to the anterior dentition (y'Edynak, 1992).

CRANIOFACIAL GROWTH

In order to better analyze evolutionary changes in the human cranium and face, it is vital to understand the growth process at both the individual and the population levels. The importance of growth is reflected in the extraordinary amount of material that has been published on this topic in general (Eveleth and

TABLE 4. Yugoslav Mesolithic and Neolithic Mandibular Measurements

Measurements	Mesolithic			Neolithic			
	X	N	S.D.	X	N	S.D.	Sig.
Condylar breadth	22.5	25	1.61	20.6	5	0.89	0.0112
Condylar thickness	11.2	26	1.20	10.4	5	0.89	0.0618
Height mand. canine	33.9	31	3.75	33.6	10	3.24	0.6909
Mand. symph. thickness	17.7	32	2.82	16.1	10	2.02	0.0900
Gonial thickness	6.6	31	1.28	6.4	10	1.51	0.0887
Min. ramus width[a]	37	25	2.47	33.6	7	2.15	0.0007
Mand. ramus length	65.8	20	7.97	61.6	7	3.29	0.0761
Min. height ramus[a]	52.6	23	5.88	45.3	7	2.81	0.0017
Bigonial breadth	104.8	15	11.37	97	3	5.29	0.3236

[a]Condylar thickness is almost significantly different at $P < 0.05$ level; minimum width of the ramus and minimum height of the ramus (posterior) are significantly reduced at $P < 0.01$ level. These three measurements are roughly proportional to muscle size and function of the masseter and pterygoid muscles, and represent statistically significant reduction between the Mesolithic and Neolithic.

TABLE 5. Nonmetric Variants of the Yugoslav Mesolithic and Neolithic Mandible

Trait	Mesolithic		Neolithic	
	Freq. %	N	Freq. %	N
Overbite	absent	0/19	absent	0/3
Alveolar torus	42	14/33	absent	0/10
Palatine torus	13	2/15	25	2/8

Tanner, 1976; Bogin, 1988; Sinclair, 1989), and specifically on the facial region (Hellman, 1932; Scott, 1957; El-Nofely, 1972; Enlow, 1975; Krogman, 1979; Vercauteren, 1990; van der Beek et al., 1991; Farkas et al., 1992a,b). However, most research on facial growth centers on orthodonture (Genecov et al., 1990; Moorrees et al., 1991; Tallgren and Solow, 1991). While it would be counterproductive to cover all of these studies, a brief review of the ontogenetic development in the face can enhance our ability to carry out craniofacial reconstruction.

The Human Face

The human face goes through a series of changes so drastic during the first years of life that an infant might not be recognizable if not seen for even a few months. A simple approach to observing the metamorphosis of the human face from infancy to adulthood was demon-

strated by Todd and associates (1980). They based their study on the relationship between the perception of growth and actual growth. Figure 6A illustrates their model: cardioidal-strain transformation. It is readily apparent that the face is the most actively enlarging region of the head. A test of their model revealed a close association between perceived and actual growth. The authors also applied the same geometric model to investigate the similarity between growth and evolution. The results appear in Figure 6B. The center drawing represents a Neanderthal and the outside a futuristic human being. They concluded that, like growth, evolutionary transitions in the skull follow an established path of morphological change.

Cranial and facial growth. Facial growth follows a different pattern from that of the cranium. Cranial growth, including the orbits, is more advanced from infancy to middle childhood and closely related to the development of the nervous system (Sinclair, 1989). Growth of the face and base of the cranium is independent from that of the brain case and is linked to the development of the jaws and teeth, tongue, and masticatory system. Facial growth reaches its peak in the early years, then slows gradually with age.

Facial growth analyzed. Farkas and associates (1992a) analyzed facial growth in North

American white children from ages 1 to 18 years. They found that by 1 year, mandibular width reached 80.2% of its adult size, while mandibular height was only 66.6% of the total. As one might expect, mandibular height and width expanded fastest from ages 1 to 5, probably to accommodate dental eruption. Facial width, height, and depth accelerated after age 5, and the face reached maturity by about 10 to 13 years in girls and two years later in boys. El-Nofely's (1972) study of Nubian children indicated that between the ages of 6 and 12 years, cephalic length increases continually in both sexes and breadth reaches peak velocity at 9 to 10 years in boys and a year later in girls. Facial breadth is gradual and peaks at 10–11 in boys, and total facial height growth follows a similar pattern. Females are, however, characterized by two slow periods, at 8–9 and 10–11 years. El-Nofely concluded that facial height growth proceeds at a different rhythm from breadth—the former is faster and does not have the periodic slowing seen in the latter. Farkas et al. (1992b) also analyzed cephalic dimensions in the North American white children. They observed that 87.1% of adult head circumference size is reached by age 1, and adult size was nearly attained by age 5. Full maturity in head length, breadth, and circumference occurred at age 10 in females and 14 in males. Final head height in both sexes reached adult size at about 13 years.

The adolescent growth spurt also alters facial dimensions. The mandible shows the greatest enlargement, beginning with ramus and chin height and gonion symphyseal length (Tanner, 1962). This process goes faster in boys, resulting in larger, more projecting jaws. A similar spurt in the nose increases its anterior projection and length. Tanner suggests that growth of the face and skull fall under different genetic controls and do not significantly influence each other. Genecov et al. (1990) investigated facial tissue development in 7–9-, 11–13-, and 16–18-year age groups and observed that nasal projection and facial depth (anterior–posterior) increased in both boys and girls continuously until age 17 in males and 12 in females. Moreover, he noted that the proportional relationship of the nose, lips, and chin was not influenced by the changes in the bony tissue and remained constant during the developmental period.

Relatively little has been published about the postadolescent years. Vercauteren (1990) investigated postmaturity changes in four head dimensions in Belgian adults (25 to 54 years). He uncovered statistically significant differences between age groups for head, bizygomatic, and bigonial breadths, but not head length. Interestingly, the head breadth dimension decreased, while the others increased. Tanner (1988) stated that cephalic and facial dimensions increase continuously throughout the life span, although only a 2–4% change can be expected after age 20.

In addition to genetics, human facial growth is also modified by environmental factors. To illustrate this, Hunt (1959) reported on the experimental work of Watts and Williams (1951), which gives insight to the role of the texture of food in the ontogenetic development of the mandible. They found that weanling rats reared on the hard diet had more dental wear, more alveolar bone, especially in the mandibular molar region, the mandible weighed more than those fed gruel, the ramus was wider in the former group, the condyle was more mineralized, and the maxillary dental arch was wider. Hunt (1959) got similar results in a cross-sectional series of aboriginal skulls ranging from 2 years to adult from a single location in Australia. He measured the nasal breadth, minimum breadth between the greater palatine foramina, and maximum breadth of the dental arch. These measurements showed an average increase of 7 mm in the cross-sectional growth period, whereas in a modern sample, the growth averaged only 2–5 mm. Hunt (1959) proposed that the narrow maxillary dental arch in modern humans results from an inhibition of transverse growth at the median palatine suture. The result produces crowded maxillary arches. Furthermore, he suspects that reduced masticatory function is responsible for the excessive downward growth of the modern face that, in turn, produces a higher face in modern humans. Finally, reduced masticatory function apparently causes the nar-

A   **B**

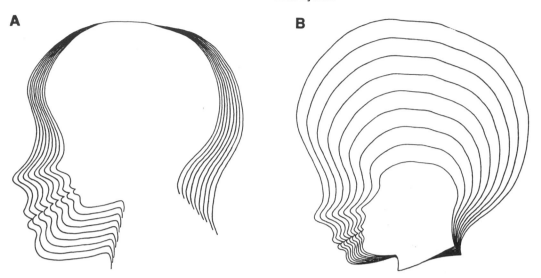

Fig. 6. Cardioidal-strain transformation profiles of craniofacial growth of an infant (innermost profile) into an adult (outermost profile) (**A**) and Neanderthal (innermost profile) to a "futuristic" man (outermost profile) (**B**) (Todd et al., 1980).

row ramus and gracile gonial region of the mandible.

CONCLUSIONS

The process of microevolutionary change in the craniofacial skeleton since the Ice Age is fairly well understood, whereas the underlying mechanisms of biological change are not. It is clear that culture and human behavior provide the theater or stimulus for biological change. Cultural or life-way changes occur first that somehow bring about phenotypic changes in the individual, and possibly genetic change in the population over generations. Both phenotypic and genetic change constitute adaptation on thc level of the individual and the population, respectively. These phenomena have occurred throughout human evolution, after the Ice Age and down to the present day.

The period after the last Ice Age in Europe, which ended about 10,000 years ago, is characterized by remarkable cultural changes. The first effects of these life-way changes on the skeleton (including craniofacial) are biome-chanical or phenotypic. As a result of less biomechanical stress on the masticatory apparatus, facial–mandibular robusticity declined, which led to craniofacial and dental reduction. All dimensions of the mandible, especially those related to the attachments of the muscles of mastication, decreased. The facial skeleton, which absorbs the forces of mastication, decreased in forward projections.

Two changes followed the reduction in facial–mandibular robusticity: brachycephalization and malocclusion. Both of these processes are continuing today. The process of brachycephalization probably involves genetic as well as secular or environmentally induced mechanisms. Brachycephalization may have had some selective advantage, as suggested by sibling studies, and therefore genes for round-headedness probably have been increasing in human populations since the Mesolithic. Brachycephalization may be related to an ongoing increase in cranial base flexure. This would account for the subtle inferoposterior descent of the face under the vault since the Mesolithic. On the other hand, rapid historical secular trends in brachycephalization in many populations argue for an environmentally induced ontogenetic process as well. Reductions in facial projections and skull length (which have low heritability) have more to do with reduced muscular activity than with genetics.

Malocclusion, and ultimately dental reduction, is easier to explain, although currently the topic is highly debated. Teeth are more genetically canalized in their growth (size) than the mandible. There will naturally be a time lag between tooth size and a reducing maxilla and mandible. This maladjustment between dental and osseous tissue (malocclusion) may occur in one or several generations within a population. In fact, malocclusion is a common problem in modern populations who eat a soft-textured diet, and may also lead to dental pathology. Some types of malocclusion (e.g., crowding, chipping, and rotation) probably contribute to alveolar resorption, caries, abscess, and antemortem tooth loss.

Both evolutionary forces and individual human ontogenetic influences also contribute to the formation of craniofacial morphology. The growth of the face, influenced primarily by the masticatory system, is independent of the brain case, whose development is linked to the neural system. Brain growth is nearly completed by middle childhood. Facial growth peaks later and features remain in the same proportions throughout life (barring tooth loss or other major deterioration).

Understanding human evolution and craniofacial growth offers a different perspective in the study of craniofacial anatomic relationships. In this way, we trace the roots of human facial variation.

ACKNOWLEDGMENTS

The National Museum of Health and Medicine, Washington, D.C., provided a supportive environment for this work. We wish to thank Dr. Richard Potts of the Smithsonian Institution for his critical reading of the manuscript and contributions to the "prehistoric connection." We are also grateful to Susan R. Loth for her editorial assistance. The research for this article was supported by the National Science Foundation grant BSN-7813033 A01 and the International Research and Exchange Board (G.J.y'E.).

REFERENCES

Biegert J (1963) The evolution of characteristics of the skull, hands, and feet for primate taxonomy. In SL Washburn (ed): Classification and Human Evolution. Chicago: Aldine, pp 116–145.

Bielicki T, and Welon Z (1966) The operation of natural selection on human head form in an east European population. Homo 15:22–30.

Boas F (1912) Changes in the bodily form of descendants of immigrants. Am Anthropol 14:530–563.

Bogin B (1988) Patterns of Human Growth. Cambridge: Cambridge University Press.

Brace CL (1962) Cultural factors in the evolution of the human dentition. In MFA Montagu (ed): Culture and the Evolution of Man. New York: Oxford University Press, pp 343–354.

Brace CL (1963) Structural reduction in evolution. Am Nat 97:39–49.

Brace CL (1967) Environment, tooth form, and size in the pleistocene. J Dent Res 46(Suppl, 5):809–816.

Brace CL (1978) Tooth reduction in the orient. Asian Perspectives 19:203–219.

Brace CL (1979) Krapina, "classic" Neanderthals, and the evolution of the European face. J Hum Evol 8:527–550.

Brace CL, and Mahler PE (1971) Post-Pleistocene changes in the human dentition. Am J Phys Anthropol 34:191–204.

Calcagno JM, and Gibson KR (1988) Human dental reduction: Natural selection or the probable mutation effect. Am J Phys Anthropol 77:505–517.

Carlson DS (1976) Temporal variation in prehistoric Nubian crania. Am J Phys Anthropol 45:467–484.

Carlson DS, and van Gerven DP (1977) Masticatory function and post-Pleistocene evolution in Nubia. Am J Phys Anthropol 46:495–506.

Clark PJ (1956) The heritability of certain anthropometric characters as ascertained from measurements of twins. Am J Hum Gen 8:49–54.

y'Edynak G (1974) Demographic change and population continuity in central Yugoslavia from prehistoric through medieval times. Unpublished Ph.D. dissertation, Harvard University, Cambridge, Mass.

y'Edynak G (1978) Culture, diet, and dental reduction in mesolithic forager-fishers of Yugoslavia. Current Anthropol 19:616–618.

y'Edynak G (1989a) Yugoslav Mesolithic dental reduction. Am J Phys Anthropol 78:17–36.

y'Edynak G (1989b) Disease and dimensional compensation during Yugoslav dental reduction. Am J Phys Anthropol 78:327 (abstr).

y'Edynak G (1992) Dental pathology: A factor in post-Pleistocene Yugoslav dental reduction. In JR Lukacs (ed): Culture, Ecology and Dental Anthropology. Delhi: Kamla-Raj Enterprises, pp 133–144.

y'Edynak G, and Fleisch S (1983) Microevolution and biological adaptability in the transition from food-collecting to food-producing in the Iron Gates of Yugoslavia. J Hum Evol 12:279–296.

Eleveth PE, and Tanner JM (1976) Worldwide Variation in Human Growth. Cambridge: Cambridge University Press.

El-Nofely A (1972) Anthropometric study of growth changes of some head and face measurements in an Egyptian group. Egyptian Dental J 18(2):141–150.

Endo B (1966) Experimental studies on the mechanical significance of the form of the human facial skeleton. J Fac Sci, Univ Tokyo, sec 5, Anthropol vol 3, pt 1, pp 5–106.

Enlow DH (975) Handbook of Facial Growth. Philadelphia: WB Saunders.

Farkas LG, Posnick JC, and Hreczko TM (1992a) Growth patterns of the face: A morphometric study. Cleft Palate-Craniofacial J 29(4):308–315.

Farkas LG, Posnick JC, and Hreczko TM (1992b) Anthropometric growth study of the head. Cleft Palate-Craniofacial J 29(4):303–308.

Frayer DW (1978) The Evolution of the Dentition in Upper Paleolithic and Mesolithic Europe. Univ Kansas Publ Anthropol, 10.

Frayer DW (1984) Biological and cultural change in the European late pleistocene and early holocene. In FH Smith and F Spencer (eds): The Origins of Modern Humans. New York: Alan R Liss, pp 211–250.

Garn SM, and Burdi AR (1971) Prenatal ordering and postnatal sequence in dental development. J Dent Res 50:1407–1414.

Garn SM, Lewis AB, and Kerewsky R (1965) Genetic, nutritional and maturational correlates of dental development. J Dent Res 44:228–242.

Garn SM, Lewis AB, and Kerewsky R (1967) Buccolingual size asymmetry and its developmental meaning. J Dent Res 37:186–193.

Garn SM, Osborne RH, Alvesalo L, and Horowitz SL (1980) Maternal and gestational influences on deciduous and permanent tooth size. J Dent Res 59:142–143.

Garn SM, Osborne RH, and McCabe KD (1979) The effect of prenatal factors on crown dimensions. Am J Phys Anthropol 51:665–78.

Genecov JS, Sinclair PM, and Dechow PC (1990) Development of the nose and soft tissue profile. Angle Orthodontist 60(3):191–198.

Goose, DH (1971) The inheritance of tooth size in British families. In AA Dahlberg (ed): Dental Morphology and Evolution. Chicago: University of Chicago Press, pp 263–269.

Guagliardo MF (1982) Tooth crown size differences between age groups: A possible new indication of stress in skeletal samples. Am J Phys Anthropol 58:383–389.

Hanna BL, Turner ME, and Hughes RD (1963) Family studies of the facial complex. J Dent Res 42:1322–1329.

Hellman M (1932) An introduction to growth of human face from infancy to adulthood. Int J Orthodont Oral Surg Radiol 18:777–798.

Henneberg M (1988) Decrease in human skull size in the Holocene. Hum Biol 60:395–405.

Holloway PJ, Shaw JH, and Sweeney EA (1961) Effects of various sucrose: Casein ratios in purified diets on the teeth and supporting structures of rats. Arch Oral Biol 3:185–200.

Howells WW (1973) Cranial Variation in Man: A Study by Multivariate Analysis of Patterns of Difference Among Recent Human Populations. Papers of the Peabody Museum, vol 67, Harvard University, Cambridge, Mass.

Hunt EE Jr (1959) The continuing evolution of modern man. Genetics and Twentieth Century Darwinism, Cold Spring Harbor Symposium on Quantitative Biology. Cold Spring Harbor, NY: 24:245–254.

Krogman WM (1979) Craniofacial growth: Prenatal and postnatal. In HK Cooper, RL Harding, WM Krogman, M, Mahazeri, and RT Millard (eds): Cleft Palate and Cleft Lip. Philadelphia: WB Saunders, pp 23–107.

Larsen CS (1983) Deciduous tooth size and subsistence change in prehistoric Georgia Coast populations. Curr Anthropol 24:225–226.

Lombardi AV (1976) A factor analysis of morphogenetic fields in the human dentition. Am J Phys Anthropol 42:99–104.

McKee JK (1984) A genetic model of dental reduction through the probable mutation effect. Am J Phys Anthropol 65:231–241.

Molnar S (1972) Tooth wear and culture: A survey of tooth functions in some prehistoric populations. Curr Anthropol 13:511–526.

Moore WJ, and Lavelle CLB (1974) Growth of the Facial Skeleton in the Hominoidea. London: Academic Press.

Moorrees CF, Efstratiadis SS, and Kent RL Jr (1991) The mesh diagram for analysis of facial growth. Proceedings of the Finnish Dental Society 87(1):33–41.

Osborne RH, and DeGeorge FV (1959) Genetic Basis of Morphological Variation: An Evaluation and Application of the Twin Study Method. Cambridge: Harvard University Press.

Paynter KJ, and Grainger RM (1956) Relation of nutrition to the morphology and size of rat molar teeth. J Can Dent Assoc 22:519–531.

Perzigian AJ (1976) Natural selection on the dentition of an Arikara population. Am J Phys Anthropol 42:63–70.

Potter RH, and Nance WE (1976) A twin study of dental dimension: I. Discordance, asymmetry, and mirror imagery. Am J Phys Anthropol 44:391–396.

Potter RH, Nance WE, Yu P-L, and Davis WB (1976) A twin study of dental dimension: II. Independent genetic determinants. Am J Phys Anthropol 44:397–412.

Potter RH, Yu P-L, Dahlberg AA, Merrit AD, and Connally PM (1968) Genetic studies of tooth size factors in Pima Indian families. Am J Hum Gen 20:89–100.

Potts R (1988) Early Hominid Activities at Olduvai. New York: Aldine De Gruyter.

Rak Y (1986) The Neanderthal face: A new look at an old face. J Hum Evol 15:151–164.

Scott J (1957) Growth in width of the facial skeleton. Am J Orthodont 43:366–371.

Shaw JH, and Griffiths D (1963) Comparison of a natural and purified diet with respect to reproductive ability and caries susceptibility. J Dent Res 43:1198–1207.

Sinclair D (1989) Human Growth After Birth. Oxford: Oxford University Press.

Smith P (1988) Changing rates of dental reduction in *Homo sapiens*. Am J Phys Anthropol 75:273 (abstr).

Sofaer JA (1973) A model relating developmental interaction and differential evolutionary reduction of tooth size. Evolution 27:427–434.

Sofaer JA, Balit HL, and MacLean CJ (1971) A developmental basis for differential tooth reduction during hominid evolution. Evolution 25:509–517.

Tallgren A, and Solow B (1991) Age differences in adult dentoalveolar heights. Eur J Orthodontics 13(2):149–156.

Tanner JM (1962) Growth at Adolescence. Oxford: Blackwell.

Tanner JM (1988) Human growth and constitution. In GA Harrison, JM Tanner JM, Pilbeam DR, and Baker PT (eds): Human Biology. Oxford: Oxford University Press, pp 337–435.

Tenczar PK, and Bader RS (1966) Maternal effect in dental traits of the house mouse. Science 152:1398–1400.

Todd JT, Mark LS, Shaw RE, and Pittenger JB (1980) The perception of human growth. Sci Am 242(2)132–144.

Townsend GC, and Brown T (1978) Heritability of permanent tooth size. Am J Phys Anthropol 49:497–504.

Trinkhaus E (1987) The Neanderthal face: Evolutionary and functional perspectives on a recent hominid face. J Hum Evol 16:429–443.

van der Beek MC, Hoeksma JB, and Prahl-Andersen B (1991) Vertical facial growth: A longitudinal study from 7 to 14 years of age. Eur J Orthodontics 13(3):202–208.

Vercauteren M (1990) Age effects and secular trend in a cross-sectional sample: Application to four head dimensions in Belgian adults. Hum Biol 62(5):681–688.

Watts DG, and Williams CHM (1951) The effects of the physical consistency of food on the growth and development of the mandible and maxilla of the rat. Am J Orthodont 37:895–928.

Waugh LM (1937) Influence of diet on the jaws and face of the American Eskimo. J Am Dent Assoc 24:1640–1647.

Weidenreich F (1945) The brachycephalization of recent mankind. Southwestern J Anthropol 1:1–54.

Weijs WA, and Hillen B (1986) Correlations between the cross-sectional area of the jaw muscles and craniofacial size and shape. Am J Phys Anthropol 70:423–431.

Chapter 3

Identification of Skulls: A Historical Review and Practical Applications

Oskar Grüner

Abteilung Rechtsmedizin, Christian-Albrechts-Universität, D-2300 Kiel 1, Germany

In medico-legal and anthropological work, the identification of human remains is a problem of growing importance. Like no other part of the skeleton, the skull—being the matrix of the form of the head and face—allows one to draw conclusions about the face of the deceased. Thus we gain important clues for the identification of an individual.

Here we will not consider the philosophical, mathematical, or any other problems of identity, but we deal with a question that played an important role in forensic medicine more than 150 years ago: Which methods of examination can be applied to the identification of a person (cf. Mende, 1829)?

It is small wonder that, even in those days, the form of the skull and the face was thought to be of particular importance and that the skull has been the center of interest in all identification work since that time. Not only the 19th-century anatomists' work on the skulls of the famous bears evidence to this interest but also all those subsequent attempts at identification by criminalists and forensic scientists.

HISTORICAL CONSIDERATIONS

One has to admire the way in which researchers like Welcker (1883), His (1895a,b), Schaaffhausen (1875, 1883), von Froriep (1913), and others painstakingly worked with (somewhat dubious) material for comparison—and one has to admire their dedication. We are in their debt not only for results of socio-historical importance but also for the system of measurement they devised, as it can be applied to all

subsequent work. Welcker (1883) and His (1895a,b) in particular made innumerable measurements of soft tissue thickness and of the relationships between the bony foundations of the external features. In fact, all of the methods of craniofacial identification are based on their studies.

Basically, the conclusiveness of all methods depends on whether the examiner can make a comparison with a suitable portrait, bust, death mask, etc., of the person in question. His's (1895a,b) method is to model a bust on a plaster cast of the skull in accordance with the measurements of the soft tissue. Portraits of the individual in question that are thought to be most characteristic are used for comparison (Figs. 1 and 2). In this way the anatomist His of Leipzig succeeded in identifying the skull of Johann Sebastian Bach. First, he examined the skeleton belonging to the skull (Fig. 3). As early as 1894, His (1895a,b) followed the procedure that should be applied as rigorously as possible to all attempts at identification: determining all characteristics of the skeleton that could help establish age, sex, and stature, as well as estimates about the time since death. This method was also applied to the reconstruction of 'portraits of different races' and was later frequently recommended by criminalists (e.g., Gross, 1899, 1901).

If death masks of men of historical importance were available, Welcker's (1883) method could be used to draw more reliable conclusions. In this method, outline drawings of the skull and the death mask are made in precise orthogonal perspective by means of Lucae's (1873) apparatus, with the two subjects held in

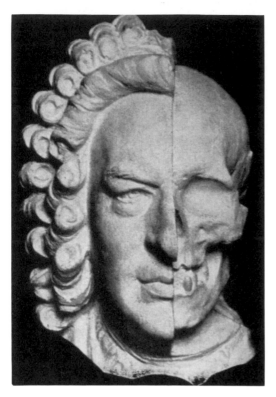

Fig. 1. Facial reconstruction of J.S. Bach (His, 1895).

exactly corresponding positions (Fig. 4). When allowance is made for soft tissue, the two drawings should match (Fig. 5). In this way, Welcker (1883) succeeded in proving the identity of Immanuel Kant's skull (Fig. 6). However, it was not as effective on a skull thought to be Schiller's, possibly because of the inadequacy of the death mask (cf. Hildebrandt, 1950; Fikentscher, 1978).

The anatomist Tandler (1909) also used Welcker's (1883) method when examining a skull preserved in the museum of the Vienna Society of the Friends of Music. In 1909, he succeeded in identifying Josef Haydn's skull, and in 1954 the skull was transported to Eisenstadt, where, at Haydn's bicentenary in 1932, Prince Paul Esterhazy erected a mausoleum in the Bergkirche with a marble sarcophagus to receive the great composer's bones.

Completely new possibilities resulted from the development of photography on one hand

and from new systems of identifying criminals on the other. Even more avenues were opened when the French criminalist Bertillon (Fig. 7) developed the system of description and characterization named after him, the so-called 'Bertillonage' (Fig. 8). Since his system could be used with photographs, one may even say that the introduction of photography marked the birth of forensic skull identification. The anatomist Stadtmüller of Göttingen gained merit by adapting Welcker's (1883) method to the use of photographs (Stadtmüller, 1932). In one of his cases, he used enlargements of forensic photographs and tried to match them with photographs of the skull taken with a lens of the same focal length at the standard distance laid down for the Bertillon (1895) system (Fig. 9). Instead of the orthogonal drawing (i.e., a drawing in parallel projection), the central projection of photographs was used. As precise as Stadtmüller's method is, it has its limitations— it cannot be used when profile and full-face photographs are not available. Stadtmüller knew of this shortcoming and tried to avoid it by attempting to reconstruct the 'pure line of profile' out of the 'lost profile' shown on oblique photographs. The resulting picture, in central projection, was regarded as an orthogonal projection (Fig. 10). Apart from the fact that this requires a dioptrograph (an improved version of Lucae's apparatus), discrepancies between the two profiles are unavoidable. Depending on the point from which the photograph is taken, the drawing is either flattened or in exaggerated relief. The drawbacks of this method are especially regrettable because developments in photography make it almost always possible to find a photograph of a missing person, if only an amateur snapshot.

TECHNICAL PROBLEMS

Several authors proceeded by using life-sized enlargements of the missing person and then taking a photograph of the skull positioned on a device that places it in a position corresponding to that of the portrait. The photograph of the

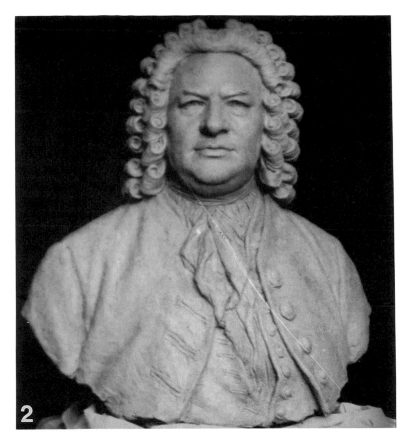

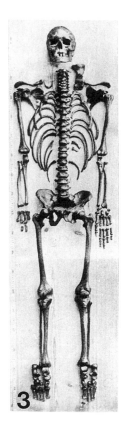

Fig. 2.   Bust of J.S. Bach (His, 1895)   **Fig. 3.**   Skeleton of J.S. Bach.

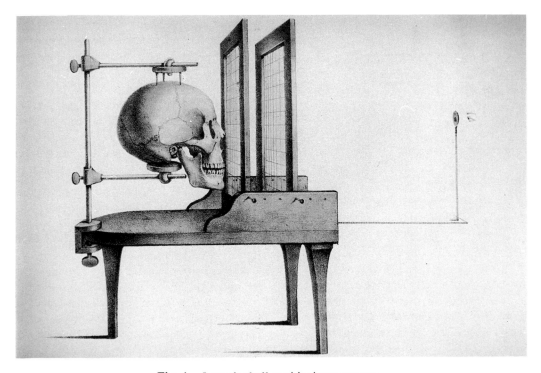

Fig. 4.   Lucae's skull-positioning apparatus.

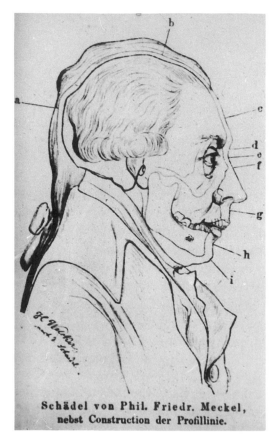

Schädel von Phil. Friedr. Meckel,
nebst Construction der Profillinie.

Fig. 5. Superimposed drawings of skull and face (Welcker, 1883).

skull is then also enlarged to life size. After outline drawings are made and compared, the two pictures are superimposed. This was done successfully by Brash and Smith in the Ruxton murder case (cf. Blundell et al., 1955, 1956). The 'superimposition technique' was also employed by other researchers (e.g., Webster and Basauri, quoted in Chandra Sekharan, 1971). Chandra Sekharan noted problems with this method that can result in one skull being matched to different persons if life-sized photographs aren't used.

The following problems arise:

1. To determine the actual size of the head in the photograph, there have to be objects for comparison.

In the Ruxton case, there was a diadem (Fig. 11). As Chandra Sekharan pointed out, other objects in the photograph, e.g., a chair or spectacles, might serve this purpose, as long as they are available for identification (which will not always be the case).

2. It is particularly difficult to position the skull as shown in the photograph. The angles of rotation and tilting play a decisive role, and without instruments it is not easy to precisely position the skull to match the picture.

3. The photographic superimposition technique is rather time-consuming because of the search for objects for comparison and the preparation of various negatives and enlargements.

Therefore, in 1959, the author (with Reinhard) devised a strictly photographic method of skull identification in which the skull can be projected onto an existing photograph and then be photographed itself. This method requires an optical bench, a perspex pane, and a sighting device (Fig. 12).

1. On an enlargement of a portrait (size 18 × 24 cm), the appropriate cephalometric measuring points (e.g., nasion, gnathion, gonion, etc.) are found. These form the basis for a system of guide lines (Fig. 13).

2. Mark the corresponding craniometric measuring points on the skull with India ink.

3. Adjust the rubber bands on the sighting device—taken off the optical bench for this purpose—so that they coincide with the guide lines on the photograph (Fig. 14).

4. Take the perspex pane off the optical bench, drawing the outlines of the skull and the guide lines (Fig. 15).

5. Position the skull:

a. With the sighting device;

b. With the sighting device and drawing on the perspex pane, taking into account the thickness of soft tissue (Fig. 16).

6. Take the photograph:

a. Fasten the enlargement (without marker points and guide lines) onto the perspex pane, and take the portrait.

b. Remove the sighting device and perspex pane from the optical bench. Take a photograph of the positioned skull (double exposure, Fig. 17).

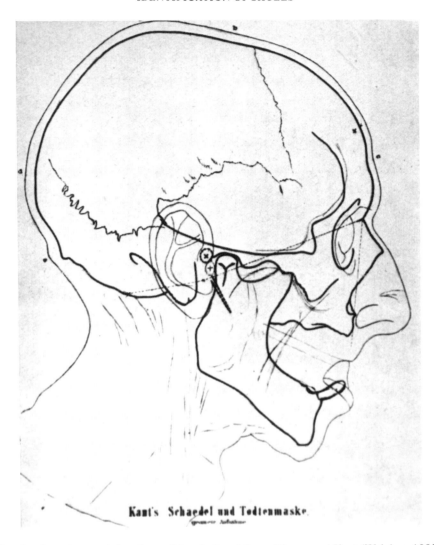

Kant's Schaedel und Todtenmaske.

Fig. 6. Superimposed drawings of the skull and face of Immanuel Kant (Welcker, 1883).

With the help of outline drawings, marking points, and the system of lines, while taking soft tissue thickness into account, it is possible to precisely position the skull to correspond with the photograph without first determining its natural size. Errors caused by the angles of rotation and tilting without lines of orientation are also avoided (cf. Grüner and Reinhard, 1959).

This method can be simplified by using a large-format camera, with its large focusing screen on which outlines and marking points can be drawn. In this case, an optical bench is not necessary, but to improve precision it is recommended that the soft tissue thickness be marked at the marking points with a corresponding layer of plasticine or wax (Fig. 18) (Grüner and Schulz, 1969).

Thus the 'superposition technique' (or superimposition technique) was superseded by the superprojection technique. The technique, developed by Grüner and Reinhard (1959), was modified by Leopold (1978), using a large-

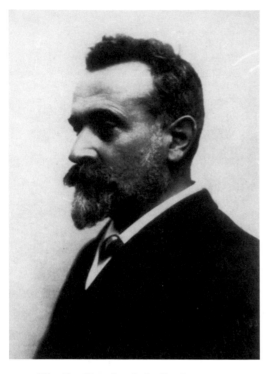

Fig. 7.   French criminalist Bertillon.

positor. This even applies to details. Pictures similar to plastic reconstructions are produced and the contours of soft tissue and bone can be precisely compared (Figs. 21, 22) (Helmer and Grüner, 1977b). With the electronic superprojection technique, too, the adjustment is made by lines of orientation on the photograph and rubber bands on a frame corresponding to the monitor. The great advantage of this method is that one can project any point on the bone surface to the surface of the soft tissue or vice versa, as already described. Congruency of the superprojection can also be controlled with the use of a video-animation compositor. This allows precise scrutiny of the congruency of the soft tissue model on the skull with the soft tissue in the photograph, as well as that of all decisive proportions of skull, face, and soft tissue.

With all superposition and superprojection techniques, the main problem is the matching of skull and photograph. All experts know that this is not a matter of 'putting the skull into the photograph of the head' but of 'fitting it in' correctly. Some apparently successful identifications by superposition show the mistakes that result from not following the most important rules of this procedure. They are as follows:

1. A precise determination of soft tissue thickness;

2. A precise topographical attribution of important morphological points and shapes to the corresponding forms of the head on the photograph (eye–orbits; nose–nasal bone; mouth–jaw and teeth; earhole–auditory meatus);

3. Together with these conditions, accounting for the rotation and tilting of the head with its consequences of changed proportions on photographs taken in central perspective.

After Stadtmüller's (1948) constructive-geometrical method did not turn out to be as successful as hoped, Leopold (1978), with the help of a special method, tried to find the desired angle on the photographs used for comparison by means of a calibration curve.

As valuable as these preliminary determinations are, the congruency of the topographical

format camera and a projection screen between the skull and camera.

Completely new techniques were made possible by the use of a video monitor and a video-animation compositor (Helmer and Grüner, 1977a,b; Grüner and Helmer, 1980). Two video cameras, adjusted to each other simultaneously, take pictures of the skull and a suitable photograph of any size. The picture signals, having gone through the video-animation compositor, are superprojected on the monitor screen (Figs. 19, 20). The infinitely variable video-animation compositor allows any desired degree of intensity in the picture of either skull or portrait. By varying the intensity, any point on the surface of the bone can be projected on the surface of the soft tissue, and vice versa (Helmer and Grüner, 1977b). Precise control of the proportions of the skull and soft tissue, as well as the contours, is made possible by the video-animation com-

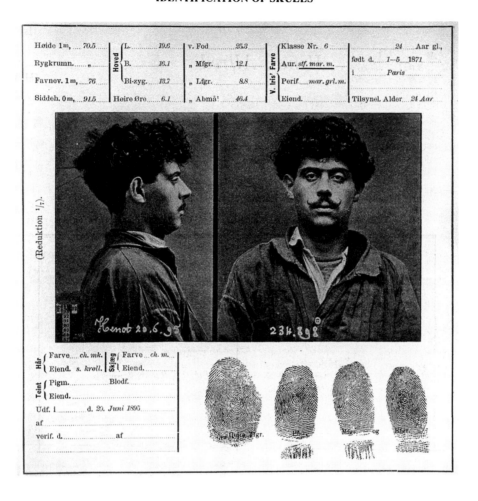

Fig. 8. 'Bertillonage' identification form.

points mentioned under 2 (above) and the comparison of contour lines are as important in the end. Soft tissue thickness plays an important role here. Several authors have pointed out the problems involved: the difficulties determining tissue thickness of corpses, its variability depending on age, sex, nutritional status, and constitution, as well as the possibility of radiological determination (cf. Leopold, 1978). Helmer (1984) paid particular attention to soft tissue measurements of the skull. He laid the foundation for a far-reaching individualization of measurement values by measuring 34 points on the head and face of 61 males and 62 females via the ultrasound impulse echo technique. If these

measurement values are transferred to the markers of soft tissue thickness on the skull, the contour lines of the face and head can be easily reconstructed.

Evaluation of the reconstruction depends on whether the points or shapes of the skull chosen for the external 'covering' correspond to the topographic proportions. The topography of the regions of the nose, eyes, and ears are as important for orientation as the jaws, teeth, and mouth.

The bony structure can also be shown on appropriate X-rays. Leopold (1978) has pointed out that they can be used for superprojection with photographs for comparison. On the other hand, more frequently, radiographs of the skull

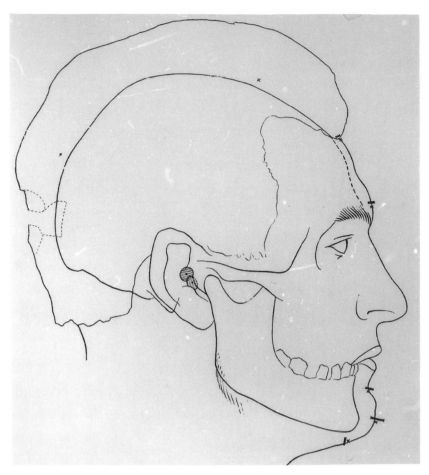

Fig. 9. Stadtmüller's attempt at skull-to-photo superimposition.

will be used for identification in the future, making use of all the advantages of radiological identification that Neiss (1968, 1976) noted 25 years ago. With this method, soft tissue thickness, with all of its variability, will play no role, and other means of comparison (e.g., the configuration of the frontal sinus) will be available. One of our skull identifications proved that odontological X-rays or those used for oral surgery can be of great importance. In this case, a cyst in the mandible X-rayed during the individual's lifetime conformed precisely with the postmortem radiograph (Fig. 23). This idiosyncratic finding contributed considerably to

a positive identification. Here, as in other cases, it was shown that careful examination of certain individual or characteristic traces in the bones or teeth can be the last link in the chain of evidence for identification (cf. Grüner, 1961; Holczabek, 1955; Riepert and Rittner, 1988).

CONCLUSIONS

It remains to be seen whether nuclear spin tomography will play a decisive role in skull identification in the future. Helmer and his col-

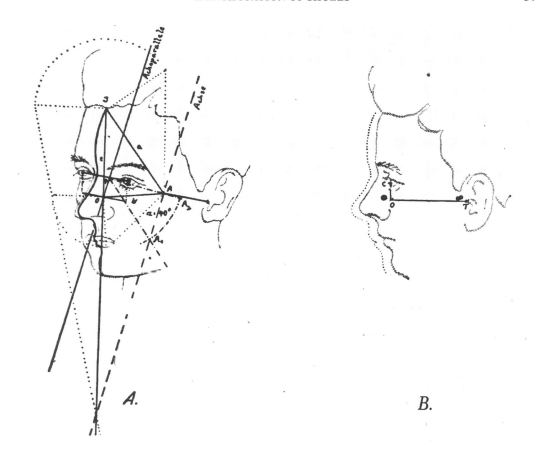

Fig. 10. Stadtmüller's attempt to reconstruct the profile from an oblique photograph.

laborators (1986) have done some interesting research in this field. Undoubtedly, the new computer-aided methods will provide new possibilities. If all the necessary preliminary findings, like determining sex, age, and blood group, are taken into account (Grüner and Helmer, 1975; Hunger and Leopold, 1978), and if individual particularities of the skull and postcranial skeleton are painstakingly examined, then modern techniques will certainly lead to proof or disproof of identity in most cases. Of course, suitable photographs must be available for comparison.

I would like to end with a quotation from Carl Gustav Carus (1962), doctor of medicine and natural philosopher (1789–1869): "Infinite proportions are here [on the skull] imaginable, an infinity which alone is reason for the miracle, that among so many million people, living and dead, because of some higher law no two human beings ever had heads of identical shape." May these words encourage us to continue our research.

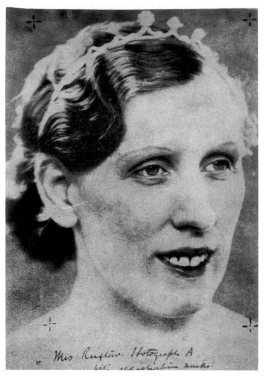

Fig. 11.   The Ruxton case photograph.

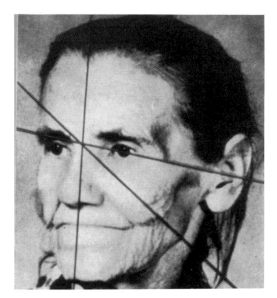

Fig. 13.   Cephalometric landmarks.

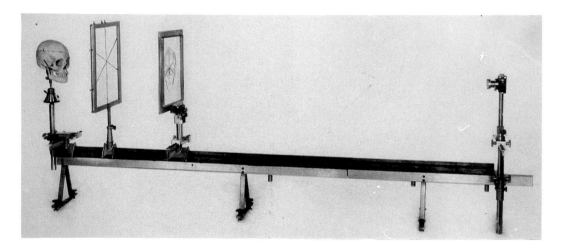

Fig. 12.   Optical apparatus of Grüner and Reinhard (1959).

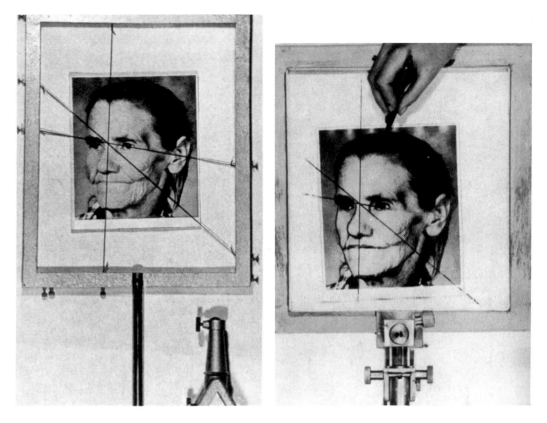

Fig. 14. Placement of photograph on the Grüner and Reinhard apparatus.

Fig. 15. Drawing outlines of the head and guide lines.

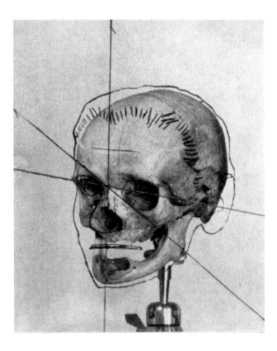

Fig. 16. Positioning the skull on the drawing.

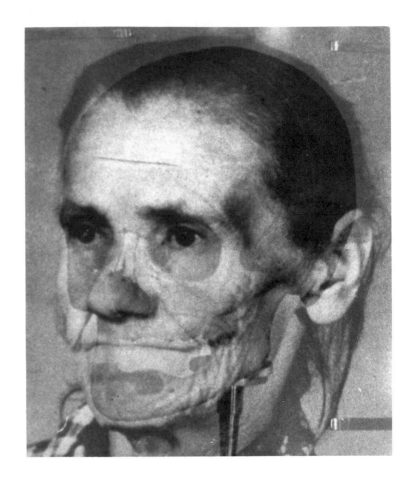

Fig. 17. Double exposure of the skull and photograph.

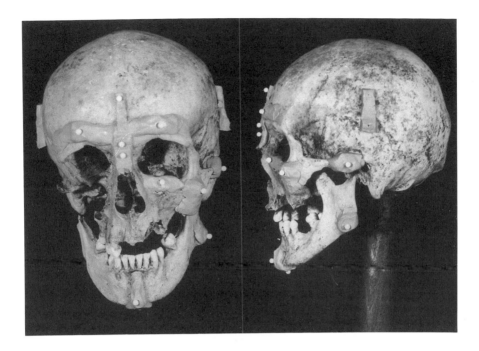

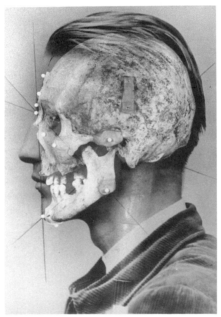

Fig. 18. Soft tissue thickness marking points.

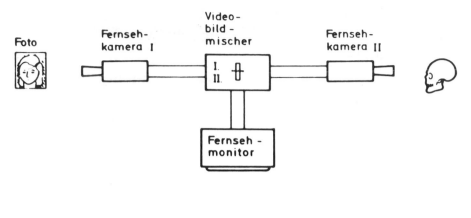

Fig. 19. Video apparatus.

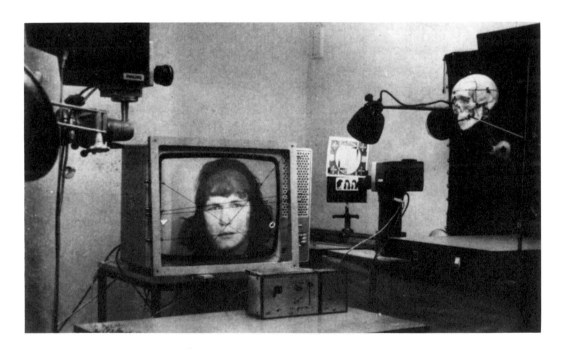

Fig. 20. Photo superprojected on monitor screen.

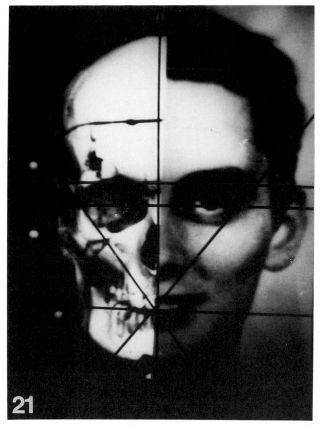

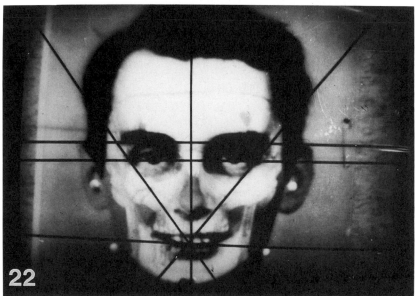

Fig. 21. Video comparison of skull to face.
Fig. 22. Video superimposition.

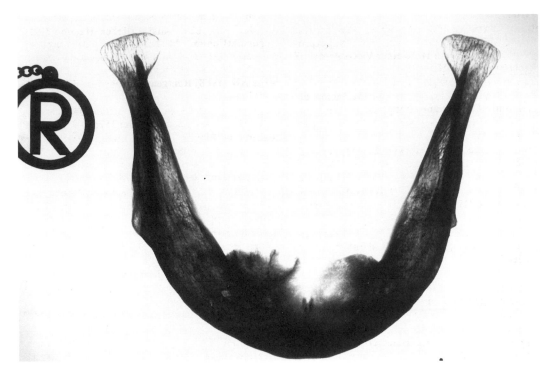

Fig. 23.   Mandibular cyst used for positive identification.

REFERENCES

Bertillon A (1895) Das anthropometrische Signalement (2 Aufl). Dtsch Ausgabe v Dr Sury Bern u Leipzig: Verlag v A Siebert.

Blundell RH, Wilson GH, and Engelhardt L (1955) Der Mordfall Ruxton. Arch Krim 115:73–83, 121–127.

Blundell RH, Wilson GH, and Engelhardt L (1956) Der Mordfall Ruxton. Arch Krim 116:30–40, 92–106.

Carus CG (1962) Symbolik der menschlichen Gestalt (2 vielf vermehrte Aufl), Leipzig 1858. Nachruck: Darmstadt: Wissenschaftl Buchges.

Chandra Sekharan P (1971) A revised superimposition technique for identification of the individual from the skull and photograph. J Crim Law, Criminol Police Sci 62:107–113.

Fikentscher H (1978) Der heutige Stand der Forschung über Friedrich Schillers sterbliche Reste. Personal communication.

Froriep A von (1913) Der Schädel Friedrich von Schillers und des Dichters Begräbnisstätte. Leipzig: JA Barth

Gross H (1899) Die His'sche Regenerationsmethode. Arch Krim Anthropol Kriminalistik 1:120–127.

Gross H (1901) His'sches Reconstructionsverfahren. Arch Krimin Anthropol Kriminalistik 7:164–165.

Grüner O (1961) Bemerkungen zur photographischen Identifizierung menschlicher Schädel. Beitr Gerichtl Med 21:149–155.

Grüner O, and Helmer R (1975) Identifizierung. In B Mueller (ed): Gerichtliche Medizin (2 Aufl). Berlin: Springer-Verlag, pp 156–206.

Grüner O, and Helmer R (1980) Identification d'un crâne par superimposition à l'aide du mixage électronique des images. Acta Med Legal Soc 30:159–165.

Grüner O, and Reinhard R (1959) Ein photographisches Verfahren zur Schädelidentifizierung. Dtsch Z Gerichtl Med 48:247–256.

Grüner O, and Schulz G (1969) Über eine Vereinfachung der photographischen Schädelidentifizierung. Beitr Gerichtl Med 26:132–137.

Helmer R (1984) Schädelidentifizierung durch elektronische Bildmischung. Zugleich ein Beitrag zur Konstitutionsbiometrie und Dickenmessung der Gesichtsweichteile. Heidelberg: Kriminalistik

Verlag.

Helmer R, and Grüner O (1977a) Vereinfachte Schädelidentifizierung nach dem Superprojektionsverfahren mit Hilfe einer Video-Anlage. Z Rechtsmedizin 80:183–187.

Helmer R, and Grüner O (1977b) Schädelidentifizierung durch Superprojektion nach dem Verfahren der elektronischen Bildmischung, modifiziert zum Trickbild-Differenz-Verfahren. Z Rechtsmedizin 80:189–190.

Helmer R, Koschorek F, Terwey B, and Frauen T (1986) Dickenmessung der Gesichtsweichteile mit Hilfe der Kernspin-Tomographie zum Zwecke der Identifizierung. Arch Krim 178:139–150.

Hildebrandt FL (1950) Die zwei Schiller-Schädel zu Weimar. Berlin: Hildebrandt-Verlag.

His W (1895a) Johann Sebastian Bach. Forschungen über dessen Grabstätte, Gebeine und Antlitz. Bericht an den Rath der Stadt Leipzig. Leipzig: FCW Vogel.

His W (1895b) Anatomische Forschungen über Johann Sebastian Bach's Gebeine und Antlitz nebst Bemerkungen über dessen Bilder. Abh Math-Physikal Kl Kgl Sächs Ges Wiss.

Holczabek W (1955) Ein Beitrag zur Identifikation durch vergleichende Röntgenuntersuchung. Beitr Gerichtl Med 20:35–36.

Hunger H, and Leopold D (1978) Identifikation. Berlin: Springer-Verlag.

Leopold D (1978) Personenerkennung durch Superprojektion. In H Hunger and D Leopold (eds): Identifikation. Berlin: Springer-Verlag, pp 263–286.

Lucae JCG (1873) Noch Einiges zum Zeichnen naturhistorischer Gegenstände. Arch Anthropol 6:1–12.

Mende LIC (1829) Ausführliches Handbuch der gerichtlichen Medizin für Gesetzgeber, Rechtsgelehrte, Aerzte und Wundärzte. Leipzig: Dyk'sche Buchhandlung.

Neiss AW (1968) Röntgenidentifikation. Stuttgart: G Thieme.

Neiss AW (1976) Röntgenidentifikation als Ergänzung der Daktyloskopie. Arch Krim 157:87–92.

Riepert T, and Rittner C (1988) Zur Röntgenidentifizierung unbekannter Leichen und lebender Personen. Vortr auf d 67. Jahrestagung d Dtsch Ges Rechtsmedizin. Kloster Banz, September 20–24.

Schaaffhausen H (1875) Über die Totenmaske Shakespeares. Jahrb Dtsch Shakespeare Ges 10:26–49.

Schaaffhausen H (1883) Der Schädel Raphaels. Zur 400 jährigen Geburtstagsfeier Raphael Santi's. Bonn: Max Cohen and Son.

Stadtmüller F (1932) Identitätsprüfung bei vorliegendem Erkennungsdienst-Photogramm des vielleicht als ehemaliger Träger in Frage kommenden Individuum. Dtsch Z Ges Gerichtl Med 20:33–52.

Stadtmüller F (1948) Über Schädelidentifikation, insbesondere die zeichnerische Zugehörigkeitsprüfung. Grenzgeb Med 1:63–68.

Tandler J (1909) Über den Schädel Haydns. Mitt Anthropol Ges 39:260–279.

Welcker H (1883) Schiller's Schädel und Todtenmaske, nebst Mittheilungen über Schädel und Todtenmaske Kant's. Braunschweig: F Viehweg and Son.

Chapter 4
Determination of Body Constitution Type From the Face

Dieter Leopold, H.J. Hammer, and Holle Greil*

Medizinische Akademie Erfurt, Institut für Gerichtliche Medizin, Erfurt (D.L.); Karl-Marx-Universität Leipzig, Bereich Medizin, Institut für Gerichtliche Medizin, Leipzig (H.J.H.); Humbolt-Universität zu Berlin, Bereich Medizin (Charite), Institut für Anthropologie, Berlin, Germany (H.G.)

Since Hippocrates, physicians have observed differences in the physical appearance of humans that were later expressed in the fine arts (Leonardo da Vinci, Dürer) and literature (Homer, Shakespeare). Though there is great variability in the physical manifestations of humans, only a few pivotal features characterize our phenotype. Certain combinations of features make many people appear the same or very similar (see theory of proportion, below), yet in the same vein, variations in these features allow us to differentiate one individual from the next. Until now, features of build were used for the classification of body structure type in adults (Flügel et al., 1986).

CONSTITUTIONAL TYPES

Years ago, experts restricted themselves to literal descriptions of somatoscopic appearance. Gross somatotyping was later supplemented by systematically defined measuring methods (Martin, 1928). Experienced investigators relied on careful visual analysis (Kretschmer, 1921; Höhne, 1947). Methods by Kretschmer (1921), Sheldon (1940), and Conrad (1941) predominated those that spread through Europe. Traditionally, physicians and trainers have been aware of the connection between constitutional (body) type and physical performance. Until 1960, Olympic specialists in sports medicine stated that good results were obtained for the assessment of adult performance using Kretschmer's principles (Klaus, 1960). When examining 131 university students, Kretschmer himself found 40% leptosomes, 30% athletes, and 30% pyknics. On the other hand, when Sheldon examined 4,000 students, he found only 28% fit into Kretschmer's pure constitutional types. This result mirrors our forensic experiences that the majority of adults cannot be neatly incorporated into Kretschmer's scheme.

Concerning habitus, many internists noted that certain individuals were disposed to particular diseases. Kretschmer originally linked this data on character types and disposition to psychiatric diseases with his somatotypic theory. However, mainstream modern anthropology has disproved and generally discarded this approach. The biological growth and development of an individual, his or her physical constitution, and body structure are, to a certain extent, genetically conditioned.

In his classification of human growth patterns, Conrad (1941) proceeded from two mutually exclusive, polar types, the leptomorph and pyknomorph (primary variants). During the postmaturity aging process, physical development can change from leptosomatic to pyknosomatic. Conrad only published graphs of Strömgren's (1937) so-called metrics index of body height, and of the breadth and depth of the chest used to monitor this transformation. Conrad, too, did not reveal his own mathematical considerations. He varied his constitutional typologies according to the second type of hypoplastic or hyperplastic development (second-

---

*H.G. contributed the Appendix beginning on page 53.

ary variants). The combination of these two series of variations gave rise to a two-dimensional system of coordinates into which everyone can be objectively incorporated (Greil, 1988; also see Appendix). Conrad's "typical" body types are actually rare in the population. The constitution during growth may be varied and is subject to change during adolescence (secondary variation) (Conrad, 1941). The investigator must differentiate between constitution and the effect of diet (e.g., fatness or thinness) (Johnsen and Scholz, 1989).

However, according to our own experience, the influence of age as well as population specificity (race or ethnicity) must also be considered. Strömgren studied Danes, and Conrad examined Saarland miners. According to Tittel and Wutscherk (1971), constitution type can be established as early as the 12th year. This was confirmed by recent investigations in Germany (Kallmeyer and Weidhase, 1986). Since the fundamental research of Bertillon (1895), it has become possible to identify an individual through a description of external characteristics and measurements of certain regions of the body. In the "*signalement*" (description) theory, which is as important as ever in forensic practice worldwide, features of the face play a crucial role. Because faces contain so much information, they are often used for the description and identification of missing persons. In the experience of many specialists in forensic medicine and anthropology, descriptions are frequently colored by the subjective influences of the witness, the victim, another criminalist, or an inexperienced expert. Therefore, when an investigation is conducted, it must be characterized by systematic, objective analysis.

According to Kretschmer, a pyknic has a relatively large, rounded head with frail hair and an inclination to baldness, as well as a short, massive neck. A leptosome, on the other hand, is characterized by a relatively small head with a long, thin neck and thick hair. In Conrad's (1941) view, there are no special features or forms that designate constitution, but rather a particular degree of progression that is type-specific. The frequently tall leptomorph is dis-

tinguished by long, slim extremities, a long, slender neck, a small face with thin, sharp nose, small zygomatic arches, and distinct, angular facial contours. The pyknomorph has a tendency to form fatty layers about the trunk with advancing age. His neck is relatively short and thick, and the head is disproportionately large for the body and has a broad face with little distinct relief. The chin is well proportioned. Conrad correlates the hypoplastic constitution with a small, retreating chin and weak supraorbital arch. The hyperplastic individual has noticeably projecting zygomatic arches, a large, strong nose, and a prominent chin (Table 1).

QUANTIFICATION OF BODY CONSTITUTION

More recently, multivariate statistical methods have been used to quantitatively identify complexes of features that could be used to objectively distinguish one individual from another. However, Bach (1987/88) warns that we still do not fully understand the basic genetic and other multifarious influential factors that determine physical appearance. According to Leopold's (1968, 1976) earlier craniometric measurements of adult skulls of both sexes, Kretschmer's scheme of classifying constitutional differences could be verified from the maximum length and breadth of the skull and width of the mandibular angle. This was confirmed in later investigations by Hammer (1986) on the basis of comprehensive genetic analysis.

Years ago, physicians sometimes used height and weight as the sole criteria for determining body type (Kohlrausch, 1926). As recently as the 1968 Olympic Games in Mexico, super athletes were arbitrarily classified by these two attributes. However, these parameters are sufficient neither for anthropological consideration nor for the assessment of performance. On the basis of Conrad's (1963) constitutional scheme, Tittel and Wutscherk (1971) worked out a detailed characterization for the biotypology of the athlete and his physical powers that also

TABLE 1. Features of the Face and Head Associated With Different Constitutions[a]

Constitution	Line of Profile	Middle of the Face	Nose	Chin	Lower Jaw
Leptomorph	Forehead plain	Distinct facial relief	Accentuated, large	Accentuated	Mandibular angle obtuse
Metromorph	Equalized	Even	Middle, straight, or back little entered	Even	Shape middle
Pyknomorph	Forehead steep	Even, broad	Back straight or thick or broad	No specialty	Mandibular angle rectangular

[a]From Conrad (1963).

considered sex differences and environmental influences.

We agree with the concept that the constitution of humans is to be understood as a total structure of appearance, function, and performance based on genetic preconditions and environmental modifiers of shape. Thus, we made a point of using modern statistical approaches derived from anthropometric studies to assess methods of determining constitutional typology (hitherto used in medical practice) for their application in forensic medicine. We know from routine investigations, and Lenz's (1982) study, that the more specific the types of constitution corresponding to the rules of biological variability become, the more infrequently they are found. Walter (1974) pointed out that the forms of the human body structure and the underlying anthropometric parameters are subject to geographic heterogeneity. The influence of growth must also be considered, not only when establishing the sex and age of an unknown skeleton but also in the diagnosis of constitution type.

In an earlier investigation, Hunger et al. (1978) performed a factor analysis of 25 important physical features on a sample of 265 females and 475 males. The adults examined showed high loading of the breadth of the head, zygomatic arch, and hand (breadth factor). High loadings were also obtained for head height, hand length, and body height (length factor). As Greil (1987, 1988) confirmed on the basis of more comprehensive studies, variations in breadth and length are frequently interdependent.

The above-mentioned factor analysis led to the establishment of a gradation of 10 metric variables as influential quantities in the two sexes concerning body height. Breadth of the mouth and nose length were not found to be dependent on the form of the skull. Schick (1953) had already referred to several factors that influence constitution. According to Hunger and associates (1978), in males, head height is in second place after hand length, followed by the morphological height of the face, breadth of the zygomatic arch, height of the nose, length of the head, breadth of the nose, breadth of the head, and the distance from one inner canthus to the other.

In his anthropologic studies, Gerasimov (1955) pointed out that the bony structure forms and influences the soft tissue covering. The results of our factor analysis of adult females included high loadings and first-place ranking for head height and length, and morphologic height of the head. These were followed by nose breadth and height. In Vienna, Macho (1986) used multidimensional regression to analyze X-rays of 199 females and 154 males. He found that the height and length of the nose are the most discriminating characteristics on the human skull.

During his 23 years as an expert in genetics, Hammer (1986) compiled anthropologic data on 539 females (average age 38 years) and 609 males (average age 33.7 years). He focused on 24 measurements and 82 descriptive morphologic features. Tables 2 and 3 contain some of his results.

Using discriminant analysis (Vahle, 1986), 26 cephalic measurements of 866 adults (295 females, 609 males) were first subjected to correlation and regression analysis. In the stepwise analysis, high loadings were obtained for the breadths of the forehead, head, zygomatic arches, and bigonial breadth, maximum length of the head, and length and breadth of the ear. Examination of head and facial characteristics for reclassification according to Kretschmer's constitutional type resulted in false diagnoses for more than 75% of females and 65% of males. Of those classified as leptosomes, 80% of the males were correctly assigned, but this dropped to only 44% in females. Only 25% of so-called athletes were diagnosed.

For further analysis we relied on the fundamental statement of Günther (1950) that the skull continues growing and changing well into the sixth decade. This was also pointed out by Martin and Saller (1957) and confirmed by Leopold's (1968) extensive dimensional analyses. Grimm (1966) emphasized that Conrad's constitutional types may well be applied here. In preliminary investigations for superimposition, Helmer (1980, 1984), as well as Leopold (1968) and Helmer and Leopold (1984), found that the relationship of soft tissue thickness to the skull be assessed based on Conrad's growth tendencies. Furthermore, they determined that, as emphasized also by Krogman and İşcan (1986), essential characteristics of the face exist on the skull.

The authors then conducted a stepwise discriminant function analysis of 16 parameters of the face and head of living adults, using Hammer's (1986) data. In this case, 52.4% of the 609 males and 63% of the 531 females were correctly classified. The sexes overlapped both in the leptomorph and in the pyknomorph categories. Continuing the factor analysis, we were

TABLE 2. Percent Distribution of Facial Features in Males and Females[a]

Features	Females			Males		
	Small	Middle	Broad	Small	Middle	Broad
Back of the nose	14.6	63.5	15.9	10.2	75.2	14.6
Root of the nose/breadth	14.6	59.0	26.4	21.0	60.3	17.9
	Low	Middle	High	Low	Middle	High
Wing of the nose/height	26.8	53.4	19.8	13.3	62.7	24
	Straight or bowly	Concave	Convex	Straight	Concave	Convex
Back of the nose/profile	63.8	29.6	6.6	67.2	18.2	14.6
	Thin	Middle	Thick	Thin	Middle	Thick
Wing of the nose/thickness	15.6	73	11.4	11.2	75.5	13.3
	Low	Middle	High	Low	Middle	High
Chin height	20	62.9	17.1	20.4	61.7	17.9
	Small	Middle	Broad	Small	Middle	Broad
Chin breadth	14.5	65.5	20	4.1	55.3	40.6

[a]From Hammer (1986).

TABLE 3. Percent Distribution of Features of the Lip and Nose
in Males and Females[a]

Features	Females			Males		
	Low	Middle	High	Low	Middle	High
Skin, upper lip/height	36.1	53.2	10.7	24.3	55.5	20.2
Skin, lower lip/height	42.5	46.8	10.7	29.2	50.4	20.4
	Straight	Concave	Convex	Straight	Concave	Convex
Skin, upper lip/shape	20.8	75.5	0.7	42.6	53.9	3.5
Skin, lower lip/shape	42.3	55.1	2.6	49.8	46.3	3.9

ultimately left with seven stable characteristics: location of the ear; breadths of the zygomatic arch, mandibular angle, and oral fissure; and length, depth, and breadth of the nose. As a result, female pyknomorphs were correctly determined with 78% accuracy, and in males that figure was 61%. For male leptomorphs, however, 45% were misdiagnosed.

In the final discriminant analysis, we primarily used descriptive features of the face. As is generally known, it is difficult to quantify purely morphologic characteristics so that they can be assessed statistically. In his dissertation, Hammer (1986) has attempted to accomplish this for the features of the head and face. Table 4 shows the frequency distribution of several characteristics of the face (in both sexes) that are important to anthropologic and forensic experts. Discriminant analysis of the breadth of the forehead, breadth and profile of the bridge of the nose, height of the wing of the nose, and form and height of the chin found significant differences between the sexes that can be utilized in several constitution types (Table 5).

DISCUSSION AND CONCLUSIONS

The characteristics of the human face are not only of forensic but also of anthropologic interest. Bernhard and coworkers (1979) used metric traits in their study of the influence of environment and genetics on the formation of the face. Like Schwidetzky (1971) and ourselves, they also included standard photographs in their investigations.

They made it clear that photographic analysis, which is also performed by forensic specialists (Hammer et al., 1981; Helmer, 1986), can lead to exact delineation of the fine structures of the eye, nose, mouth, and ear region. Once adulthood is reached and aging progresses, a number of changes occur. The nose more prominently emerges from the profile of the face. Compared with the thickness of the mucosa and lips, the height of the region between the nose and mucosa of the upper lip increases as the mucosal lips become narrower (Ziegelmayer, 1969). Studies by Leopold (1968) also confirmed that the quantitative analysis of the soft parts of the face allows us to draw significant conclusions and is thus important for identification (see Leonhard, 1976).

Besides age, sex, and genotype, body constitution is of importance for establishing individualization. Although several studies of living adults indicate that the face can also be altered by disease, the essential properties of the underlying bony structure of the skull remain. Nevertheless, when photographic comparisons are performed, false diagnoses can still occur (see İşcan, Chapter 5, this volume). On the whole, in the preliminary research for the determination of constitutional type on the basis of the formation of the face, one must also consider the position of the head and the technique of the photographer. Therefore, Hammer et al. (1981) referred to the fact that photos made by professional photographers or amateurs should be standardized and analyzed anthropologically as well as technically (in terms of lighting, depth of focus, retouching, devel-

TABLE 4.   Anthropometry of the Face in Males and Females[a]

Features	Females				Males			
	Mean	Min.	Max.	v (%)	Mean	Min.	Max	v (%)
Forehead breadth	114	95	137	5.6	119	101	145	6.0
Bigonial breadth	103	85	127	5.6	109	84	132	5.4
Nasal height	47	37	60	9.0	51	39	67	8.5

[a]From Hammer (1986).

opment, film material, and shading) before being relied upon for identification.

Special representations of a face sometimes bring out characteristics of form and individual peculiarities. It has yet to be decided whether constitutional type can thus be diagnosed more clearly, since no suitable studies have been conducted. Special techniques — photostereometry or moire photography — require experience on the part of the expert. Furthermore, this has not yet been used in criminalistic practice, because there were no comparative pictures.

In forensic examinations of fatal accidents or mass disasters, it is necessary to provide the police not only with information about sex and age but also body build or constitution type. We were also able to use our new knowledge of individualization from the face for live but unconscious individuals as well as intact bodies. Following our initial examination of the face and head, we compared identity cards with our findings.

TABLE 5.   Determination of Constitution From Morphological Landmarks and Test of Significance Between the Three Constitutional Types[a]

	Lept. vs. Metro.		Lept. vs. Pykn.		Pykn. vs. Metro.	
			Males			
Chin/shape	Bowly	Elliptic	Bowly	Oval	Oval	Elliptic
Back of the nose/profile	Straight	Bowly*	Straight	Straight,* Bowly		
Wing of the nose/height	Middle	Middle-high*				
Chin/height	High	Middle*				
Skin, upper lip/height	Low	Middle	Low	High*		
			Females			
Back of the nose/profile	Straight	Concave*	Straight	Wavy*	Wavy	Concave
Chin/shape	Oval	Elliptic*	Oval	Bowly		
Skin, lower lip/shape			Straight	Concave*	Concave	Straight*

[a]Males, *N* = 309 leptomorph, 206 metromorph, 75 pyknomorph; Females, *N* = 194 leptomorph, 181 metromorph, 131 pyknomorph.
*Indicates statistical significance.

When further information was needed to make an identification, we included the condition, form, and size of the ears. Knussmann (1988) and Schwarick (1991) repeatedly referred to the influences of age and sex on the condition of the ears. The whole form of the ear is preponderantly environmentally variable, whereas according to the data of Bernhard et al. (1979) individual anatomic segments of the ear are, to a high degree, genetically determined.

Apart from the characteristics of the face and skull, we included dimensions of other parts of the skeleton to make the definitive diagnosis of constitutional type. The epicondylar breadths of the humerus and femur serve not only as measurements of robusticity but also for the determination of constitution (Greil, 1987, 1988). Bones of the lower leg (Leopold et al., 1986), the femur (Weigel et al., 1977), and the arm (Vollmüller, 1989) have also been used for this purpose. Despite numerous assessments of mandibular measurements for all age groups of adults, Pfeiffer (1989) could not isolate any unequivocal constitutional differences in the sexes, apart from bigonial breadth (Leopold et al., 1988).

APPENDIX: SOMATOTYPING BASED ON FACTOR ANALYSIS
Holle Greil

Assessment of the variability of body structure is one of the essential tasks of anthropology (Sigaud, 1914; Kretschmer, 1921; Strömgren, 1937; Sheldon, 1940; Conrad, 1941; Cohen, 1943; Knussmann, 1961, 1988). From 1982 to 1984, members of the Institute of Anthropology at Humboldt University performed anthropometric studies of 96 measurements from 6,000 adults between the ages of 18 and 60 years. The aim of this investigation was the development of an objective and practicable typology of constitution on the basis of factor analysis (Rees and Eysenck, 1945; Burt, 1947; Howells, 1952; Fricke and Knussmann, 1978; Greil, 1988).

First, a sex-specific linear correlation analysis was performed. This statistical evaluation indicated that all vertical measurements showed high to very high positive correlations. The same was true for all horizontal measurements. However, there were only slightly positive or even negative correlations between vertical and horizontal dimensions. On the basis of this analysis, 43 of the 96 measurements were found to generally consider the whole body in all of the three dimensions and to be significant for constitution. These measurements were subjected to principle component analysis with the aim of tracing the incalculably great number of more or less interdependent features back to a few influential and possibly independent quantities. In this way, about 80% of the determined variance was traced back to only three factors in both sexes.

When the factor loadings were entered into a coordination system, the measurements of body structure in the developing three-dimensional factor space arranged themselves into four complexes of features that can be interpreted as growth tendencies. In a two-dimensional projection of the factor loadings to the levels of factors 1 and 2 in males (Fig. 1), all linear measures entered into the analysis form a complex of features with high loadings for factor 2. This tendency to growth in length was seen as clearly in small measuring segments such as length of the middle finger or foot as by body height or arm spread. Nearly independent of this complex of features for "body height" with high loadings, a complex of "corpulence" features is revealed in factor 1. These include such dimensions as chest girth and depth, and neck girth.

Between these two complexes of features, a third complex can be differentiated in which all of the measurements of skeletal robusticity lie close to each other (e.g., hand breadth, elbow breadth, or bicondylar breadth). Biacromial breadth and pelvic breadth unequivocally belong to the complex of robusticity features. On the other hand, the closely related dimensions of bideltoid breadth and maximum hip breadth are associated with measurements of corpulence.

By the position of the features in the three-dimensional factor space, skeletal robusticity

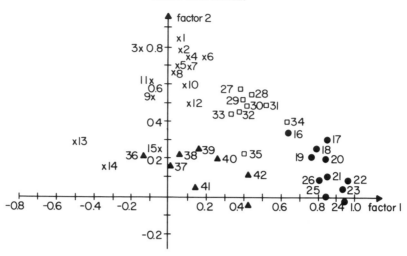

Fig. 1. Two-dimensional projection of 18–60-year-old males (N = 2,933): 1, arm stretch; 2, hand length; 3, stature; 4, middle finger length; 5, forearm length; 6, foot length; 7, upper arm length; 8, lower leg length; 9, thigh length; 10, dorsal trunk height; 11, sitting height; 12, pelvic height; 13, neck length; 14, nape length; 15, malleolare; 16, hip breadth; 17, weight; 18, lower arm girth; 19, bideltoid breadth; 20, hip girth; 21, chest breadth; 22, thoracic girth; 23, chest girth; 24, chest depth; 25, girth at waist; 26, girth of neck; 27, hand breadth I; 28, hand breadth II; 29, foot breadth; 30, elbow breadth; 31, hand thickness; 32, biacromial breadth; 33, bicondylar breadth; 34, pelvic breadth; 35, hand circumference; 36, height of forehead; 37, auricular height; 38, head length; 39, total head height; 40, interpupillary distance; 41, transverse head arc; 42, head circumference; 43, head breadth.

can be characterized as a third growth tendency. Although it is certainly not independent of the development of length and corpulence, it can be clearly differentiated from them. A fourth and final complex of features is composed of length, breadth, and girth measurements of the head. Thus the head is—at least anthropometrically—a relatively independent and self-contained part of the body.

These four complexes of features also remain in a two-dimensional projection into the levels of factors 1 and 3 as well as 2 and 3. A nearly corresponding constellation is the result in the females.

The next step to creating a typology of constitution is the selection of important features in which one factor is distinctly characterized. For this purpose, individual features as well as indices formed from them can be scaled. In the developing typological groups, the changes in all other measuring segments show a steady increase. The individual measure or index functioning as a sig-

nificant feature can then be investigated. The primary features that allow the greatest separation are most suitable for this exercise. For the complex of "corpulence" features, the neck index is calculated as the quotient of neck length × 100/girth of neck. The "robusticity" complex relies on the humeral index—the quotient of elbow breadth × 100/upper arm length. As the neck index increases, a primary hyperplastic–hypoplastic series of variations with increasing measurements of length and decreasing measurements of breadth, depth, and girth develop. This series of variations is similar to the classical series of variations between a low broad-built and high-leptosomatic types. As the humeral index decreases, a secondary series of variations between a robust and gracile pole develops.

The robust type is characterized by relatively small length dimensions, along with large skeletal breadths and high values for the measurements of corpulence. The gracile type shows greater length with relatively insignificant values for measurements of skeletal breadth and corpulence. This new series of variations permits excellent separation.

A two-dimensional coordinate system consists of the primary hyperplastic–hypoplastic series of variations as the *x* axis and the secondary robust–gracile series of variations as the *y* axis. Based on neck girth, elbow breadth, and upper arm length, as well as calculations of the neck and humeral indices, this system allows every possible characterization of the corpulence and skeletal robusticity of adult males.

If an even more detailed determination of constitution type is wanted in an actual case, the two-dimensional system can easily be expanded by a tertiary series of variations. For this purpose, the proportionality of length measured by the leg length to trunk length index (the quotient of leg length × 100/dorsal trunk height) offers itself as an independent criterion that provides very effective separation. The tertiary series of variations is entered into the coordinate system as the *z* axis between a short-legged and long-legged pole. In practice, a relatively rough scaling of three types within a series of variations in every case is recommended—a two-dimensional application yields only nine types, while in a three-dimensional application, there will be 27 possible types.

ACKNOWLEDGMENTS

The editors of this volume are grateful to S.R. Loth for editing this chapter.

REFERENCES

Bach H (1987/88) Normvarianten aus anthropologischer und humangenetischer Sicht. In H Bach and U Jaeger (eds): Tagungsbericht "Normvarianten aus anthropologischer und humangenetischer Sicht" Jena, pp 10–18.

Bernhard W, Bräuer G, Chopra A, and Hancke A (1979) Quantitative genetische Analyse morphologischer Merkmale der Weichteilregionen des menschlichen Kopfes. Homo 30:26–43.

Bertillon A (1895) Das anthropometrische Signalement (2 Aufl); Dtsch Ausgabe v Dr Sury Bern u Leipzig: Verlag v A Siebert.

Burt C (1947) Factor analysis and physical types. Psychometrika 12:171–188.

Cohen J (1943) Physique size and proportions. Br J Med Psychol 18:323–337.

Conrad C (1963) Der Konstitutionstypus. Seine Genetische Grundlegung und Praktische Anwendung(2 Aufl). Berlin: Springer.

Flügel H, Greil H, and Sommer K (eds) (1986) Anthropologischer Atlas. Grundlagen und Daten. Berlin: Tribüne.

Fricke R, and Knussmann R (1978) Intercorrelations of growth and maturity characters in the male sex: A factor analysis. In L Gedda and P Parisi (eds): Auxology: Human Growth in Health and Disorder. London: Academic Press.

Gerasimov MM (1955) Wiederherstellung des Gesichtes aufgrund des Schädels. Moscow: Akademie Nauk (in Russian).

Greil H (1987) Der Korperbau im Erwachsenenalter—DDR—repräsentative anthropologisch Querschnittsstudir (1982/1984), Promot B, Humbolt-Univ, Berlin.

Greil H (1988) Mehrdimensionale Variabilität von Körperbaumassen im Erwachsenenalter. Wiss Z Humboldt-Univ Berlin, R Med 37:212–221.

Grimm H (1966) Grundriss der Konstitutionsbiologie und Anthropometrie. Berlin: Volk und Gesundheit.

Günther H (1950) Die physiologische Akromegalie. Endokrinologie 27:253–258.

Hammer H-J (1986) Die metrischen und deskriptiven morphologischen Merkmale des Menschen—eine Studie über ihre Verteilung in einer DDR—Population und ihre Bedeutung fur die forensische Praxis. Promot B, Bereich Medizin, Karl-Marx-Univ Leipzig.

Hammer H-J, Hunger H, and Leopold D (1981) Zur Anwendbarkeit morphologischer Gesichtsmerkmale bei der Identifikation. Kriminalistik Forens Wiss 44:111–120.

Helmer R (1980) Schädelidentifizierung durch elektronische Bildmischung-Habilschr, Univ Kiel.

Helmer R (1984) Schädelidentifizierung durch elektronische Bildmischung. Heidelberg: Kriminalistik Verlag.

Helmer R (1986) Bildanalyse per elektronischer Bildmischung. Heidelberg: Kriminalistik Verlag.

Helmer R, and Leopold D (1984) Neuere Aspekte zur Schädelidentifizierung. Kriminalistik Forens Wiss 55/56:82–88.

Höhne K (1947) Schnell—und Reihendiagnostik der Kretschmer'schen Konstitutionstypen. Arztl Forsch 1:219–222.

Howells WW (1952) A factorial study of constitutional type. Am J Phys Anthropol 10:91–118.

Hunger H, Leopold D, and Rother P (1978) Statistik brauchbarer Masse bei Lebendbegutachtungen. In H Hunger and D Leopold (eds): Identifikation. Leipzig: Barth, pp 416–423.

Johnsen D, and Scholz C (1989) Anthropometrische

Methoden zur Ermittlung und Beurteilung des Ernährungszustandes des Menschen. Wiss Z Humboldt-Univ R Med 38:218–226.

Kallmeyer F, and Weidhase R (1986) Körpermessungen und Konstitutions-typenbestimmung an Leipziger Schülern—ein Beitrag zur Akzeleration. Dissertation A, Med Akademie Erfurt.

Klaus EJ (1960) Die Konstitutionsbestimmung in der sportärztichen Praxis. In F Heiss (ed): Praktische Sportmedizin. Stuttgart: Enke.

Knussmann R (1961) Zur Methods der objektiven Körperbautypognose. Z Vererb Konst 36:1–44.

Knussmann R (ed) (1988) Anthropologie: Handbuch der Vergleichenden Biologie des Menschen. Vol 1: Wesen und Methoden der Anthropologie. Stuttgart: Gustav Fischer.

Kohlrausch W (1926) Sporttypen. Mitt Gymn Ges Bern 6:139–154.

Kretschmer E (1921) Körperbau und Charakter. Berlin: Springer.

Krogman WM, and İşcan MY (1986) The Human Skeleton in Forensic Medicine. Springfield, Ill: Charles C Thomas.

Lenz JG (1982) Neue daten zur Körpergrussa. Med Klin 77:37–40.

Leonhard K (1976) Der Menschliche Ausdruck in Mimik. Leipzig: Gestik und Phonik.

Leopold D (1968) Identifikation durch Schädeluntersuchungen unter besonderer Berücksichtigung der Superprojektion. Habilitations—Schrift, Med Fak, Karl-Marx Univ, Leipzig.

Leopold D (1976) Identifikation durch Kraniometrie an Fernröntgenaufnahmen. Wiss Z, Karl-Marx-Univ, Leipzig, Math—Naturw R 25:507–512.

Leopold D, Minuth I, and Krüger G (1986) Zum Sexualdimorphismus der Unterschenkelknochen—ein Beitrag zur Identifikation. Kriminalistik Forens Wiss 63/64:62–66.

Leopold D, Pfeiffer H, and Beckert G (1988) Neuere Untersuchungen zur Geschlechtadiagnostik an der Mandibula. Kriminalistik Forcns Wiss 71/72:111–114.

Macho G (1986) An appraisal of plastic reconstruction of the external nose. J Forensic Sci 31:1391–1403.

Martin R (1928) Lehrbuch der Anthropologie. Jena: Fischer.

Martin R, and Saller K (1957) Lehrbuch der Anthropologie. Stuttgart: Fischer.

Pfeiffer H (1989) Untersuchungen zum Geschlechtsdimorphismus an der Mandibula—ein Beitrag zur Identifikation. Promot A, Med Akad Erfurt.

Rees WL, and Eysenck HJ (1945) A factorial study of some morphological and psychological aspects of human constitution. J Ment Sci 91:8–21.

Schick C (1953) Zur Faktorenanalyse der Konstitutionstypen. Z Menschl Vererb-u Konstit Lehre 32:1–31.

Schwarick J (1991) Zur Morphologie der Ohrmuschal bei Neugeborenen und Sauglingen. Dissertation A, Med Akad, Erfurt.

Schwidetsky I (1971) Hauptprobleme der Anthropologie. Freiburg: Breisgau Rombach.

Sheldon WH (1940) The Varieties of Human Physique. New York: Harper.

Sigaud C (1914) La Forme Humaine. Paris: Maloine.

Strömgren E (1937) Über anthropometrische Indizes zur Unterscheidung von Körperbautypen. Z Ges Neurol Psychiatr 159:75–81.

Tittel H, and Wutscherk H (1971) Sportanthropometrie. Leipzig: Barth.

Vahle H (1986) Semidefinite Faktorprobleme—ihre softwaremassige Lösung und Anwendung. Promot B, Math—Naturw Fak, Karl-Marx-Univ, Leipzig.

Vollmüller J (1989) Untersuchungen zur Geschlechts—und Altersbestimmung an Humerus, Radius und Ulna unter Berücksichtigung der Akzeleration und des Konstitutionstypus. Promot A, Med Akad Erfurt.

Walter H (1974) Gedanken zur geographischen Variabilitat der menschl. Körperform Anthropol Közl 18:219–227.

Weigel B, Leopold D, and Krüger G (1977) Beziehungen zwischen Ausbildung des Humerus, Femur, der Scapula sowie der Konstitution. Wiss. Z Ernst-Moritz-Arndt-Univ Greifswald, Med Reihe 26:53–55.

Ziegelmayer G (1969) Mund-Kinn-Region. In PE Becker (ed): Humangenetik. Stuttgart: Georg Thieme, pp 56–81.

Chapter 5

Introduction of Techniques for Photographic Comparison: Potential and Problems

Mehmet Yaşar İşcan

Department of Anthropology, Florida Atlantic University, Boca Raton, Florida 33431

As crime levels increase, anthropologists are more frequently being called upon to express expert opinions on many aspects of human biology in an attempt to identify both victims and criminals. Their expertise has ranged from the identification of skeletal remains and footprint analysis to facial recognition, comparison, and reconstruction. Photographic comparisons are becoming particularly important. Surveys of diplomates of the American Board of Forensic Anthropology indicated the number of requests for this type of analysis rose from 8 in 1987 to 20 in 1991—and these figures are just for the United States. One must also consider that there are cases of this sort in other parts of the world. The demand for photographic comparisons is no doubt fueled by the proliferation of surveillance cameras. This technology can catch criminals in the act, but the images caught on film are of little value unless they can be linked with an acceptable degree of certainty to a particular individual.

In 1981, İşcan and Charney compared two- and three-dimensional facial reconstructions using measurements from their photographs. They found that the two forms of facial reconstruction produced dimensional similarities but very different morphological features. Kerley (1982) briefly presented his experience with photographic comparison. Both studies outlined problems associated with this process and introduced measurements that might allow valid comparisons. In a recent study attempting to determine if a skull in Salzburg belonged to Mozart,

Kritscher and Szilvássy (1991) compared their facial reconstruction from the skull with known portraits of Mozart and his parents and sister. These authors used standard anthroposcopic characteristics obtainable from living individuals to compare with the photographs. Law enforcement agencies also conducted experiments to determine the value of using measurements from photographs for facial comparisons (Catterick, 1992).

Called to Israel as an expert witness for the trial of accused Nazi concentration camp guard John (Ivan) Demjanjuk, İşcan (1987, 1988a) used this approach with additional criteria. The focus of this trial was an old I.D. photograph of a Nazi guard who resembled a retired auto worker from Cleveland. İşcan was faced with comparing the features from that photo with pictures of Demjanjuk at different ages. The author continued his attempts to determine if a definitive match could be made or an individual excluded on the bases of photographic comparisons with trials in Toronto, Canada, and in Florida (İşcan, 1990, 1992). He realized that carefully developed scientific standards were necessary for acceptance in a court of law.

In general, positive identification from the skeleton depends upon isolating factors that make one person unique from the rest. Evidence from dentition and antemortem radiographs are probably the most effective (Krogman and İşcan, 1986; Clark, 1992). General characteristics like age, sex, race, and stature can either suggest or rule out a match, but they can never be absolutely conclusive in and of themselves (İşcan, 1988b).

Although it seems deceptively simple, the comparison of two or more photographs remains one of the most difficult types of identification. As yet, no standard procedures have been developed for the analysis of photographs or video images. In most cases, each expert "reinvents" a method to fit the case at hand. Some situations that call for this type of analysis include the comparison of two or more photographs taken at different ages (e.g., a child's photograph with that of a young adult), and identification from images recorded by a video surveillance camera and the actual suspect or his photograph.

The purpose of this chapter is to develop, summarize, and evaluate the effectiveness of techniques that have been attempted in the last few years. These techniques can be divided into three types: morphological analysis of facial structures, photo-anthropometry of the face, and photo-to-photo video superimposition.

MORPHOLOGICAL ANALYSIS

The face is the most individually recognizable part of the human body (with the exception of gross postcranial deformities). It also reacts to stresses arising from the environment, the physiological process of aging, and genetic determinants. There is no doubt that these and many other factors lead to the differences and similarities seen in facial physiognomy (see Leopold et al., Chapter 4, this volume).

Populations isolated geographically or socially are bound to reflect morphological similarities that can be traced to inbreeding. Assessment of these phenotypic similarities formed the basis for the development of racial typologies (Hooton, 1946; Coon and Hunt, 1965; Molnar, 1992). Population affinities go beyond the traditional classifications of Mongoloid, Negroid, and Caucasoid to subdivisions marked by high concentrations of certain features in, for example, diverse geographic regions. Hooton

(1946) devised a system that included numerous subgroups. Alpines (concentrated in the central zone of Europe), for one, were described as "basic brunet round-heads with medium broad noses" whose primary sorting criteria include dark to medium dark brown hair and eye color, globular heads with high foreheads, and a mesorrhine nose with a slightly concave or straight profile and fleshy, "blobby," often elevated tip (Hooton, 1946:578). Other characteristics include olive to brunet white skin color, abundant hair and beard, and round or square face with prominent gonial angles.

The systematic, feature-by-feature approach used by 19th- and 20th-century anthropologists has become a very important tool in forensic facial analysis. Along this line, some recent forensic studies subdivide the face into components to obtain a thorough analysis (e.g., Hammer, 1978; Kritscher and Szilvássy, 1991). The author assembled Table 1 to serve as a compilation of the entire range of morphological features. This table is intended for use as a data collection form for photographic analysis and comparisons. It promotes a consistent, systematic, and scientifically comparable evaluation of facial features. It is also designed to make individual variation and population differences emerge from a seemingly unremarkable visage, and thus can be used to guide the expert in making a decision about the viability of a match.

As a supplement to Table 1, Figures 1 and 2 illustrate a variety of facial forms and features listed in the table. These schematic drawings emphasize such characteristics as facial outline shapes, hairlines, and mouth and chin shapes (Fig. 1). The caricature-type sketches in Figure 2 exaggerate a range of profiles.

One of the biggest problems in this type of analysis is that the appearance of facial features can be altered by even the most subtle changes in expression or photographic angle. Emotions such as anger, fear, happiness, curiosity, concern, worry, or surprise all alter facial expression. To these temporary variations, one must also consider permanent changes due to aging, disease, changes in lifestyle, and exposure to the elements. The aging factor is a serious issue because one is often called upon to compare pictures taken years apart—and even a year or less can make a significant difference. Figure 3 displays a series of pictures from age 11 to 49 taken professionally (except for the last one at 49). Some changes are obvious—graying hair, beard, deepening cheek furrows—others are more subtle. Although a slight asymmetry in the opening height of the eye may first be noted in the early years, this becomes more conspicuous with increasing age. By the time the subject is in his thirties, the right eyelid appears "droopy." On the other hand, there is little change in mouth shape and lip thickness. The general facial outline and chin form vary little, even with some thickening from weight gain in his early forties. A pronounced "widow's peak" was traceable until a change in hairstyle obscured it.

The development of facial wrinkles illustrates but one of the many factors resulting from the aging process (Hammer, 1978; Adams, 1991; Doual et al., 1991). Figure 4 shows some of the wrinkles of the face. Those around the eyes and chin show earliest evidence of aging. Wrinkles may also develop as a result of disease, exposure to the sun, and even smoking (Burke 1990; Kadunce et al., 1991; Warren et al., 1991; Grady and Ernster, 1992). The creases and folds in these schematic drawings are observable in some form in all individuals at every age. However, their shape, form, and degree of development can vary greatly from one individual to the next. With advancing age, furrows deepen, folds sag, and new wrinkles form. All of these events can significantly alter appearance.

The manifestations of aging are so varied that it is very difficult to predict the rate of change for a given individual. This is complicated by the fact that each feature may change independently within and among individuals. For example, the lateral epicanthic fold of the eye may develop in middle age in some people, becoming more pronounced with increasing age. On the other hand, this feature may never develop in others.

So with this seemingly endless list of problems, the question remains: What features are valid indicators of individuality? As noted above, members of isolated populations exhibit many common features as a result of inbreeding. Therefore, these commonalities are not useful in discriminating one person from another. To complicate matters further, a set of features that easily distinguish individuals in one group may be of no use in other groups. For example, hair color and form are very uniform in Asian Mongoloids, but exhibit a wide range of variation in whites. Thus, there must be some scientific basis for the selection of these key features. Most would agree that structures such as the nose and mouth vary enough to be used to exclude a large number of candidates. It is obvious that an individual with thick, everted lips cannot be matched to a thin-lipped photographic image.

Another concern is the relationship of one feature to another. Ideally, one would wish to determine which features are independent and which structural configurations are genetically ordered and dependently related. There is, however, no known scientific study that can explain if a hereditary relationship exists for a particular set of structures or the features within them. Some attributes are often found in association with others to present a properly proportioned face with regular, ordinary features. For example, snub noses tend to occur in conjunction with concave nasal profiles. Therefore, it would be notable if a person with a snub nose had a convex profile. Deviations from the "norm" such as a disproportionately large nose or protruding ears also create a distinctive appearance. Therefore, the selection of standards for facial comparison must be based on *a priori* knowledge of the conditions mentioned above. It is also advisable to choose structures that are most resistant to the ravages of time.

PHOTO-ANTHROPOMETRIC APPROACH

Photo-anthropometry can be defined as the analysis of anthropometric landmarks, dimensions, and angles to quantify facial characteristics and proportions from a photograph. This technique involves measuring similar dimen-

**TABLE 1.   Morphological Characteristics of Human Head and Face That Can Be Observed
From Photographs[a]**

Name_____	Sex___	Age___	Birthdate_____	Birthplace_____
Ancestry_____	Occupation_____		Purpose _____	Case No._____
Illness_____	Peculiarities_____		Asymmetry_____	Date_____

Facial forms	Texture	Small
Elliptical	Fine	Medium
Round	Moderate	Large
Oval	Coarse	Upper lid
Pentagonal	Wiry	Low
Rhomboid	Baldness	Medium
Square	Absent	High
Trapezoid	Slight	Eyebrow thickness
Wedge-shaped	Advanced	Slight
Double concave	Complete	Small
Asymmetrical	Beard quantity	Average
Facial profiles	Very little	Large
Jutting	Small	Concurrency
Forward curving	Average	Absent
Vertical	Hairy	Slight
Concave	Hair color: Head and beard	Average
Lower jutting	Black	Continuous
Upper jutting	Brown	Eyebrow shape
Forehead height	Red bright	Straight
Low	Golden	Wavy
Medium	Red	Arched
High	Gray	Eyebrow density
Forehead width	White	Sparse
Small	Iris color	Thick
Medium	Black	Bushy
Broad	Brown	Nasion depression
Skin color	Green-brown	Trace
Pale	Blue-brown	Slight
Brunet	Green	Average
Brown	Gray	Deep
Chocolate	Blue	Very deep
Black	Other	Bony profile
Vascularity	Eyefolds	Straight
Slight	Absent	Concave
Average	Internal	Wavy
Extreme	Slight	Convex
Freckles	Average	Bridge height
None	Developed	Small
Few	Median	Medium
Moderate	Slight	High
Extreme	Average	Bridge breadth
Moles	Developed	Very small
None	External	Small
Few	Slight	Medium
Moderate	Average	Large
Extreme	Developed	Tip thickness
Hair form	Palpebral slit	Very small
Straight	Down	Small
Low waves	Horizontal	Average
Deep waves	Up slight	Thick
Curly	Up moderate	Tip shape
Frizzy	Up extreme	Pointed
Woolly	Opening height	Bilobed

TABLE 1. Morphological Characteristics of Human Head and Face That Can Be Observed From Photographs[a] *(Continued)*

Angular	Philtrum shape	Gonial eversion
Rounded	Flat	Compressed
Blobby	Deep	Slight
Snub	Sides parallel	Moderate
Septum tilt	Sides divergent	Everted
Up	Upper lip notch	Very everted
Up slight	Absent	Ear size
Horizontal	Wavy	Small
Down slight	V-shape	Medium
Down	Mouth corner	Large
Nostril form	Straight	Ear projection
Slit	Upturn	Slight
Ellipse	Downturn	Medium
Intermediate	Alveolar prognathism	Large
Round	Absent	Helix
Nostril visibility	Slight	Flat
Lateral	Medium	Slight roll
None	Pronounced	Average
Slight	Chin projection	Very rolled
Medium	Negative	Anti-helix
Visible	Neutral	Slight
Frontal	Slight	Medium
None	Forward	Developed
Slight	Protruding	Darwin's point
Medium	Malars	Absent
Visible	Anterior projection	Present
Nasal alae	Absent	Lobe
Compressed	Slight	None
Slight	Medium	Soldered
Flaring	Pronounced	Attached
Extended	Lateral projection	Free
Lip thickness	Compressed	Long and free
Very thin	Slight	Other features
Thin	Medium	Birth marks:
Average	Pronounced	Moles:
Thick	Chin projection	Wrinkles:
Eversion	Negative	Asymmetry:
Slight	Neutral	Fatness:
Small	Slight	Mustache:
Average	Average	Beard:
Everted	Pronounced	Sideburns:
Lip seam	Chin type	Trauma:
Absent	Median	Surgery:
Slight	Triangle	Scars:
Average	Bilateral	Glasses:
Present	Chin from front	
Integument lips	Small and round	
Thin	Wide and round	
Average	Pointed	
Thick	Chin shape	
Philtrum size	Dimple	
Small	Cleft	
Wide	Double chin	

[a]Modified from J. Lawrence Angel's unpublished Anthropometry and Morphology data collection form, and Hammer (1978).

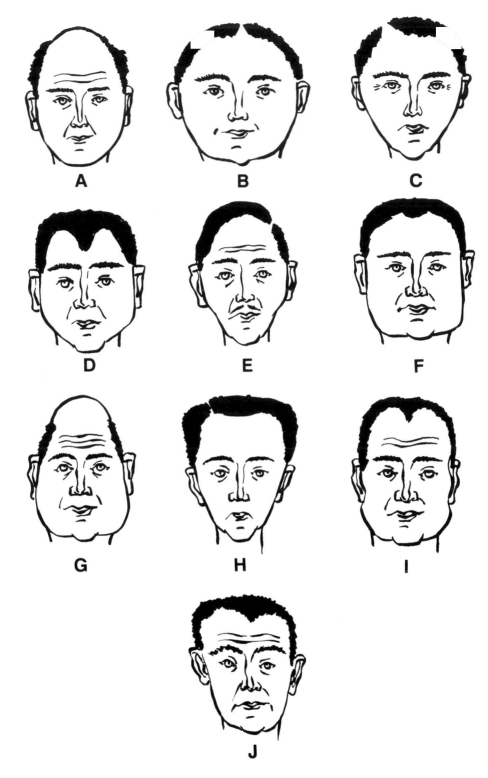

Fig. 1. Full-face schematic drawings: **A**: Elliptical; **B**: round; **C**: oval; **D**: pentagonal; **E**: rhomboid; **F**: square; **G**: trapezoid; **H**: wedge-shaped; **I**: double concave; **J**: asymmetrical. (Modified from Hammer, 1978, Fig. 276.)

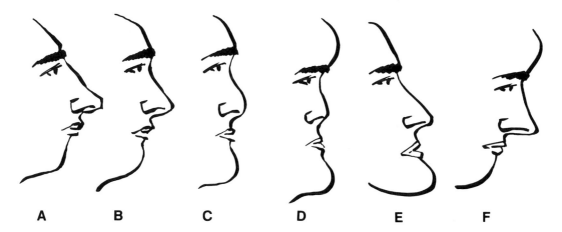

Fig. 2. Caricature-type profiles: **A**: Jutting; **B**: forward curving; **C**: vertical; **D**: concave; **E**: lower jutting; **F**: upper jutting. (Modified from Hammer, 1978, Fig. 177.)

sions of a known person's photographs with those of the individual in question. It differs from the anthropometry of the living because the landmarks are not easily identifiable or visible on the photograph. However, if a photograph is of good quality, and shows facial features clearly, then landmarks can be defined and measurements obtained.

In the past, this type of analysis has been attempted for a number of purposes (Brothwell et al., 1972; Bernhard et al., 1979; Knussmann, 1988). The study by Brothwell and associates was designed to assess the biological affinities and history of the people of Tristan da Cunha, the Ainu, and compare them with populations of Mongoloid, Negroid, and Caucasoid stocks. The intention of Bernhard et al. (1979) was to determine genetic difference between family members from a German sample. In both studies, as many as 29 measurements, and 21 angles and indices generated from them were used. Knussmann's (1988) emphasis was on forensic facial comparison and the estimation of body size using photographs and video images.

In order to begin a photographic analysis, the pictures must be copied and enlarged to 8 × 10" prints. (The use of smaller pictures is not recommended because it will be much more difficult to tag landmarks, take accurate measure-

ments, and present findings in court.) The originals themselves must not be altered. Once the landmarks have been chosen, they must be marked with a very fine-tipped pen on both photographs to be compared. Suggested sites visible (some in full face, others in profile, some in both, as indicated below) when the picture is oriented in the Frankfort horizontal plane appear in Figure 5 and are described as follows:

A. Trichion: Midpoint of the hairline (full face and profile)

B. Metopion: Most anterior point of the forehead (profile only)

C. Glabella: Midpoint between the eyebrows on the median plane (profile only)

D. Nasion: Deepest point of the nasal root (profile only)

E. Midnasal point: Midpoint between the endocanthions (full face only)

F. Pronasale: Most anterior point of the nose tip (profile only)

G. Subnasale: Point where the nasal septum meets the philtrum (can be located in both full and profile if the nose tip is horizontal or elevated)

H. Superior labiale: Midpoint of the vermilion seam of the upper lip (full face and profile)

I. Stomion: Midpoint of the occlusal line between the lips (full face and profile)

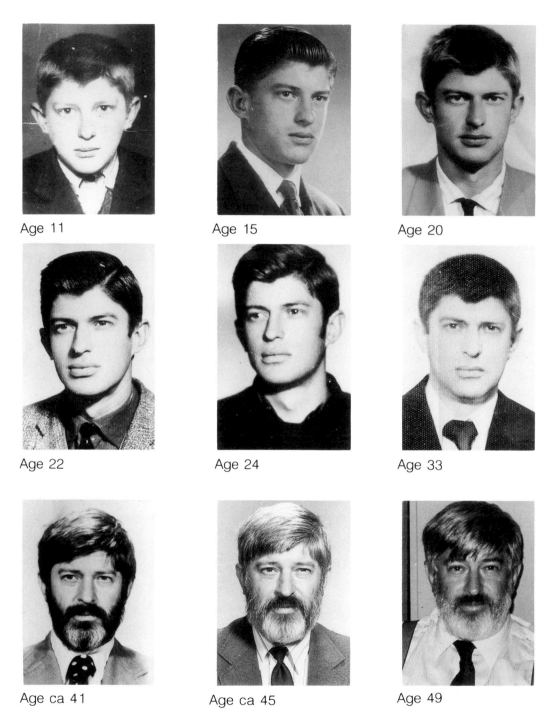

Age 11   Age 15   Age 20

Age 22   Age 24   Age 33

Age ca 41   Age ca 45   Age 49

Fig. 3. Facial growth and aging over a nearly 40-year span. Observe the consistencies in facial outline, nose shape, and lip and hair form. Note how longer hair covers distinctive "widow's peak" obvious in younger photos. Though the face thickened with added weight, the general shape was not lost.

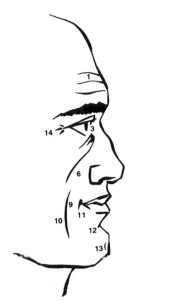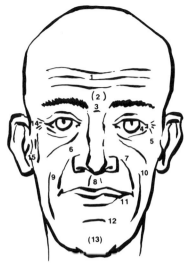

Fig. 4. Wrinkles of the face: 1: Horizontal forehead wrinkles; 2: vertical wrinkles of the glabella; 3: wrinkles of the nasal root; 4: eye fold below the orbit; 5: eye–cheek fold; 6: nose–cheek wrinkle; 7: nose–lip fold; 8: nose–lip fold; 9: cheek–chin wrinkle; 10: cheek–chin fold; 11: mouth corner fold; 12: lip–chin fold; 13: chin cleft; 14: temporal wrinkles; 15: ear wrinkles. (Modified from Hammer, 1978, Fig. 206.)

J. Inferior labiale: Midpoint of the vermilion seam of the lower lip (full face and profile)

K. Pogonion: Most anterior point of the chin (profile only)

L. Gnathion: The most inferior point of the chin (full face and profile)

M. Cheilion: Corner of the mouth (full face and profile)

N. Alare: Most lateral point of the nasal wings (full face and profile)

O. Superaurale: Most superior point of the ear (full face and profile)

P. Tragion: Most anterior point of the tragus (profile only)

Q. Subaurale: Most inferior point of the ear (full face and profile)

R. Postaurale: Most posterior point of the ear (profile only)

Numerous measurements can be taken from these two views. If trichion is clear, it can be the starting point for most of the vertical measure-ments. Therefore, one may use A–D (A–E), A–G (or A–F), A–H, A–I, A–J, A–L, N–N, and P–P. If trichion is not available or the head is balding, then D (or E) can be the starting point. Some of the facial width measurements include A–P, B–P, D–P, F–P, G–P, and O–Q.

Additional landmarks can be used if necessary and if clearly visible from both photographs. Although many dimensions can be taken, a particular set cannot be standardized because their availability depends on the quality of the evidence in each case. Dimensions must be measured with a precision caliper with vernier accurate to at least one decimal place. Keep in mind that the investigator is not limited to these landmarks and may choose others as long as they are clearly defined on both photographs.

Finally, in order to make the values truly comparable, indices must be calculated from these measurements. Although objects in the photo may be of known size and can be used as a scale, this is not usually the case. More often

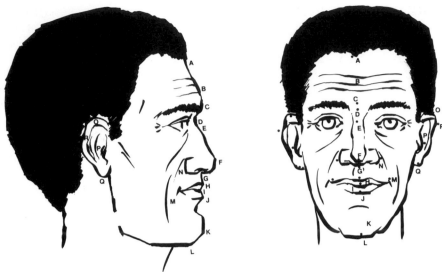

Fig. 5. Photographic landmarks of the face: A: Trichion; B: metopion; C: glabella; D: nasion; E: midnasal point; F: pronasale; G: subnasale; H: superior labiale; I: stomion; J: inferior labiale; K: pogonion; L: gnathion; M: cheilion; N: alare; O: superaurale; P: tragion; Q: subaurale; R: postaurale.

than not, it is impossible to determine the actual dimensions of the face and its features. Therefore an index must function to eliminate the effects of absolute size differences between individuals or objects. An index is formed as follows: Small dimension × 100/Large dimension. The result quantifies the proportion of the small dimension to the large dimension and thus the problem of scale is eliminated. As many indices as necessary can be generated. For linear dimensions, it is best to use the maximum dimension as a constant denominator (e.g., D–G/A–L, D–H/A–L, D–H/A–L, etc.). Facial width can also be assessed in relation to height or other dimensions. These calculations can be done easily on any computer spreadsheet program.

The marked photographs must be used for the investigation and submitted to the court as evidence. If more copies are needed, this can be done by making extra prints, but only after the photographs have been marked, otherwise it is very difficult to exactly duplicate the positioning of the marks. Photocopies may be used for less crucial purposes.

Photo-anthropometry is a technique that at-

tempts to metrically compare the proportional relationships of one photo to another rather than determine absolute visual similarities, as is done in morphological comparisons. Although quantification reduces the subjectivity of photographic comparison, one cannot always reach a definite conclusion regarding the matching of two images. Some of the obvious problems are: (1) The photographs may have been taken under different conditions (e.g., lighting); (2) the angle of the lens and the distance between the camera and subject alter the apparent proportions of the face (see Lan and Cai, Chapter 10, this volume); (3) some photographs may have been retouched to improve the appearance of the subject; in this case the facial features may not match those of the unretouched photographs even if it is the same individual; (4) weight and age differences may bring about changes in the location and appearance of landmarks; and (5) differences in facial expression may result in different values. This is especially true when a picture with a laughing or smiling face is compared with a serious or frowning one. Laughter, for example, may widen the mouth, shorten the nose-to-mouth distance, and lengthen the face.

PHOTOGRAPHIC VIDEO SUPERIMPOSITION

Many chapters in this volume explain the technical aspects of video superimposition in great detail. Advances in video technology have eliminated the laborious work of photographic enlargement and orientation of the object (e.g., the skull) to duplicate the pose of the picture (Krogman and İşcan, 1986). In photographic superimposition, two comparably enlarged photographs are superimposed over each other using video cameras, a mixer, and a monitor. The procedure can be done easily if one has the right equipment.

The aim of this technique is to determine if facial features and dimensions can be correctly superimposed on each other. Once the cameras are properly positioned and photographic distances are adjusted until the images are the same size, a mixer will allow different types of visual comparisons. A "fade" will make one face appear to disappear into another, with the second image eventually replacing the first. A "horizontal wipe" will result in one face passing laterally across the other. The wipe can also be in a vertical direction from top to bottom and vice versa. Additional superimpositions can be carried out to emphasize a particular region of the face. One may focus on a particularly telling feature (e.g., an obvious asymmetry or dimples) to emphasize its difference or similarity.

When an expert opinion is requested, the qualified scientist must demonstrate in detail how the superimposition technique was carried out. The simplest approach to satisfy the concerns of law enforcement and the court is to allow plenty of time to show and explain how one photo is superimposed over another. In most cases superimpositions do not match exactly, although a very slow fade may give the illusion of a perfect match as one image is almost imperceptibly replaced by the other. Such an approach must be avoided in order to maintain objectivity. Following a complete initial wipe, the process of dissolving one image into the next should be repeated, with pauses to demonstrate important areas where there are marked differences or perfect matches. The expert should literally point out and trace these areas on the screen during pre-trial deposition or testimony in court.

The ideal approach is to superimpose a photograph on a living person. As demonstrated in this volume, the best possible alignment can be obtained when one of the objects (a skull or living person) is three-dimensional and readily adjustable. If the suspect is willing to pose, or is under court order to do so, the head can be oriented to the same position as that of the photograph. Another important advantage is that the living person can duplicate the facial expression in the photograph. This is not possible in photo-to-photo superimposition because the positions and expressions are fixed.

There are a number of problems with this type of superimposition, including many that are associated with morphological and anthropometric comparisons. Photo-to-photo superimposition is the least accurate method of comparison. A problem unique to this technique is the rarity of finding photographs that are taken under the exact same conditions and in identical poses. In various trials, the author has observed that only a few features rather than the face as a whole have been superimposed. For example, some witnesses draw attention to agreements in ear or nose length while ignoring obvious discrepancies in the chin and forehead. An expert should not be content or even defend an identification based on merely a few general features like facial roundness, projecting ears, and receding hairline. One also must not lose sight of the fact that, for example, an open mouth is dissolving into a closed one or a smile disappears. Camera "tricks" may either enhance or minimize the actual differences and similarities between pictures.

Recent advances in superimposition by computer digitizing may offer an even more objective mode of comparison. A computer can quantify and judge the characteristics that differentiate one face from another without the blending that can obscure differences in video superimposition. Majumdar and Sinha (1989) have developed a program that digitizes projective symmetry in photographs and uses the patterns thus obtained to assess the comparability of two individuals. The software generates a composite image containing sections of each photograph. If the pieces from both pictures fit together precisely, it is likely that one is dealing with a single individual. This has even shown success when a disguise is used. Thus it is effectively demonstrated that symmetry should remain fairly constant even if visual appearance is altered.

To end on a more positive note, a video or computer system allows the expert to develop and demonstrate a series of visual effects and to focus on morphological details and anthropometric measurements. In this way the viewers (e.g., the jurors, attorneys, and law enforcement officers) can see the entire procedure and visualize exactly how the expert came to his or her conclusions.

CONCLUSIONS

The three methods described in this chapter that have been used to compare one photograph with another (or videotape frame) are (1) morphological: detailed comparison of facial features following the form in Table 1; (2) photoanthropometry: quantitative analysis based on measurements of facial dimensions and generation of indices; and (3) photographic video superimposition: superimposition of one photograph or videotape frame on another.

There is no question that photographic identification is plagued with many problems—some related to the physiognomy of the persons in the photographs, others arising from the quality of the evidence. One must often deal with materials of the most marginal nature. Any comparison based on photographs taken under differing conditions (e.g., light, exposure, camera–subject distance and angle, expression, and pose) may affect how one image is seen in relation to another. Old photographs may be torn, creased, and faded. Surveillance videotapes have their own built-in problems. The images tend to be fuzzy, making it impossible to delineate sharp

borders; further clarity is lost when transferring a frame to a photographic print for analysis; and camera location is usually far from ideal in terms of lighting, position, etc. (especially in outdoor automatic bank tellers). It is imperative to have the most advanced, high-quality equipment. It will definitely hurt a court case if opposing counsel contests evidence based on inadequacies of the apparatus used to make the comparison.

Physiognomic differences that can affect appearance range from facial expression to hairstyle (Koury and Epker, 1991; Wogalter and Hosie, 1991). One must be prepared for the challenge of comparing a bearded chin to one that is clean-shaven, the bald pate of an older man to his younger, curly-haired visage, or a smooth face to a wrinkled one. Loss of teeth makes the nose and chin appear more pronounced, and also reduces both the mouth-to-nose and mouth-to-chin distances. Cartilage in both nose and ears continues to grow throughout life, lengthening these structures. Eyelids can sag, creating epicanthic folds or asymmetries. Trauma and surgery may leave scars. Moles may develop or be removed; freckles vary seasonally. Cosmetic changes range from plastic surgery to modifications of hair color or style, makeup, and facial hair. Glasses may make the eyes appear larger or smaller and may obscure surrounding features. All of these conditions may alter the appearance both morphologically and metrically to the extent that even two pictures of the same individual may not match!

Because the morphological approach may identify obvious factors of individualization, this type of analysis of the face is most likely to lead to a positive identification or to rule out a match, as in skeletal analysis (Krogman and İşcan, 1986). However, there remain many indeterminate areas, especially when dealing with an "average-looking" person. What makes one individual different from all others is the complexity of variation possible in many features. Interpretations and conclusions must be made with caution because certain characteristics may be common to a specific racial or ethnic group.

To reiterate, the literature does not contain

scientific studies that offer precise standards for photo-anthropometric comparisons. Research in this area must lead to methods that can account for mensural variations arising from differences in pose and angle by experimenting with control subjects. To be of real value, studies of this type should follow exacting scientific protocols and include rigorous testing of empirical data. Attempts are being made in this direction. In a new study, an image-processing system using a video camera was devised and used to analyze passport-sized photographs (good quality, $N = 27$ photographs) and magazine photographs (poorer quality to simulate those taken under less ideal conditions, $N = 27$ photographs) (Catterick, 1992). Computerized measurements were taken from co-planar facial segments between the eyes and chin and two indices were generated. The computer performed 351 pairwise permutations and revealed that 72% of the good-quality photographs and 66% of the magazine copies showed at least two standard deviations of difference: These pairs were considered distinguishable. This means that less than 1 in 4 randomly selected pairs of photographs cannot be distinguished by this procedure. The outcome was significantly poorer if the photographs were taken at different camera angles. The main value of this procedure is to narrow the range of possible matches.

As the least reliable and most subjective technique, photo-to-photo superimposition in its present form cannot result in a positive identification. From a technical point of view, this approach can only provide support for photo-anthropometry by allowing visualization of dimensional and morphological discrepancies. Furthermore, in order to make use of the myriad of surveillance evidence now available, two things must change: The quality of these films must be greatly improved, and analytical methods must be perfected.

In their present state of development, the techniques discussed in this chapter have the potential to lead to a definitive decision regarding identity or a match. This is especially true if the comparative materials have unusual features, or at least have those not common to their population. However, in most cases the results will be indeterminate, at best—and thus cannot stand alone as evidence to convict or exonerate a suspect. The expert witness must be cautious and responsible in his or her conclusions. Areas of conjecture must either be avoided or clearly enunciated as such. Finally, the expert must know and be able to communicate to others the potentials and limitations of current technology in this field.

ACKNOWLEDGMENTS

The author is grateful to S.R. Loth for critically editing this chapter. Appreciation also goes to W.N. Watkins, J. Turner, K. Gutierrez, S. Kika, and S. Von Heartman for their photographic and art work.

REFERENCES

Adams D (1991) Age changes in oral structures. Dental Update 18(1):14–17.

Bernhard W, Bräuer, Chopra VP, and Hancke A (1979) Quantitativ genetische Analyse morphologischer Merkmale der Weichteilregionen des menschlichen Kopfes. Homo 30:26–43.

Brothwell DR, Healy MJR, and Harvey RG (1972) Canonical analysis of facial variation. J Biosoc Sci 4:175–185.

Burke KE (1990) Facial wrinkles: Prevention and nonsurgical correction. Postgraduate Med 88(1):207–222.

Catterick T (1992) Facial measurements as an aid to recognition. Forens Sci Int 56:23–27.

Clark DH (ed) (1992) Practical Forensic Odontology. Oxford: Wright.

Coon CS, and Hunt EE (1965) The Living Races of Man. New York: Alfred A Knopf.

Doual JM, Doual-Bisser A, Crocquet M, and Laude M (1991) Contribution à l'étude du vieillissement facial: Evolution des tissus mous. Bull Groupement Int Rech Sci Stomatol Odontol 34(1):11–15.

Grady D, and Ernster V (1992) Does cigarette smoking make you ugly and old? Am J Epidemiol 135(8):839–842.

Hammer HJ (1978) Körperliche Merkmale. In H Hunger and D Leopold (eds): Identifikation. Leipzig: Barth, pp 391–404.

Hooton AE (1946) Up from the Ape. New York: Macmillan.

İşcan MY (1987) Transcripts of the State of Israel vs John Ivan Demjanjuk. Jerusalem, Israel.

İşcan MY (1988a) The use of video superimposition for the identification of photographs. Paper presented at the International Symposium Advances in Skull Identification via Video Superimposition, 3–5 August, Kiel, Abstr 9.

İşcan MY (1988b) Rise of forensic anthropology. Yrbk Phys Anthropol 31:203–230.

İşcan MY (1990) Transcripts of Regina vs Collie Williams, Toronto, Canada.

İşcan MY (1992) Transcripts of the State of Florida vs Jeffrey Bellamy, Orange County Courthouse, Orlando.

İşcan MY, and Charney M (1981) Two-dimensional versus three-dimensional facial reconstruction. Am Acad Forens Sci Prog, p 47 (abstr).

Kadunce DP, Burr R, Gress R, Kanner R, Lyon JL, and Zone JJ (1991) Cigarette smoking: Risk factor for premature facial wrinkling. Ann Intern Med 114(10):840–844.

Kerley ER (1982) Faces in the crowd. Am Acad Forens Sci Prog, p 102 (abstr).

Knussmann R (1988) Methoden des anthropologischen Vergleichs in der forensischen Anthropologie. In R Knussmann (ed): Anthropologie: Handbuch der Vergleichenden Biologie des Menschen. Stuttgart: Gustav Fischer Verlag, pp 368–407.

Koury ME, and Epker BN (1991) The aged face: The facial manifestations of aging. Int J Adult Orthodont Orthognath Surg 6(2):81–95.

Kritscher H, and Szilvássy J (1991) Zur Identifizierung des Mozartschädels. Annalen des Naturhistorischen Museums in Wien, vol 93, ser A. Selbstverlag Naturhistorisches Museum, Vienna.

Krogman WM, and İşcan MY (1986) The Human Skeleton in Forensic Medicine. Springfield, Ill: Charles C Thomas.

Majumdar T, and Sinha P (1989) Photographs of the human face and broken projective symmetry. J Forens Sci Soc 29:387–395.

Molnar S (1992) Human Variation: Races, Types, and Ethnic Groups. Englewood Cliffs, NJ: Prentice Hall.

Warren R, Gartstein V, Kligman AM, Montagna W, Allendorf RA, and Ridder GM (1991) Age, sunlight, and facial skin: A histologic and quantitative study. J Am Acad Dermatol 25(5 Pt 1):751–760.

Wogalter MS, and Hosie JA (1991) Effects of cranial and facial hair on perceptions of age and person. J Soc Psychol 131(4):589–591.

Chapter 6

Morphologic and Osteometric Assessment of Age, Sex, and Race From the Skull

Vladimír Novotný, Mehmet Yaşar İşcan, and Susan R. Loth

Department of Anthropology, Faculty of Science, Masaryk University, Brno, Czech Republic CZ-611 37 (V.N.); Department of Anthropology, Florida Atlantic University, Boca Raton, Florida 33431-0991 (M.Y.İ., S.R.L.)

The three most vital determinations that must be made when dealing with skeletal remains are age, sex, and racial affinity. It would be nearly impossible to attempt to identify, much less reconstruct, the face of an individual without this information. There is no question that all of these factors have a significant bearing on appearance and also serve to narrow the range of possible matches. If the face of someone who dies at age 80 is reconstructed with the characteristics of a 25-year-old, few who knew him only in his later years would be able to see a resemblance. An even more egregious error would be to construct a male countenance on a female skull, or to assign Negroid features to a Swede.

In a complete, undamaged skeleton, experts can often determine sex with nearly 100% accuracy, estimate age at death to within about five years, and assign membership to one of the three major race groups—Caucasoid, Mongoloid, or Negroid—with a fairly high degree of certainty in the absence of admixture. Unfortunately, these conditions are rarely met, and the odds go down appreciably if one has only the skull or part of it.

In just the last 10–15 years, a great deal of new research has been published that introduced new methods and modified older ones (Krogman and İşcan, 1986). Although no system is perfect and many problems remain, these contributions have significantly improved our chances of correctly judging age, sex, and race from the skeleton.

Of the demographic parameters discussed here, only the determination of race is best made from the skull and face. Age and sex are much better assessed from the postcranial skeleton, but because of the nature of this book, the present chapter details only techniques for all determinations from the skull. However, since other remains are available in many cases, references and suggestions for the best postcranial sites and methods have also been included.

AGE

Estimation of age at death has always been one of the most difficult assessments to make, especially from the adult skeleton. Fortunately, many advances have been made in the last decade, and the current array of aging techniques is detailed in several recent books (e.g., Krogman and İşcan, 1986; İşcan, 1989; Seta and Yoshino, 1990). A critical review of age estimation methods with a focus on forensic application can be found in İşcan (1988), and İşcan and Loth (1989) offer an overview and critical analysis of the development and application of skeletal aging methods.

It is always hoped that the skeletal biologist has access to as many bones as possible from

TABLE 1.   Emergence Dates (in Months) for Deciduous Teeth[a]

Population[a]	A	B	C	D	E
Maxilla					
Egypt	9.4	11.2	19.1	14.1	24.7
Tunisia	9.3	12.5	18.3	15.7	22.0
U.S.	7.5	8.0	18.0	14.0	25.0
Canada	9.0	10.2	18.0	15.2	27.5
New Guinea	10.6	11.9	18.2	16.0	24.1
Mandible					
Egypt	8.3	12.2	19.1	14.1	24.7
Tunisia	6.0	14.0	19.0	15.7	21.7
U.S.	6.5	7.0	18.0	14.0	25.0
Canada	7.1	12.0	18.2	15.3	26.5
New Guinea	8.2	13.0	18.8	16.6	23.9

[a]Modified from El-Nofely and İşcan (1989, Table 10.1).

which to estimate age, because only the roughest assessment can be made from the skull itself once adulthood is reached. As a matter of fact, the progression of suture closure and dental wear are the only indicators of age in the adult skull.

Dentition can pinpoint age with great accuracy, but only for about the first 12 years of life. The formation, eruption, and loss of deciduous teeth followed by replacement with permanent dentition occurs in a consistent, predictable sequence, although the exact ages of these events vary by population. These rates have been calculated for children from many groups, some of which appear in Tables 1 and 2 (El-Nofely and İşcan, 1989; Ubelaker, 1989).

Adulthood is marked in some cases (though not consistently) by the eruption of M_3, and postmaturity aging by widely variable patterns of attrition. Researchers have found that tooth-wear rates and patterns show significant interpopulational variation and are affected by diet, jaw size, sex, and chewing stresses (Molnar, 1971; Brothwell, 1981; Lovejoy, 1985). According to Brothwell (1989), standards must be population-specific and based on the wear rates for a subadult sample within each group. This method is not recommended for assessing individuals over age 50 (Brothwell, 1989).

Although Brothwell's (1981) standards for tooth wear remain the most popular, Lovejoy (1985) has reported successful application of standards he derived from the archaeological American Indian Libben population. To his surprise, Lovejoy obtained a high correlation with age when the Libben standards were tested on the racially, geographically, and temporally diverse Hamann-Todd collection (of American whites and blacks). His progression of dental

TABLE 2.   Eruption of Permanent Dentition in Various Groups[a]

Country	Upper			Lower		Upper
	I_1	I_2	C	Pm_1	Pm_2	M_2
Boys						
Czechoslovakia	7.2	8.1	11.2	10.4	11.0	12.1
Egypt	8.0	9.1	12.1	11.3	12.1	12.7
England	8.1	8.9	12.4	11.4	12.1	12.4
Hungary	7.3	8.5	11.4	11.8	11.9	12.4
U.S.	7.5	8.7	11.7	10.8	11.4	12.7
Japan	8.0	9.2	11.6	10.8	11.6	12.9
Girls						
Czechoslovakia	6.9	7.7	10.6	9.4	10.6	11.7
Egypt	7.3	8.6	11.8	10.8	11.2	11.7
England	7.7	8.7	11.0	11.4	12.0	12.1
Hungary	7.1	8.0	11.6	10.0	11.3	12.0
U.S.	7.2	8.2	11.0	10.2	10.9	12.3

[a]Modified from El-Nofely (1982, Table 2, and Hurme, 1957).

wear is illustrated in Figure 1, along with the age range per phase (Lovejoy, 1985).

One must be cautious in applying these standards meant for assessment on the population level to individual forensic cases. Lovejoy (1985:54) states that in this situation "assignment of age on the basis of dental wear alone, would allow only a gross approximation at best." Therefore, this technique not should be used in forensic cases unless the skull is the only site available.

If necessary, teeth can also be examined histologically. However, this type of analysis should never be the method of choice in forensic cases, especially when reconstruction is being attempted, because it involves destruction or modification of the remains. This approach was introduced by Gustafson (1950), who studied cross sections of teeth and observed age-related changes in six areas: attrition, periodontosis, secondary dentin, cementum, root resorption, and root transparency. He ranked their progres-

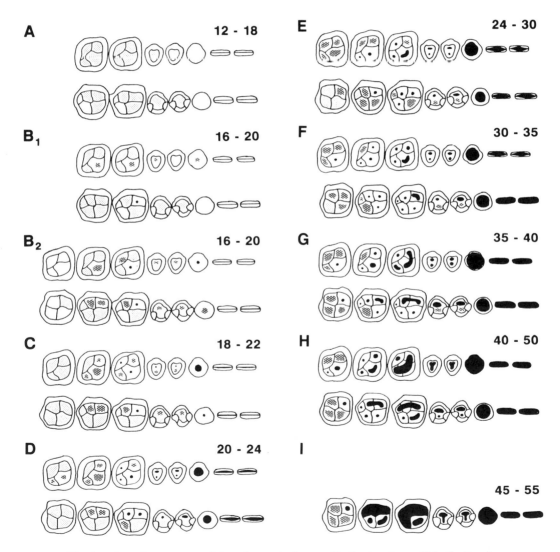

Fig. 1. Age-phase ranges of dental wear in the maxilla (top) and mandible (bottom). (Modified from Lovejoy, 1985.)

sion on a scale of 0 to 3, added the resultant scores, and used the total in a regression formula to calculate the age of the individual.

Many modifications of this technique have made since then. Bang and Ramm (1970) tested Gustafson's method on a large sample ($N = 265$) and found that one criterion, root transparency, was adequate to use alone. They measured the length of the transparent section of the root and developed three regression formulae from them. Kilian and Vlček (1989) recently tested existing techniques and concluded that Kilian's method

yielded the best overall results. They reported that more than 75% of their estimates were within a range of ±5 years, and, unlike most other procedures, an acceptable assessment was possible from a single tooth. However, these authors advise using "intact front teeth"—something to be avoided if facial reconstruction is planned. Because of the complex preparation and long, detailed analysis these techniques require, we suggest consulting the original sources when attempting to apply them.

Taking a different approach, Wei and associ-

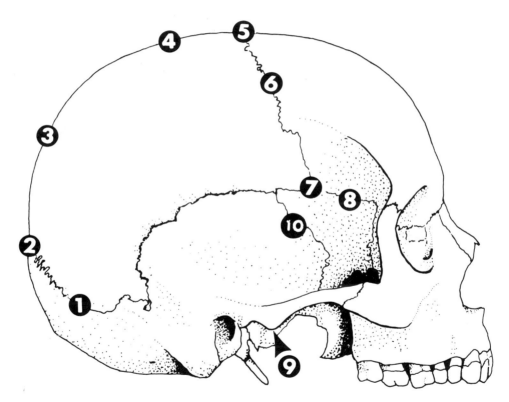

Fig. 2. Vault suture sites: 1: Midlambdoid, midpoint of each half of the lambdoid suture; 2: Lambda, at pars lambdica of both the sagittal and lambdoid sutures; 3: Obelion; 4: Anterior sagittal, point on the sagittal suture at the juncture of the anterior one-third and posterior two-thirds of its length; 5: Bregma, on both sagittal and coronal sutures; 6: Midcoronal, midpoint of each half of the coronal suture at pars complicata; 7: Pterion. **Lateral–anterior suture sites**: 8: Sphenofrontal, midpoint of the sphenofrontal suture; 9: Inferior sphenotemporal, point on the sphenotemporal suture lying at its intersection with a line connecting both articular tubercles of the temporomandibular joint; 10: Superior sphenotemporal, point on the sphenotemporal suture lying 2 cm below its juncture with the parietal bone. (Modified from Meindl and Lovejoy, 1985, Fig. 1, Table 1.)

TABLE 3. Ages Calculated for Composite Scores From Lateral–Anterior Sutures[a]

Composite Score	N	Mean Age	S.D.	Interdecile Range
0 (open)	42			x–43
1	18	32.0	8.3	21–42
2	18	36.2	6.2	29–44
3–5	56	41.1	10.0	28–52
6	17	43.4	10.7	30–54
7–8	31	45.5	8.9	35–57
9–10	29	51.9	12.5	39–69
11–14	24	56.2	8.5	49–65
15 (closed)	1			

[a]Modified from Meindl and Lovejoy (1985, Table 7).

ates (1983) thin-sectioned (to 0.5 mm) the maxillary M_1 buccolingually through the center of the tooth. Using a microscope with micrometer, they measured the height and width of the pulp chamber and dentin in a sample of 97 Chinese people. They found an age-related relationship between the maxillary molar pulp cavity and dentin size and created a pulp–dentin index as follows: Pulp–dentin index = [(Height + width of pulp chamber)/(Height + width of dentin)] × 100.

Noting a negative correlation between the index and age, they developed the following regression formula: Y (age) = -1.01 × (pulp–dentin index) + 82.82.

All researchers cautioned that many factors can affect age estimation from this site. Neglected teeth may look older (Gustafson, 1950). Estimates can be affected by the type of occlusion, degree of abrasion, malocclusion, missing teeth, caries, fillings, trauma, disease, antemortem treatment, and method of extraction (Kilian and Vlček, 1989). Finally, all of these methods require considerable technical expertise, specialized equipment, and a great deal of time to apply.

Cranial suture closure has always been associated with extreme, inherent variability (Krogman and İşcan, 1986). It is not uncommon to find complete sutural obliteration in the twenties, and conversely, unfused sutures are often found in elderly individuals. Some have noted

significant differences between the sexes and even from one cemetery population to the next (e.g., Masset, 1989), while others have not (e.g., Meindl and Lovejoy, 1985).

The first data-based technique to assess suture closure was presented by Todd and Lyon in 1924, and many modifications have been offered in hopes of improving accuracy (e.g., Nemeskéri et al., 1960). These have culminated in the most recent attempt by Meindl and Lovejoy (1985), who tested several sutural loci from lateral anterior and vault sites illustrated in Figure 2. The degree of suture closure at each 1-cm segment of suture was evaluated on a scale of 0 to 3, as follows:

Score 0: Completely open. No ectocranial closure.

Score 1: Minimal to moderate closure, from a single bony bridge to about 50% synostosis.

Score 2: Significant but not complete closure.

Score 3: Complete obliteration and fusion.

The scores for each site noted above were added by region and plotted against age. Table 3 lists the ages calculated for composite scores from the five lateral anterior sutures which were found to have the best correlation with age.

Although Meindl and Lovejoy claim that their modifications of Todd and Lyon have reduced error significantly, inaccuracy remained substantial. These authors found that correlation of suture closure with age was still inferior to most other methods and do not recommend using this site as the only age indicator (Meindl and Lovejoy, 1985).

In the last few years, attention has turned to the maxillary sutures (Belli, 1991; Mann et al., 1991). The four sites studied are all located on the hard palate and are thus easily accessible. Earliest closure was observed in the incisive suture for both males and females at the age of 20 years. This was followed by the posterior median palatine about six years later. The sexes diverge greatly in both the transverse and anterior median palatines, with figures of 33 and 40 years for males and 84 and 67 years, respectively, for females. In males, complete obliteriation of all sutures was noted as early as 40 years, but in females this was not found until 84. Findings to date indicate that this process in the maxilla is highly variable and can only allow categorization as a "child, adolescent, young, middle-aged, or old adult" (Mann et al., 1991).

Much more reliable age assessments can be made from the postcranial skeleton. Until the last decade, attention focused first on applying, then modifying, Todd's (1920) pubic symphyseal phases. However, a number of tests indicate that pubic-based methods are not very reliable (e.g., Klepinger et al., 1992; Saunders et al., 1992). Yet, despite their problems, most techniques from this site will be more effective than sutural closure.

Aging standards from the auricular surface of the ilium have shown some success in paleodemographic population studies (Lovejoy et al., 1985; Saunders et al., 1992). However, they are not recommended for precise analysis of individual forensic cases (Murray and Murray, 1991).

Recent tests by Loth and İşcan (1989) and İşcan et al. (1992), as well as other evaluations (e.g., Masset, 1990; Dudar, 1992; Saunders et al., 1992), indicate that the most consistently accurate age marker (especially for modern humans) may be the sternal end of the rib. The rib-phase method, first introduced by İşcan and associates in 1984, features sex-specific standards and narrow 95% confidence intervals (İşcan et al., 1984, 1985). Race differences were also reported (İşcan et al., 1987). The rib phases were found to be at least twice as accurate as those from the pubic symphysis (Loth and İşcan, 1989; İşcan et al., 1992). Unlike most other methods, interobserver error is minimal and is negligibly affected by experience (İşcan and Loth, 1986a,b).

If only long bones are available, one must resort to radiographic or histomorphometric approaches, but these are fraught with technical problems that greatly reduce their effectiveness (Uytterschaut, 1985; Drusini, 1987; Stout, 1989). Furthermore, histologic examinations such as a cross section of femur or tooth involve destruction of the skeletal remains; thus their use is discouraged in forensic cases.

Finally, age estimation is further complicated by as yet unexplainable discrepancies in physiologic vs. chronologic aging. Just as living persons may not "look their age," their skeletons may not either. No matter how accurate age assessment is from the bones, a reconstruction expert can only guess if the owner of a skeleton judged to be 50 years old looked his age, 10 years younger, or 20 years older.

RACE

Through the years, the term race has been used in nonbiological connotations to describe ethnicity, religious groups, and nationalities. No one can deny that significant, genetically based physical differences exist between Caucasoids, Mongoloids, and Negroids. There is nothing wrong with using these terms in that context as a classificatory mechanism to convey necessary information.

In the forensic context, the approach to race must be a pragmatic one. The identification of unknown individuals is one of the most important justifications for maintaining biologically based racial typologies. Forensic interests have refocused research efforts on this subject, despite attempts in some anthropological circles to eliminate these classifications. Even though not all skeletons fit neatly into established categories, designating remains as white, Mongoloid, or black significantly decreases the number of possible candidates and facilitates physical description, especially after sex and age are considered. This classification is also essential to facial reconstruction, where recognizability is a major aim. Furthermore, most standards for tissue thickness and so forth are race-specific. Several sources offer helpful guides for determining race from the skeleton (Stewart, 1979; Krogman and İşcan, 1986) and discuss their value in forensic applications (İşcan, 1988).

As mentioned previously, the skull is the best part of the skeleton to use for the determination of racial affinity, both morphologically and osteometrically. A number of newer publications on race discuss approaches from both the cranial and postcranial skeleton (e.g., St. Hoyme and İşcan, 1989; Gill and Rhine, 1990). These studies favor the use of morphological criteria over osteometric assessment, but discriminant function analysis does play an important role, especially when morphological differences are not clear. However, the myth persists in legal circles that quantitative analysis is more definitive and reliable even though a weak score standing alone is basically indeterminate. Ideally, both approaches should be utilized whenever possible.

Traditional morphological characteristics of the skull are listed in Table 4. In general, blacks have a longer, lower skull, wider nose with guttered nasal sills, wider interorbital distance, and greater alveolar prognathism than other groups. Mongoloids are best differentiated by the presence of shovel-shaped incisors, a round head, and laterally and anteriorly projecting malar bones. Most Caucasoids exhibit a long,

narrow nose with sharp sills, a high cranial vault, and orthognathic profile. Of course, these classic descriptions are most accurate for groups with little or no admixture and do not adequately account for extremes of intraracial variation.

Other less obvious traits have been discerned. Post (1969) determined that black males have shorter, wider nasolacrimal canals than whites. Minute observations have been made of racial differences in the auditory canal. Napoli and Birkby (1990) discerned variation in the visibility of the oval or vestibular window of the middle ear, slightly superior to the cochlear opening, from the external auditory meatus. Using a Caucasoid and American Indian forensic sample, they scored their observation as visible, not visible, or partially visible. Their results indicated that the window was visible in 94% of Caucasoids, while this figure was only 13% in Mongoloids. For Caucasoid–Mongoloid admixtures, 69% were visible.

Brues (1990) considers the nose to be the most diagnostic area for race determination.

TABLE 4.   Racial Characteristics of the Face and Skull[a]

Dimensions	Caucasoid			Mongoloid	Negroid
	Nordic	Alpine	Mediterranean		
Skull length	Long	Short	Long	Long	Long
Skull breadth	Narrow	Broad	Narrow	Broad	Narrow
Skull height	High	High	Moderately high	Middle	Low
Sagittal contour	Rounded	Arched	Rounded	Arched	Flat
Face breadth	Narrow	Wide	Narrow	Very wide	Narrow
Face height	High	High	Moderately high	High	Low
Orbital opening	Angular	Rounded	Angular	Rounded	Rectangular
Nasal opening	Narrow	Moderately wide	Narrow	Narrow	Wide
Lower nasal margin	Sharp	Sharp	Sharp	Sharp	Troughed or guttered
Nasal profile	Straight	Straight	Straight	Straight	Downward slant
Palate shape	Narrow	Moderately wide	Narrow	Moderately wide	Wide
General impression of skull,	Massive, rugged, elongated, ovoid	Large, moderately rugged, rounded	Small, smooth, elongated, pentagonoid to ovoid	Large, smooth, rounded	Massive, smooth elongate, constricted oval

[a]From Krogman (1955, Table 13).

She observed three types of nasal bridge shapes around the naso-maxillary suture: (1) Negroid: "quonset hut"—low and rounded; (2) Mongoloid: "tented"—low to moderate with relatively straight sides; and (3) Caucasoid: "church with steeple"—high and pinched. In a study of Terry and forensic collection blacks and whites of both sexes, Angel and Kelley (1990) found that black males have mandibular ramus inversion 65% more often than whites, but this differentiation was less distinct in females.

Obvious differences in the head morphology of American whites and blacks led Todd and Lindala (1928) to attempt to determine if any of these could be quantified anthropometrically. A selected group from the 32 measurements they took from the head and face of Todd collection cadavera appears in Table 5. In the head, the most apparent disparities between whites and blacks were in maximum length in both sexes, and in maximum breadth and auricular height in males. In the face, the most outstanding differences were in nasal breadth and interlabral height in both sexes, and in mouth breadth in females. Bizygomatic and maximum ear breadth were the same in males, as was the case for the nasion–stomion dimension in females.

Race differences in the skull can also be detected metrically using discriminant function statistics (Giles and Elliot, 1962; Howells, 1970; Snow et al., 1979). Even though it is actually a continuous variable, biological race is amenable to this type of analysis because two races can be expected to produce a bimodal curve despite obvious overlapping. The first discriminant function race formulae were developed by Giles and

TABLE 5. Selected Cephalic Dimensions of 19th-Century American Whites and Blacks[a]

Dimensions	Males				Females			
	White		Black		White		Black	
	Mean	S.D.	Mean	S.D.	Mean	S.D.	Mean	S.D.
Head								
Maximum length	188	7.5	193	6.1	182	6.5	186	7.7
Maximum breadth	154	6.5	149	6.1	145	5.6	144	6.2
Min. forehead breadth	106	6.6	107	6.5	100	6.0	103	5.9
Auricular height	120	5.1	124	5.3	118	5.3	120	4.8
Face								
Bizygomatic breadth	139	6.7	139	6.1	130	7.0	132	8.7
Bigonial breadth	110	7.4	109	8.7	103	8.9	105	11.9
Interocular breadth	33	3.5	35	2.7	31	2.8	34	2.3
Interpupillary breadth	63	4.2	68	4.4	61	3.9	65	3.8
Palpebral fissure breadth	30	3.0	33	3.6	28	2.3	31	3.3
Trichion-gnathion	189	12.0	194	9.8	172	11.9	179	10.3
Nasion-gnathion	122	9.7	125	7.6	113	9.5	116	11.6
Nasion-prosthion	69	6.3	71	5.6	66	6.2	67	4.5
Nasal height	54	4.7	52	4.8	52	3.8	50	4.4
Nasal breadth	35	3.7	43	3.7	32	4.9	40	4.1
Nasal depth	21	3.0	16	3.0	19	3.0	15	3.2
Nasion-stomion	74	5.7	75	5.9	71	6.3	71	6.1
Mouth breadth	53	4.6	57	4.1	45	4.8	52	5.5
Interlabral height	12	3.7	21	4.9	9	4.2	18	6.5
Max. ear length	67	4.9	62	4.6	61	6.9	60	5.6
Max. ear breadth	38	3.4	38	3.0	34	4.1	36	3.3

[a]From Todd and Lindala (1928:114–118).

Elliot (1962). They analyzed racial differences in the skulls of American whites and blacks from the Hamann-Todd and Terry collections, along with various American Indian samples. Their formulae were calculated from 75 skulls from each sex and race group (total $N = 450$). The craniometric dimensions and discriminant function equations derived from them are shown in Table 6.

This table also contains another discriminant equation that Giles and Elliot (1962) calculated for cases in which neither sex nor race are known. The sex of the specimen must be determined first using the formula in the last column of Table 6. A score lower than the sectioning point would classify as female, a higher score as male. For racial classification, the sectioning points are treated as pairs of coordinates. Each pair denotes a point on the graph in Figure 3, and race is assigned based upon the sector in which the point lies. The accuracy of this method

ranged from 80% to 95% for the base sample and 77% to 100% for the test samples.

The Giles and Elliot (1962) method has been reassessed by a number of anthropologists. Several earlier studies criticized the method because it was found that the formulae did not work as well on other samples from the same race groups (Birkby, 1966; Snow et al., 1979). However, the basic soundness of their approach is reflected in the fact that several researchers have been carrying out similar studies on different skeletal assemblages. Rigorous testing on more modern skeletons and other Indian samples have produced mixed results (Ayers et al., 1990; Fisher and Gill, 1990). Ayers and associates (1990) obtained acceptable results for whites of both sexes and for black females. However, black males and Indians of both sexes remained problematic. These authors suggested that the sectioning point for the black/white ordinate be reduced from 89.27 to 62.89 in order to increase

TABLE 6. Race Determination From the Skull in American Whites, Blacks, and Indians by Discriminant Function Analysis[a]

	Discriminant Function Coefficients				
	Males		Females		
	White vs.		White vs.		Male vs.
Variables	Black	Indian	Black	Indian	Female
Basion-prosthion	3.06	0.10	1.74	3.05	-1.00
Glabella-occipital length	1.60	-0.25	1.28	-1.04	1.16
Maximum cranial breadth	-1.90	-1.56	-1.18	-5.41	
Basion-bregma height	-1.79	0.73	-0.14	4.29	
Basion-nasion length	-4.41	-0.29	-2.34	-4.02	1.66
Max. bizygomatic breadth	-0.10	1.75	0.38	5.62	3.98
Prosthion-nasion height	2.59	-0.16	-0.01	-1.00	1.54
Nasal breadth	10.56	-0.88	2.45	-2.19	
Sectioning point	89.27	22.28	92.20	130.10	891.12
Percent correct	**Base**	**Test**	**Base**	**Test**	**82.9**
Whites	80.0	87.9	88.0	100.0	
Blacks	85.3	92.1	88.0	81.8	
Indians	94.7	76.9	93.3	87.1	

[a]Modified from Giles and Elliot (1962, Table 1).

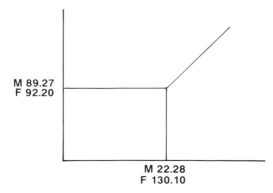

Fig. 3. Racial classification is based upon the sector in which the discriminant scores fall when treated as pairs of coordinates on this graph. The x axis represents the white–Indian continuum and the y axis represents the white–black continuum. For example, scores of $x = 20$, $y = 106$ classify either sex as black. (Modified from Giles and Elliot, 1962.)

classification accuracy, but their sample was not large enough to make similar adjustments for other groups. Fisher and Gill's (1990) findings of considerable inaccuracy for whites and Plains Indians led them to conclude that extensive intrapopulational variation cannot be accounted for by this type of metric analysis. This is an inherent weakness in the system that limits its application outside the original base sample.

Focusing on the midfacial skeleton of three major racial groups, Gill and Gilbert (1990) discovered that the formation of indices produced better results than discriminant function analysis. They were also easier to apply. The method involves the quantification of naso-maxillary projection from the anterior lacrimal crest and zygomaticomaxillary suture at the inferior orbital margin and the line between the two nasomaxillary sutures. The resultant indices separated one race from another with 82% to 88% accuracy in males and 91% to 95% in females. However, tests by Curran (1990) raised a number of concerns about this technique. Accuracy can be significantly impaired by mensural errors because the measurements are difficult to take and landmarks are hard to find. Furthermore, projection can only be measured with a modified caliper called a simometer that must be specially constructed for this purpose. Finally, Curran noted that this technique successfully separates whites from Indians and blacks but is not effective in distinguishing blacks from Indians.

In our experience, morphological indicators are usually adequate to distinguish one race group from another. However, in cases where this distinction is not visually clear, there are numerous craniometric techniques available to help make this diagnosis.

SEX DETERMINATION

Of all demographic characteristics, differences between the sexes have probably been studied the most—almost every human bone has been analyzed in this regard (Stewart, 1979; Krogman and İşcan, 1986; Seta and Yoshino, 1990). Apart from its obvious importance in forensic applications, an understanding of sexual dimorphism is also fundamental to the study of human growth and evolution. Theoretically, this assessment should be easy once puberty is reached and males and females diverge significantly to follow their distinct, genetically determined forms and reproductive functions.

In spite of the obvious differences and numerous studies of sexual dimorphism, sex determination from the skeleton can be problematic in some cases. The definitiveness of differences between fleshed individuals stands in stark contrast to what is seen in many bones. The problem arises from the contradiction between discrete, genetically determined sex classifications and the continuous transitions of somatic sexual characteristics in the phenotype. A simple analysis of sex differences always shows a certain overlapping of the two sexes; in the skeleton sex is not binary, even though a normal human is either a man or a woman. This diagnosis is also influenced by a number of other factors such as the environment, age differences, pathological changes, and, above all, interpopulational variation. Even various populations of the same race may exhibit different manifestations of sexual dimorphism, which may change with time. Thus, it is difficult to develop a method that would always partition a given population into males and females. These problems are still being investigated (Novotný, 1986). The applied aspect was discussed at the Workshop of European Anthropologists (Ferembach et al., 1980).

The pelvis and skull are excellent sites for sexing and it is important to make the most of both. Although sexual dimorphism is better expressed in the pelvis, this site is very often damaged. The skull, on the other hand, is usually better preserved, but its sexual differences are not quite as definitive. A long-standing argument also centers on whether morphological (i.e., visual, morphoscopic) or morphometric traits are more effective (Stewart, 1954). The evaluation of morphological traits is thought to be more subjective and depends on the experience of the investigator. Metric traits, while seemingly more objective, are also affected by inexperience. Moreover, a random set of measurements may not always be conclusive. It is possible to apply multivariate discriminant analyses *in sensu stricto* only on a reference sample of known sex from which standards have been worked out. This is also true for populations with the same sexual dimorphism as the reference sample when statistical inferences for a given probability are used. Furthermore, the dimensions of total size may be misleading: Small males may be misclassified as females, and large females as males.

To test available methods, the skulls of 151 adults (83 males and 68 females) of known sex and age from the 1930s were assessed using a blind study protocol (Solowiej, 1982). Another factor considered was the importance of experience—the tester had none. This test verified the diagnostic reliability of Acsádi and Nemeskéri's

(1970) morphologically based method.

According to Acsádi and Nemeskéri (1970), the degree of development of any sexually differentiated characteristic may be scored in one of the five following categories: hypermasculine, masculine, indifferent, feminine, and hyperfeminine by means of scoring grades: +2, +1, 0, -1, -2, respectively (see Fig. 4). The individual traits are weighted by criteria established empirically based on their significance in sexing. The score of the most significant traits is then multiplied by two or three (see Table 7).

The degree of sexualization is determined by computing weighted means from the scores of the various grades of the individual morphologic traits of the skull. To every variable investigated, a corresponding score is allocated and multiplied by the respective weight of the trait. The products obtained from individual traits are added up and the result is divided by the sum of the weights. Positive results indicate a male; negative, a female. The absolute value of this figure indicates the degree of sexualization (Acsádi and Nemeskéri, 1970).

Corresponding sexing indices, similar to those of Acsádi and Nemeskéri (1970), have been calculated for four complexes of sex characteristics of the skull recommended by different authors (Borovanský, 1936; Vlček, 1971; Ferembach et al., 1980). All attribute a specific "weight" to the individual traits, although in a different manner. The significance of the trait is evaluated either in two or three degrees of manifestation. Using this approach, 22 sexually differentiated morphological traits of the skull and mandible were evaluated. Because the mandible is often missing, sexing indices have also been computed using only traits of the skull without the mandible.

Testing of the development of morphologic traits and ascertaining their diagnostic reliability yielded the following results (see Table 8):

1. To be considered very reliable, traits must correspond with actual sex in more than 60% of cases and misclassify less than 10% of individuals. These traits include the os zygomati-

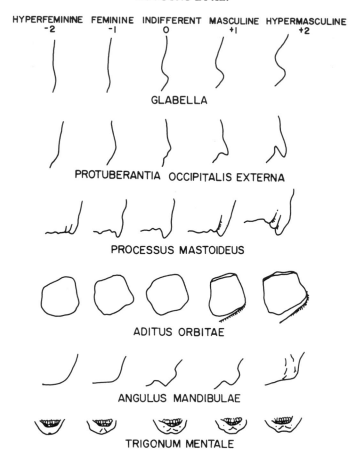

Fig. 4. Degrees of development of sexually differentiated characteristics (Acsádi and Nemeskéri, 1970).

cum, crista supramastoidea, arcus superciliaris, and glabella and arcus superciliaris (together). This group of traits is assigned triple weight.

2. Traits designated as reliable allow correct assignment of individuals in more than 50% of cases and misclassify less than 15%. They include the margo supraorbitalis and aditus orbitae (together), pons zygomaticus, glabella (alone), alveolar prognathia, and general appearance of the mandible. These traits are double weighted.

3. Traits of low reliability enable 50% correct classification, but have a 20% incidence of misclassification. They are the processus mastoideus, angulus mandibulae, inclination of the os frontale, margo supraorbitalis (alone),

trigonum mentale, and protuberantia occipitalis externa. These traits were single weighted.

4. Traits for which the number of correctly classified individuals was below 50% and/or the number of misclassified specimens extended beyond 20% were declared unreliable and were not taken into consideration. They are the processus marginalis, caput mandibulae, spina nasalis anterior, aditus orbitae, and tubera frontalia et parietalia.

Sexing indices were evaluated in a similar way. The percentage of individuals correctly classified by the index and the percentage of individuals whose index misclassified them by +0.4 to -0.4 units should be labeled "uncertain"

(Acsádi and Nemeskéri, 1970). From this point of view, the most suitable index is that for the complex of traits from the "European Recommendations" (Ferembach et al., 1980) (see Table 9). Sexing accuracy was 94.3% for females and 86.1% for males. This equaled the best results obtained metrically from the ischio-pubic index. The other groups of traits were less reliable.

Inspired by this result, we attempted to use multivariate discriminant analysis to evaluate the significance of the variables according to their statistical weights and to select the minimum number of traits yielding the maximum discriminatory effectiveness with the least possible risk of error. Each morphological trait from a given individual was scored in one of five categories (on a scale of -2 to +2) according to the strength of its development.

The morphologic trait was represented by the number reflecting the general degree of its development. This quantification of qualitative traits enables us to use them as metric variables and thus apply discriminant function analysis. The stepwise discriminant analysis of the best 14 traits selected the nine variables listed in Table 10. The function assessed sex correctly in 98.2% of cases—a surprisingly good accuracy rate, comparable to the best functions from metric traits of the pelvis.

DISCUSSION

Theoretically, only age can be considered as a continuous biological variable in the strictest sense of the word—namely, that the aging process is ongoing and there is no sharp distinction from one moment to the next. In practice, however, the skeletal overlap between the sexes and races that interferes with our ability to achieve 100% classification accuracy gives these discrete traits a certain "continuous" quality. There is no one sharp point of metric or morphologic demarcation to which there are no exceptions. Therefore, one is limited to making "estimates" of these characteristics with varying degrees of

certainty. In the last decade or so, research has developed improved methods that have enhanced our proficiency at making these estimates (Krogman and İşcan, 1986; İşcan, 1989; Gill and Rhine, 1990).

In childhood, the sequence of dental development and eruption is the most accurate indicator of age. By the teens, however, age markers in the skull cannot be relied upon for dependable estimates. In this chapter we have described the newest modifications of dentition- and suture-based techniques, but we strongly recommend that priority be given to the postcranial methods mentioned. At present, the rib phase technique is likely to give the best results, especially in forensic cases. Beyond the use of standard methods, judgment gained from years of osteologic experience often enables an examiner to "read" more subtle signs of aging—an overall loss of bone density may contradict a young-looking pubic symphysis.

As far as race is concerned, the skull is the optimal site for this determination. And while sex is best assessed from the pelvis, the skull offers a number of very good indicators. Despite the proliferation of osteometric techniques for the assessment of both race and sex, morphologically based approaches should be considered the methods of choice. This has been true in the experience of the authors and finds a great deal of support in the literature. The successful quantification of qualitative morphological sex characters of the skull and their use in discriminant function analysis has demonstrated that their effectiveness rivals osteometric sexing techniques from the pelvis.

The common denominator in the assessment of age, sex, and race in the skeleton is that they are best reflected morphologically. However, the selection of a technique and the accuracy of its application are very much a function of the experience and skill of the forensic practitioner.

Finally, it cannot be emphasized strongly enough that correct determinations of age, sex, and race are prerequisites to all aspects of craniofacial reconstruction, superimposition, and identification. A significant error in age assignment

TABLE 7. Scaling of the Skull Morphologic Characters for Sex Determination

Trait[a]	Weight	Hyperfeminine -2	Feminine -1	Indifferent 0	Masculine +1	Hypermasculine +2
Os zygomaticum	3/AN	Very low, smooth	Low, smooth	Medium high, contoured	High, well-contoured	Very high, marked contours
Crista supramastoidea	3/ER	Very slightly developed	Slightly developed	Medium	Strongly developed	Very strongly developed
Arcus superciliaris	3/ER	Smooth	Slightly delimited	Medium	Marked	Very marked, arched
Glabella + arcus superciliaris	3/AN	Smooth, showing a line occasionally	Slightly delimited	Delimited	Marked, arched	Massive, prominent
Margo supraorbitalis + aditus orbitae	2/AN	Very sharp edge, circular	Sharp edge, circular	Intermediate	Slightly rounded edge, slightly squared	Rounded edge, squared
Pons zygomaticus	2/AN	Very thin	Thin	Medium	Thick	Very thick
Glabella	2/ER	Smooth	Slightly delimited	Delimited	Marked	Massive, prominent
Prognathia alveolaris	2/B	Very oblique	Oblique	Slightly oblique	Nearly sheer	Sheer
Squama occipitalis	2/AN	Smooth	Slightly arched traces of nuchal lines	Nuchal lines + occipital crest evident	Nuchal lines + occipital crest marked	Nuchal lines + occipital crest with rough surface

Feature	Code					
Mandibula	1/ER	Very gracile	Gracile	Medium	Robust	Very robust
Processus mastoideus	1/AN	Very small	Small	Medium	Large	Very large
Angulus mandibulae	1/AN	Smooth	Incipient eminences	Moderate eminences	Marked eminences	Strongly marked eminences, laterally directed angle
Inclinatio ossis frontalis	1/ER	Vertical	Almost vertical	Little inclined	Medium inclined	Strongly inclined
Margo superaorbitalis	1/B	Very sharp	Sharp	Medium	Rounded	Very rounded
Trigonum mentale	1/AN	Rounded, smooth	Medial, slightly delimited	Medial, delimited	Inverted T-shaped, protruding	Bilateral protuberance
Protuberantia occipitalis externa	1/AN	Smooth	Hardly visible	Poor	Marked	Massive
Processus marginalis	0/B	Missing	Slightly	Medium	Marked	Well-developed
Caput mandibulae	0/AN	Very small	Small	Medium	Large	Very large
Spina nasalis anterior	0/B	Very small	Small	Medium	Large	Very large
Aditus orbitae	0/B	Round	Horizontally trapezoid	Trapezoid laterally wider	Obliquely oblong	Rhombic
Corpus mandibulae (M_2)	0/AN	Very narrow	Narrow	Medium	Thick	Very thick
Tubera frontalia et parietalia	0/AN	Marked	Medium	Moderate	Indistinct	Missing

[a]Modified from Solowiej (1982). AN refers to Acsádi and Nemeskéri (1970) method; ER, Ferembach et al. (1980); and B, Borovanský (1936).

TABLE 8. Sexing Accuracy From Weighted Morphologic Traits of the Skull[a]

Trait Groups	Percent Correct	Incorrect
I. (weight = 3x)		
Os zygomaticum	68.2	9.9
Crista supramastoidea	67.5	9.3
Arcus superciliaris	66.9	7.3
Glabella + Arcus superciliaris	63.6	7.9
II. (weight = 2x)		
Margo supraorbitalis + Aditus orbitae	64.9	12.9
Pons zygomaticus	63.6	13.9
Glabella	62.9	11.3
Prognathia alveolaris	58.8	14.7
Squama occipitalis	57.6	13.2
Mandibula	50.7	12.7
III. (weight = 1x)		
Processus mastoideus	59.6	15.9
Angulus mandibulae	56.1	15.5
Inclinatio ossis frontalis	59.6	15.9
Margo supraorbitalis	58.9	18.5
Trigonum mentale	57.7	19.7
Protuberantia occipitalis externa	55.6	19.9
IV. (weight = 0)		
Processus marginalis	51.7	23.8
Caput mandibulae	50.7	28.2
Spina nasalis anterior	49.7	13.2
Aditus orbitae	48.3	25.8
Corpus mandibulae (MP$_2$)	47.8	25.3
Tubera frontalia et parietalia	42.4	24.5

[a]Modified from Solowiej (1982).

TABLE 9. Tests of Sexing Accuracy From Morphologic Traits of the Skull[a]

Methods Tested	Percent Correct		
	Male	Female	Total
Cranium			
Ferembach et al.	86.1	94.3	90.1
Acsádi and Nemeskéri	88.9	88.6	88.7
Vlček	94.4	81.3	88.2
Borovanský	88.9	81.2	85.3
Calvarium			
Ferembach et al.	83.1	92.6	87.4
Borovanský	79.5	91.2	84.8
Acsádi and Nemeskéri	79.5	91.2	84.8
Vlček	73.5	91.2	81.5

[a]Modified from Solowiej (1982).

TABLE 10. Discriminant Function Coefficients and Accuracy of Sex Determination From the Skull

Trait	X_1 (Males)	X_2 (Females)
Glabella	-2.32308	0.24297
Arcus superciliaris	-0.66695	1.01545
Crista supramastoidea	-1.78610	0.94836
Squama occipitalis	-0.67799	0.21830
Pons zygomaticus	-0.34589	0.26312
Os zygomaticum	-2.03353	1.08861
Inclinatio ossis frontalis	1.31358	-0.58290
Mandibula	1.34310	-0.21927
Angulus mandibulae	-0.04189	0.92854
Constant	-4.59787	-2.13217

Percent Accuracy		N
Males	97.2	35/36
Females	100.0	35/35

could eliminate the actual individual in question from consideration. Diagnosing race or sex incorrectly makes identification absolutely impossible. Therefore, an experienced forensic anthropologist or skeletal biologist should always be consulted when skeletal remains are found.

REFERENCES

Acsádi G, and Nemeskéri J (1970) History of Human Life Span and Mortality. Budapest: Akadémiai Kiadó.

Angel JL, and Kelley JO (1990) Inversion of the posterior edge of the jaw ramus: New race trait. In GW Gill and JS Rhine (eds): Skeletal Attribution of Race. Maxwell Mus Anthropol Papers 4. Albuquerque: University of New Mexico, pp 33–39.

Ayers HG, Jantz RL, and Moore-Jansen PH (1990) Giles and Elliot race discriminant functions revisited: A test using recent forensic cases. In GW Gill and JS Rhine (eds): Skeletal Attribution of Race. Maxwell Mus Anthropol Papers 4. Albuquerque:

University of New Mexico, pp 65–71.

Bang G, and Ramm E (1970) Determination of age in humans from root dentin transparency. Acta Odontol Scand 2:3–35.

Belli ZP (1991) Maksiller Sütürlerin Silinme Dönemli Tam veya Eksik Maksillarin Incelenmesiyle Yas Tayini. Doctoral dissertation, Univ Istanbul Adli Tip Enstitüsü.

Birkby WH (1966) An evaluation of race and sex identification from cranial measurements. Am J Phys Anthropol 24:21–28.

Borovanský L (1936) Pohlavní rozdíly na lebce člověka. Prague.

Brothwell DR (1981) Digging Up Bones. Ithaca: Cornell University Press.

Brothwell DR (1989) The relationship of tooth wear to ageing. In MY İşcan (ed): Age Markers in the Human Skeleton. Springfield, Ill: Charles C Thomas.

Brues AM (1990) The once and future diagnosis of race. In GW Gill and JS Rhine (eds): Skeletal Attribution of Race. Maxwell Mus Anthropol Papers 4. Albuquerque: University of New Mexico, pp 1–7.

Curran BK (1990) The application of measures of midfacial projection for racial classification. In GW Gill and JS Rhine (eds): Skeletal Attribution of Race. Maxwell Mus Anthropol Papers 4. Albuquerque: University of New Mexico, pp 55–57.

Drusini A (1987) Refinements of two methods for the histomorphometrics determination of age in human bone. Z Morphol Anthropol 77:167–176.

Dudar JC (1992) Estimating Adult Skeletal Age at Death Using Morphological and Histological Rib Techniques. MA thesis, University of Guelph.

El-Nofely A, and İşcan MY (1989) Assessment of age from the dentition in children. In MY İşcan (ed): Age Markers in the Human Skeleton. Springfield, Ill: Charles C Thomas, pp 237–254.

Ferembach D, Schwidetzky L, and Stloukal M (1980) Recommendations for age and sex diagnoses of skeletons. J Hum Evol 9:517–549.

Fisher TD, and Gill GW (1990) Application of the Giles-Elliot discriminant function formulae to a cranial sample of northwestern Plains Indians. In GW Gill and JS Rhine (eds): Skeletal Attribution of Race. Maxwell Mus Anthropol Papers 4. Albuquerque: University of New Mexico, pp 59–63.

Giles E, and Elliot O (1962) Race identification from cranial measurements. J Forensic Sci 7:147–157.

Gill GW, and Gilbert BM (1990) Race identification from the midfacial skeleton: American blacks and whites. In GW Gill and JS Rhine (eds): Skeletal Attribution of Race. Maxwell Mus Anthropol Papers 4. Albuquerque: University of New Mexico, pp 47–53.

Gill GW and Rhine JS (eds) (1990) Skeletal Attribution of Race. Maxwell Mus Anthropol Papers 4.

Albuquerque: University of New Mexico.

Gustafson G (1950) Age determinations on teeth. J Am Dental Assoc 41:45–54.

Howells WW (1970) Multivariate analysis for the identification of race from the crania. In TD Stewart (ed): Personal Identification in Mass Disasters. Washington, D.C.: American Museum of Natural History, pp 111–123.

İşcan MY (1988) Rise of forensic anthropology. Yrbk Phys Anthropol 31:203–230.

İşcan MY (ed) (1989) Age Markers in the Human Skeleton. Springfield, Ill: Charles C Thomas.

İşcan MY, and Loth SR (1986a) Determination of age from the sternal rib in white males: A test of the phase method. J Forensic Sci 31:122–132.

İşcan MY, and Loth SR (1986b) Determination of age from the sternal rib in white females: A test of the phase method. J Forensic Sci 31:990–999.

İşcan MY, and Loth SR (1989) Osteological manifestations of age in adults. In MY İşcan and KAR Kennedy (eds): Reconstruction of Life from the Skeleton. New York: Alan R Liss, pp 23–40.

İşcan MY, Loth SR, and Wright RK (1984) Age estimation from the rib by phase analysis: White males. J Forensic Sci 29:1094–1104.

İşcan MY, Loth SR, and Wright RK (1985) Age estimation from the rib by phase analysis: White females. J Forensic Sci 30:853–863.

İşcan MY, Loth SR, and Wright RK (1987) Racial variation in the sternal extremity of the rib and its effect on age determination. J Forensic Sci 32:452–466.

İşcan MY, Loth SR, and Scheuerman EH (1992) Age assessment from the sternal end of the rib and pubic symphysis: A systematic comparison. Anthropologie (in press).

Kilian J, and Vlček E (1989) Age determination from teeth in adult individuals. In MY İşcan (ed): Age Markers in the Human Skeleton. Springfield, Ill: Charles C Thomas, pp 255–275.

Klepinger LL, Katz D, Micozzi MS, and Carroll L (1992) Evaluation of cast methods for estimating age from the os pubis. J Forensic Sci 37:763–770.

Krogman WM, and İşcan MY (1986) The Human Skeleton in Forensic Medicine. Springfield, Ill: Charles C Thomas.

Loth SR, and İşcan MY (1989) Morphological assessment of age in the adult: The thoracic region. In MY İşcan (ed): Age Markers in the Human Skeleton. Springfield, Ill: Charles C Thomas, pp 105–136.

Lovejoy CO (1985) Dental wear in the Libben population: Its functional pattern and role in the determination of adult skeletal age at death. Am J Phys Anthropol 68:47–56.

Lovejoy CO, Meindl RS, Pryzbeck TR, and Mensforth RP (1985) Chronological metamorphosis of the auricular surface of the ilium: A new method for the determination of age at death. Am J Phys Anthropol 68:15–28.

Mann RW, Jantz RL, Bass WM, and Willey PS (1991) Maxillary suture obliteration: A visual method for estimating skeletal age. J Forensic Sci 36:781–791.

Masset C (1989) Age estimation on the basis of cranial sutures. In MY İşcan (ed): Age Markers in the Human Skeleton. Springfield, Ill: Charles C Thomas, pp 71–103.

Masset C (1990) Ou en est la paléodémographie? Bull Mém Soc d'Anthropol Paris 2:109–122.

Meindl RS, and Lovejoy CO (1985) Ectocranial suture closure: A revised method for the determination of skeletal age at death and blind tests of its accuracy. Am J Phys Anthropol 68:57–66.

Molnar S (1971) Human tooth wear, tooth function and cultural variability. Am J Phys Anthropol 34:175–190.

Murray KA, and Murray T (1991) A test of the auricular surface aging technique. J Forensic Sci 36:1162–1169.

Napoli ML, and Birkby WH (1990) Racial differences in the visibility of oval window in the middle ear. In GW Gill and JS Rhine (eds): Skeletal Attribution of Race. Maxwell Mus Anthropol Papers 4. Albuquerque: University of New Mexico, pp 27–32.

Nemeskéri J, Harsányi L, and Acsádi G (1960) Methoden zur Diagnose des Lebensalters von Skelettfunden. Anthropol Anz 24:70–95.

Novotný V (1986) Sex determination of the pelvic bone: A systems approach. Anthropologie 24:197–206.

Post RH (1969) Tear duct size differences of age, sex and race. Am J Phys Anthropol 30:85–88.

St Hoyme L, and İşcan MY (1989) Determination of sex and race: Accuracy and assumptions. In MY İşcan and KAR Kennedy (eds): Reconstruction of Life from the Skeleton. New York: Alan R Liss, pp 53–93.

Saunders SR, Fitzgerald C, Rogers T, Dudar C, and McKillop H (1992) A Test of Several Methods of Skeletal Age Estimation Using a Documented Archaeological Sample. Can Soc Forensic Sci J 25:97–118.

Seta S, and Yoshino M (1990) Hakkotsu-Shitai no Kantei (Identification of Human Skeletal Remains). Tokyo: Reibunsha Publishing (in Japanese).

Snow CC, Hartman S, Giles E, and Young FA (1979) Sex and race determination of crania by calipers and computers: A test of the Giles and Elliot discriminant functions in 52 forensic science cases. J Forensic Sci 24:448–460.

Solowiej D (1982) Určování pohlaví podle lebky—ověření metod doporučovaných různými autory. Universitas Carolina, Prague.

Stewart TD (1954) Sex determination of the skeleton by guess and by the measurement. Am J Phys Anthropol 12:385–392.

Stewart TD (1979) Essentials of Forensic Anthropology: Especially as Developed in the United States. Springfield, Ill: Charles C Thomas.

Stout S (1989) The use of cortical bone histology to estimate age at death. In MY İşcan (ed): Age Markers in the Human Skeleton. Springfield, Ill: Charles C Thomas, pp 195–207.

Todd TW (1920) Age changes in the pubic bone: I. The male white pubis. Am J Phys Anthropol 3:285–334.

Todd TW, and Lindala A (1928) Dimensions of the body: Whites and American Negroes of both sexes. Am J Phys Anthropol 12:35–119.

Todd TW, and Lyon DW Jr (1924) Endocranial suture closure, its progress and age relationship: Part I. Adult males of white stock. Am J Phys Anthropol 7:325–384.

Ubelaker DH (1989) Human Skeletal Remains. Washington, DC: Taraxacum.

Uytterschaut HT (1985) Determination of skeletal age by histological methods. Z Morphol Anthropol 75:331–340.

Vlček E (1971) Gebräuchliche Methoden zur Geschlechtsdiagnose auf Grund des Schädels. Symposium über die Alters—und Geschlechtsbestimmung an Skeletermaterial. Symposium Anthropologicum, Národní Muzeum, Prague, pp 7–26.

Wei B, Feng J, and Fang Z (1983) The relationship between the construction of maxillary first molar and age. Acta Anthropol Sinica 2:79 (in Chinese).

Chapter 7
Craniometric Individuality
of Human Skulls

Jörg B. Schimmler, Richard P. Helmer, and Jürgen Rieger

*Data Processing Centre of the Christian-Albrechts-University, Kiel, Kiel, Germany (J.B.S.);
Institute of Experimental Forensic Medicine, University of Bonn, Bonn, Germany (R.P.H.);
Institute of Forensic Medicine, University of Kiel, Kiel, Germany (J.R.)*

The individuality of human skulls is the basis for identification from this site. A human skull can be identified as that of a missing person if its attributes are unique, or more precisely, if the probability of confusing it with another skull is very low.

It is customary to represent an object by the (ordered) set of *a priori* selected attributes, each of which can be regarded as a point in a so-called attributes space. Although a wide variety of variables might be used, it is advantageous to select those that are measured in the same unit of scale. The coordinates of craniometric points, for example, can all be expressed in millimeters relative to a fixed three-dimensional coordinate system. The following 14 craniometric points on the skull have proven to be important for identification:

1. Porion (right)
2. Porion (left)
3. Nasion
4. Intersection concha nasalis inferior/margin of maxilla (right)
5. Intersection concha nasalis inferior/margin of maxilla (left)
6. Ectoconchion (right)
7. Ectoconchion (left)
8. Gnathion
9. Prosthion
10. Zygion (right)
11. Zygion (left)
12. Vertex

13. Insertion of ligamentum palpedrale mediale (right)
14. Insertion of ligamentum palpedrale mediale (left)

A frequently used coordinate system for the skull is delimited by the frontal plane, the mediosagittal plane, and the Frankfort horizontal. The x-, y-, and z-coordinates are defined by the intersections of the Frankfort horizontal and the mediosagittal plane, the Frankfort horizontal and the frontal plane, and the mediosagittal and the frontal planes, respectively. Positive coordinates lie in the frontal, left, and upper quadrants.

Taking the coordinates of selected craniometric points generates precise information about their spatial positions for the analysis. Angles, distances, etc., can also be calculated from the coordinates of these points, although some information will be lost if derived attributes are used instead. Usually, a set of q coordinates is selected for a specific analysis and are arranged in an ordered set $(x_1, x_2, \ldots, x_q)$ that can be considered as point **x** in a q-dimensional Euclidean space. In this way, every cranium is represented by a point in this space.

Example

Let $(-61.0, 61.0, 28.5, -99.0)$ and $(-59.5, 59.5, 28.0, -79.0)$ be the respective coordinate vectors of two skulls, where the y-coordinates of right porion and left porion and the z-coordinates of nasion and gnathion are used. The number of dimensions of the appropriate Euclidean space is four.

In this framework, the similarity or dissimilarity of skulls can be defined by the principles of cluster analysis. Here, the Euclidean distance, i.e., the square root of the sum of squared coordinate differences, is a natural measure of dissimilarity. In the above example, there is a (four-dimensional) distance of 20.12 mm. Two skulls can be considered identical for selected dimensions when respective measurements are equal or the Euclidean distance vanishes.

DEFINITION OF CRANIOMETRIC INDIVIDUALITY

The reliability of skull identification on the basis of a set of craniometric points depends heavily on the individuality of skulls expressed in terms of the craniometric points entering the analysis. If different skulls have identical craniometric measurements, positive identification is impossible. As skulls randomly vary in size and shape beyond influences like age, sex, race, etc., finding equal craniometric dimensions is possible. Furthermore, the identification of human skulls is affected by unavoidable measurement errors of different origins. The vector x cannot be determined exactly. So two skulls are to be regarded as identical when their dimensions are close enough to lie within the bounds of measurement error (Helmer et al., 1989). Therefore, a probabilistic concept seems to be adequate to cope with skull identification by performing multiple measurements.

The craniometric data of a particular skull allow identification if the probability of mistaken identity for another skull is sufficiently small. That is why this probability should be used for the definition and quantification of craniometric individuality.

For the sake of convenience, it is assumed that the measurement accuracy is the same for all coordinates and measurement errors are statistically independent. There is clearly a certain simplification in assuming equal measurement accuracies for all coordinates and the independence of the measurement errors, but the gain in simplification outweighs any deviations from the perfection of the model.

In this framework, skulls s and x, which have a certain q-dimensional distance of less than Δ, have to be identified; or, in other words, all skulls within a q-dimensional hypersphere of radius Δ around the skull s cannot be recognized as different from s. The set $K_\Delta(s)$ of all skulls x thus to be identified with the skull s is given by the formula

$$K_\Delta(s) = \{ x : \|x - s\| < \Delta \},$$

which describes a vicinity of s in terms of a q-dimensional hypersphere around s. The function $\| \cdot \|$ denotes the Euclidean vector norm. A sphere is selected for practical reasons. Other choices, e.g., q-dimensional hypercubes or q-dimensional ellipsoids, in the case of correlated errors would lead to similar definitions and results. Figure 1 shows a vicinity of s in the plane spanned by the y-coordinate of right porion and the z-coordinate of nasion.

The coordinates of the craniometric points on the skulls are apparently correlated. This fact must be taken into account when probabilities are evaluated. Therefore, a joint probability distribution for the measurements of the skulls has to be assumed in the following. For fixed Δ, let $p(s) = p\{x \in K_\Delta(s)\}$, i.e., the probability that a skull x is situated in the vicinity of s. If this probability is high, the individuality is low, and vice versa. So the individuality $I(s)$ of the skull s is defined to be $1/p(s)$. By definition, the product of $I(s)$ and $p(s)$ is unity. That is why individuality can be interpreted as the number of skulls necessary so that just one skull in the population in question can be expected in the vicinity of s.

By definition, the individuality $I(s)$ of a cranium is a number greater or equal to 1, which depends on:

1. The selected attributes $x_1, x_2, \ldots, x_q$ of the skull;
2. The joint probability distribution of the q attributes;

3. The magnitude of measurement error Δ; and

4. The skull **s** under consideration.

The attributes to be used for skull identification should be selected carefully. The points on the skull should be uniquely defined, precisely determined, and the measurement of their coordinates should be easily obtained and replicated. Partial damage or missing parts, e.g., the lower jaw, will limit the selection of points. Furthermore, certain craniometric points might be selected because they can easily be related to the respective points on a photograph of a missing person. In general, it can be stated that additional points contribute more or less to a better identification by producing a higher degree of individuality; however, it is recommended that they be added selectively and with restraint.

The determination of the probability distribution is important because it greatly affects skull individuality. If a skull is situated in a region of low probability, it has a high individuality and vice versa. In other words, if only a few skulls represented by points are expected to lie in a particular area, they will be much easier to identify because of their relative uniqueness.

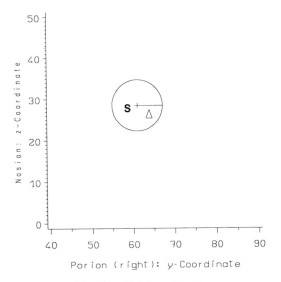

Fig. 1. Vicinity of skull s.

Even when a specific distribution type, e.g., the multivariate normal probability distribution, is chosen, different probability distributions may be adequate if different populations are to be considered. This situation occurs when the skull in question is known to belong to one of several populations, but the true parent population is unknown. For every skull an individuality value can be calculated with respect to each distribution. A discriminant analysis would be a means to decide which parent distribution is to be regarded as the true one.

Individuality with respect to a specific distribution will now be considered. In practice, this probability distribution is not known, but has to be estimated from an appropriate, sufficiently large sample. These large samples can be established by incorporating craniometric data from different populations, provided a sufficient standardization of the selected attributes and their quantification is achieved.

The choice of a realistic and suitable probability distribution type is somewhat delicate, but very important for the calculation of probabilities and individualities. With respect to the craniometric data used here, it seems to be justifiable to assume that the vectors **x** follow a regular q-dimensional normal distribution $N(\mu, \Sigma)$, where μ is the vector of expectations and Σ the variance–covariance matrix. The definition of a regular multivariate normal probability distribution can be found in textbooks, e.g., Rao (1973:36).

Although the assumption of normality is not essential for the definition of $I(\mathbf{s})$, the calculation of lower bounds for $I(\mathbf{s})$ is considerably simplified because well-known statistical methods can be applied. The true parameter matrices μ and Σ, which determine the underlying normal probability distributions, are unknown, but they can be estimated from a reasonably large sample by the sample mean vector $\bar{\mathbf{x}}$ and the sample variance–covariance matrix **S**, respectively.

The magnitude of the measurement error is crucial for skull identification. Obviously, a more precise measurement lowers the probability of an incorrect identification. As a rule, the accuracy of a univariate measurement is described in terms of a symmetric interval around the determined value. If two attributes are determined simultaneously, a two-dimensional region of accuracy is given by a square around the pair of measured values when both univariate accuracies are equal. At worst, the two-dimensional distance of a point in the region from the midpoint is half the length of the square's diagonal (Fig. 2). In a q-dimensional space, the respective value is given by the product of the univariate accuracy and the square root of q.

In order to get a realistic idea of the errors' magnitudes, the three coordinates of eight craniometric points on 52 skulls have been measured three times by the same person. After having measured all those coordinates of one skull, it was dismounted from the measuring device and then once more fixed for the second set of measurements. This procedure was repeated a third time. The intraobserver error could thus be quantified by examining the differences $x_{ij} - \bar{x}_i$ ($i = 1, \ldots 2, , 52; j = 1, 2, 3$), where $\bar{x}_i$ is the mean vector of the ith skull, obtained by averaging the three respective repetitions x_{ij} for $j = 1, 2, 3$. Thus, the lengths of 156 deviation vectors have been calculated in the appropriate

20-dimensional space. (In order to take all possible univariate measurement errors into account, the maximum dimension for all coordinates of eight points on the skull would be 24. This dimension is to be reduced by four because the x- and z-coordinates of left porion and right porion are zero by definition of the Frankfort horizontal.)

In summary, the craniometric individuality is a number greater than one that cannot be directly obtained from a skull as can volume, weight, etc. It is a number reflecting the context in which a given skull is seen.

CALCULATING INDIVIDUALITIES AND LOWER BOUNDS

The individuality of a skull is determined if the measured items, the accuracy, and the appropriate probability distribution are given. It can be calculated by integrating the probability density function over the region $K_\Delta(s)$ numerically.

However, in order to decide whether the achieved accuracy and the selected set of craniometric coordinates ensure that an erroneous identification is highly improbable, the calculation of lower bounds for the determination of individuality is sufficient and, therefore, an exact calculation of the individuality is not necessary.

The method explained below relies heavily on the assumption of the multivariate normality of the data. Obviously, the measurements are correlated, as can be seen from the respective variance–covariance matrices. So the probabilities of a coincidence of several coordinates by chance may not be multiplied in order to obtain the probability for a simultaneous coincidence. This problem can be solved by introducing statistically independent random variables instead of the original measurements. A principal components analysis (PCA) of the population variance–covariance matrix Σ yields statistically independent linear functions of the correlated measurements (Rao, 1973:590). Linear functions of normally distributed random vectors

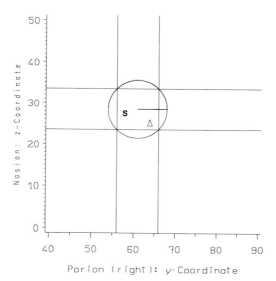

Fig. 2. Univariate and bivariate vicinities of **s**.

are normally distributed (Rao, 1973:524). So vanishing correlations imply independence.

This concept has an obvious geometrical interpretation. If two items are positively correlated, it is more probable to find skulls where both items show either large or small values rather than a combination of a large value of one item and a small value of the other one. The respective two-dimensional normal probability distribution yields concentric ellipses as lines of constant probability density, as shown in Figure 3. In selecting an appropriate coordinate system, the linearly transformed variables become independent random variates following a bivariate normal distribution.

The calculations presented here are based on measurements taken from 95 human skulls. This rather small number can easily be enlarged by additional measurements. For the sake of illustration, an artificial example from the skull data used is given below.

Example

Porion, Nasion, and Gnathion of 95 European Skulls
Number of Skulls in the Population = 95
Number of Craniometric Points on the Skulls = 4

Numbers and Names of Variables:
1: Porion(right)-y
2: Porion(left)-y
3: Nasion-z
4: Gnathion-z

Variance–Covariance Matrix

	1	2	3	4
1	8.34	-8.35	-1.29	4.93
2	-8.35	8.35	1.29	-4.92
3	-1.29	1.29	4.74	-0.04
4	4.93	-4.92	-0.04	43.84

Means
1	-57.36
2	57.36
3	29.27
4	-86.77

The PCA of **S** yields positive eigenvalues $\hat{\lambda}_i$ ($i = 1, 2, \ldots, q$), numbered in decreasing order and respective orthogonal eigenvectors $\hat{\mathbf{u}}_i$ of unit length. The eigenvalues $\hat{\lambda}_i$ and eigenvectors $\hat{\mathbf{u}}_i$ of **S** are estimates of the eigenvalues λ_i and eigenvectors $\mathbf{u}_i$ of the unknown variance–covariance matrix Σ. As the scalar random products $\mathbf{u}_i'\mathbf{x}$ are linear functions of the multivariate normally distributed random vector $\mathbf{x}$, they are univariate normal with the expectation $\mathbf{u}_i'\mu$ and variance λ_i (Rao, 1973:519). It should be noted here that the eigenvectors of Σ are constant.

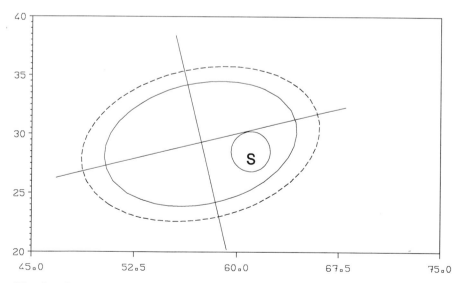

Fig. 3. Contour ellipses of the bivariate normal distribution of Porion(left)-y and Nasion-z.

Example (continued)

Eigenvalues

1	45.53
2	15.30
3	4.44
4	0.00

Eigenvectors

	1	2	3	4
1	0.1666	-0.6772	0.1154	0.7073
2	-0.1664	0.6779	-0.1144	0.7069
3	-0.0116	0.1644	0.9863	-0.0008
4	-0.9718	0.2341	-0.0276	-0.0002

The scalar products involving different eigenvectors are uncorrelated (Mardia, 1979:215). Moreover, they are statistically independent because of their normal distribution property. This fact allows an easy calculation of a lower bound for $I(s)$.

The orthogonal projection of the vector x on the one-dimensional linear subspace spanned by u_i is the point given by the coordinate $u_i'x$ with respect to the basis vector u_i. The projection of $K_\Delta(s)$ on the same linear subspace is an interval of length 2Δ centered about $u_i's$, defined by the formula

$$\{x: |u_i'(x - s)| < \Delta \}.$$

The probability $p_i(s)$ that $u_i'x$ takes a value in this interval can easily be computed using the appropriate univariate normal distribution:

$$p_i(s) = p(|u_i'(x - s)| < \Delta)$$

$$a = \Phi(\frac{u_i'(s - \mu) + \Delta}{\sqrt{\lambda_i}}) - \Phi(\frac{u_i'(s - \mu) - \Delta}{\sqrt{\lambda_i}}),$$

where Φ is the univariate standard normal cumulative distribution function.

As the scalar products of x by different eigenvectors are statistically independent, the probability that each projection of x lies in the respective projection of $K_\Delta(s)$ is given by the product of the $p_i(s)$. This is true if x is in the smallest cube containing $K_\Delta(s)$ that is parallel to the coordinate system established by the q eigenvectors u_i. We obtain the following inequality

$$p(s) < p_1(s)p_2(s) \dots p_q(s).$$

The right side of this inequality yields a lower bound for $I(s)$ that can easily be evaluated. The inequality remains valid if a subset of eigenvectors and eigenvalues of Σ is used. The loss of accuracy is of minor importance if small eigenvalues and appropriate eigenvectors are ignored.

The above considerations are exact for the population eigenvalues and eigenvectors of Σ. As Σ is unknown, the sample estimates $\hat{\lambda}_i$ and u_i calculated from S have to be taken instead. Of course, we can only get estimates of the lower bound for $I(s)$ derived above.

The definition of $I(s)$ and the assumption of a normal probability distribution allow an additional simple conclusion. The expected skull μ has the lowest individuality and it increases with growing (MAHALANOBIS-) distance from the expected skull. (For the definition of the MAHALANOBIS- distance, see Mardia et al., 1979:17.)

The expected skull μ is estimated by the mean skull $\bar{x}$ and provides a global lower bound for the individualities.

As stated above, the choice of the measurements taken from a skull greatly influences its individuality. If one takes additional measurements into account, the individuality will increase. PCA can also give an answer to the question of which measurements should be taken to obtain a sufficient individuality for the identification of skulls (see Mardia et al., 1979:242).

Example (continued)

The estimated bounds for skull individuality and the probabilities $p(s)$ for the first 10 skulls are shown below.

Delta = 0.500
Number of eigenvalues used = 4
Variance explained = 100.000%

Skull No.	Probability	Individuality
Mean	0.112624E-02	887.910
1.	0.104842E-02	953.815
2.	0.189052E-03	5289.56
3.	0.594487E-03	1682.12
4.	0.977859E-03	1022.64
5.	0.509079E-03	1964.33
6.	0.597367E-04	16740.1
7.	0.112821E-03	8863.59
8.	0.136994E-03	7299.58
9.	0.561432E-04	17811.6
10.	0.523200E-03	1911.31

RESULTS AND CONCLUSIONS

With reference to the individualities of the skulls in our collection, the calculations show that there will be remarkably high individualities if the coordinates can be measured with an accuracy within 1 mm. Ranges for the orders of magnitude of the individualities' lower bounds are reported in Table 1. If all coordinates of the eight craniometric points used for the calculations in row 1 of Table 1 are introduced in the analysis, fairly high individualities are to be expected. Assuming a measurement error of about 0.5 mm, which seems to be realistic, the skulls in our sample have an individuality of 1 billion at least, i.e., less than 1 in 1 billion skulls will show identical coordinates within the measurement error of 0.5 mm.

As the video superimposition technique relies on two-dimensional images of the skull, the individualities of the given skulls have been calculated on the basis of orthogonal projections of the points on a coordinate plane. This was easily achieved by leaving out one coordinate; e.g., leaving out the y-coordinates, say, of all points would result in an orthogonal projection on the x,z-coordinate plane. Thus, a frontal and a lateral view of the skulls is obtained. The second row of Table 1 displays the results, using a frontal view. Of course, the lacking information from the x-coordinates results in decreased individualities.

The results displayed in the third and fourth rows of Table 1 are based on five craniometric points in a lateral view. In order to obtain information about the individualities for skulls with missing lower jaw, we dispensed with the respective points. There is no severe loss of individuality if gnathion is replaced by prosthion. However, the absence of a mandible results in a

TABLE 1. Order of Magnitude of Lower Bounds for the Individualities of 95 European Skulls

	$\Delta = 0.5$	$\Delta = 1$	$\Delta = 1.5$	$\Delta = 2$	$\Delta = 4$
8 points[a] 3 dimensions	10^{13}–10^{22}	10^9–10^{15}	10^5–10^{12}	10^4–10^8	10^1–10^6
8 points[b] Frontal view	10^9–10^{16}	10^5–10^{11}	10^2–10^8	10^1–10^7	10^0–10^3
5 points[c] Lateral view	10^9–10^{14}	10^6–10^{11}	10^4–10^9	10^3–10^8	10^1–10^4
5 points[d] Lateral view (lower jaw excl.)	10^9–10^{13}	10^5–10^{11}	10^4–10^8	10^3–10^7	10^1–10^4
10 points[e] Frontal view (lower jaw excl.)	10^{10}–10^{18}	10^5–10^{12}	10^3–10^9	10^2–10^7	10^0–10^2
9 points[f] Frontal and lateral view	10^{10}–10^{17}	10^7–10^{14}	10^6–10^{12}	10^4–10^{11}	10^2–10^7

[a]Nasion, sp cni/max. l./r., ectoconchion l./r., lig. palp. med. l./r., gnathion.

[b]Nasion, sp cni/max. l./r., ectoconchion l./r., lig. palp. med. l./r., gnathion.

[c]Vertex, nasion, sp cni/max. r., ectoconchion r., gnathion.

[d]Vertex, nasion, sp cni/max. r., ectoconchion r., prosthion.

[e]Zygion l./r., nasion, sp cni/max. l./r., ectoconchion l./r., prosthion, lig. palp. med. l./r.

[f]Vertex, nasion, sp cni/max. l./r., ectoconchion l./r., lig. palp. med. l./r., gnathion.

significant loss of individuality if a frontal view is chosen. Although gnathion has been replaced by left and right zygion, and prosthion, as can be seen in rows two and four of Table 1, the individualities show nearly the same order of magnitude.

The combined information of frontal and lateral views can be used easily. This situation corresponds to a superimposition based on photographs from different angles. Row six of Table 1 displays the respective results.

Every experienced examiner knows that, for technical reasons, congruity with a tolerance of ±0.5 mm cannot be achieved in superimposition. The video superimposition technique entails additional, unavoidable inaccuracies. They might be caused, for example, by errors in relating soft tissue topography to the corresponding morphological details of the skull. Additional errors may be caused by inaccuracies of the graphical devices. However, a quantification of these error types has to be accomplished by appropriate experiments. An increased measurement error might compensate for these additional errors. Therefore, we calculated the individualities on the basis of increased measurement errors.

Of course, both an increasing delta and a limitation to frontal or lateral views result in a decreased individuality. This is implied by the definition of craniometric individuality. Furthermore, we found that the frontal view of a skull shows less individuality than a lateral one. The combined information of frontal and lateral views of a skull increases the (calculated) individuality.

It can be concluded that the craniometric individuality of a skull is as distinctive as a fingerprint, provided a measurement error of 1 mm or less can be achieved.

REFERENCES

Helmer RP, Schimmler JB, Rieger J (1989) On the conclusiveness of skull identification via the video superimposition technique. Can Soc Forensic Sci J 22:177–194.

Mardia KV, Kent JT, Bibby JM (1979) Multivariate Analysis. London: Academic Press.

Rao CR (1973) Linear Statistical Inference and Its Applications. New York: Wiley.

Chapter 8

Three-Dimensional Skull Identification via Computed Tomographic Data and Video Visualization

J. Thomas Lambrecht, F. Brix, and Helmut Gremmel

Universität Basel, Zahnärztliches Institut, PCH-4051 Basel, Switzerland (J.T.L.); Department of Radiology, City Hospital (F.B.), Christian-Albrechts-Universität Hospital (H.G.), Kiel, Germany

Obtaining sufficient information on the size and shape of an object is the key to being able to reproduce it. This information can be drawn from computed tomographic (CT) data when the model of an individual skull is desired. Several authors have reported on "three-dimensional reconstruction" by showing TV-monitor visualizations of transformed CT data (Hemmy et al., 1983; Marsh and Vannier, 1983; Vannier et al., 1984; Gillespie and Isherwood, 1986; Gillespie et al., 1987). In 1985, Brix et al. introduced a milling machine for the construction of models used for planning surgical procedures for orthopedics and trauma. We now have modified this device for surgery as well as for craniofacial identification.

MATERIALS AND METHODS

Computer Tomography

The exactness of the images and richness of detail that can be obtained in the model are dependent on the amount of CT data and its precision. Image precision is influenced by the positioning of the patient. Movement must be avoided, because it can lead to continuity disruptions or torquings in the model. A Picker Synerview is used for collecting the basic CT data.

Positioning aids and simple Bandaid fixation are helpful for the necessary bent-back position. For correct computed tomographic differentiation between the upper and the lower jaw, a splint is placed between the teeth. The quality of detail in the model grows with the number of cuts, the picture chosen, and the number of points per line. Data enrichment lengthens the examination time for the patient and the counting time of the computer tomography. One must therefore compromise to reach an optimal balance between data quality and patient comfort. All examinations should be carried out with the minimal distance between the cuts. We now prefer to make 2-mm cuts with a high-solution matrix (512×512). This means 75 to 80 CT cuts for a craniofacial identification.

Software Processing

All incoming data are fed into the internal computer system, a Hewlett Packard 310 with a Motorola 16-byte processor type 68020 for processing. The program (written in Pascal) contains more than 10,000 lines in four subprograms:

1. Data presentation (interactive program):
   a. The first part of the program makes it possible to show each CT cut on a color TV monitor. This picture can be moved with a graphic cursor, and special areas can be defined and enlarged up to eight times.

   b. The "page turning" proceeds in series following the picture sequence up or down as taken in the computer tomography.

c. Contrast and brightness can be regulated using a line change.

2. Contour search (interactive):

a. This part of the program defines the optional model profile and improves it. A starting point above the optional contour and a given limit value of Hounsfield units serve as entrance parameters. The program finds the first contour point perpendicular beneath the starting point where the given limited Hounsfield unit is exceeded. The following control points are obtained by comparison with points adjacent to this reference point. If no location of equal valence can be found, interpolation between the two adjacent points with the greater and smaller Hounsfield unit in a linear manner is performed. Thus, in each CT cut, a marked profile contour develops automatically.

b. Regional parts of a given CT cut can be excluded from processing or temporarily separated manually, using the intra-active part of the program. Thus, the inner outline can be demonstrated and modeled.

c. Finally, the parameter that controls the size of the models can be invoked in this part of the program.

3. The hypothetical three-dimensional (3-D) construction of data within the system:

a. The defined outlines in all CT cuts are integrated to a hypothetical three-dimensional model. The contour data of any interval cut can be interpolated. Instead of a linear interpolation, this procedure has the advantage that the formation of the mean takes place on a continuous "round shaping" function. Following the first derivation, a gradient is formed at any given control point. In this way the later line-up angle of the working tool can be calculated. The contour should be worked in a perpendicular manner whenever possible.

b. During this hypothetical programming procedure, that is, before the actual cutting of the skull, it is necessary to perform a collision detection, since it is possible that two or even three closed contours define one part of the model lying in one cutting level. This summation effect does not take the previous cut and the next cut into consideration. Thus, this part of the program detects overlapping contours and tries to avoid them. The easiest way to describe this feature is to have the computer simulating the cutting in the area of interest. If this simulation cannot be performed without matching all defined contours of the actual picture, the computer announces this problem and offers an alternative solution.

c. The result is a vector that defines the coordinated movements of the tool in all four working axes. A further improvement of the tool is the velocity, which can be held constant to gain a smooth surface on the model (styrodur or polyureol). Finally, around the vector, a second one will be placed at an equal distance to cover and protect the first vector. This second vector conducts the rough preparation of the styrodur and again takes into consideration the previous and coming cuts. The smooth and definitive grinding is performed as the last step, terminating the hypothetical milling within the system. To keep track of this process, the contours can be featured using either a TV monitor or a plotter.

4. Visualization (interactive):

The surface of the model can be featured on a high-resolution color TV monitor. The suitable positioning of an abstract light source and the resulting reflections allow for an accurate calculation of the color scale. Thus, a two-dimensional picture showing the third dimension in perspective can be created. The position of both the observers and the light sources can be varied. Certain model areas can be suppressed or enhanced. This option presents a pure image for monitor-operation planning and for the possibility of documentation using a camera.

Milling the 3-D Model

All data collected thus far are now stored on a standard 3.5-inch floppy disk for the actual construction of the model. These data from the cutting system are transferred into the conducting calculator (HP 150) and activate the actual model-fabricating machine. The precision of the machine is limited by the number of its axial movements and degree of freedom, as well as the method used for cutting.

A detailed description of the technical features of the cutting machine has already been published (Brix et al., 1985). The styrodur bloc is prepared manually using measurements from the conducting calculator. After this preparation, the styrodur will be cut roughly, and the fabrication maneuver started. After a second and, if necessary, third milling, the final model develops.

RESULTS

To illustrate the possibilities of individual three-dimensional skull identification using CT data and video visualization, a patient with polyostotic fibrous dysplasia of the skull and mandible is presented (Fig. 1). Multiple CT cuts (Fig. 2) first are displayed on the monitor (Fig. 3A,B) and the desired contours (hard tissue, soft tissue) are defined. The summarized contours can be viewed separately on the monitor to check for and eliminate programming failures (Fig. 3C,D). The next step is to create a picture featuring the third dimension in perspective on the monitor. Here, both soft (Fig. 4A) and hard tissues (Fig. 4B) of the same patient can be seen.

The milling machine (Fig. 5) is equipped with a styrodur block large enough to cut the desired model. After the cutting process is started, the milling device runs over the styrodur block two or three times to precut and grind the defined contours exactly (Fig. 6). The three-dimensional individual skeletal model serves as a surrogate for the patient (Fig. 7A,B). The instruments used to identify skeletal asymmetries are shown in Figure 7C. Individual three-dimensional skull identification can be performed to the millimeter (Fig. 7D).

DISCUSSION

Individual skull model fabrication through computed tomographic data and video visualization has potential for successful skull identification. It now appears that this method may be the ultimate point of the logical development in the progress of technology in this area. Grüner and Reinhard published a method for skull identification using photography in 1959; almost two decades later, Helmer and Grüner (1977) applied video technology in their superimposition technique. Again, a decade later, Pesce Delfino et al. (1986) published their results on computer-aided skull/face superimposition.

Our system contains photography (in a transformed sense), video technology, computer technology, and imaging procedures that finally lead to a real three-dimensional individual skull model. So-called "three-dimensional anatomical reconstruction" (Gillespie and Isherwood, 1986) results in two-dimensional pictures with the third dimension featured perspectively. The most important step—after TV images are generated—to obtaining an actual plastic reconstruction is accomplished by the fabrication of an individual skull model. Our system appears to offer a few important advantages. The size of the machine and its cost place it within the reach of every medical center that is equipped with a computer tomograph. Model fabrication would be an optional service for all associated integrated specialties (cranio- and maxillo-facial surgery, plastic surgery, traumatology, orthopedics), including forensic medicine, pathological anatomy, and morphology for experimental purposes.

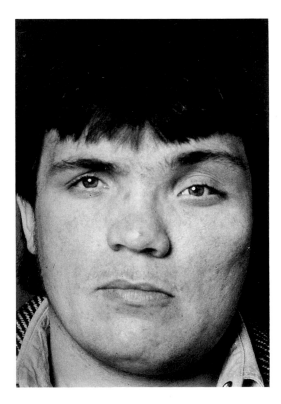

Fig. 1. Patient with polyostotic fibrous dysplasia of the left lateral skull and mandible.

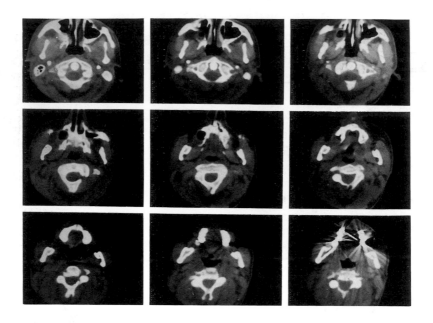

Fig. 2. CT series as usually provided by CT scan.

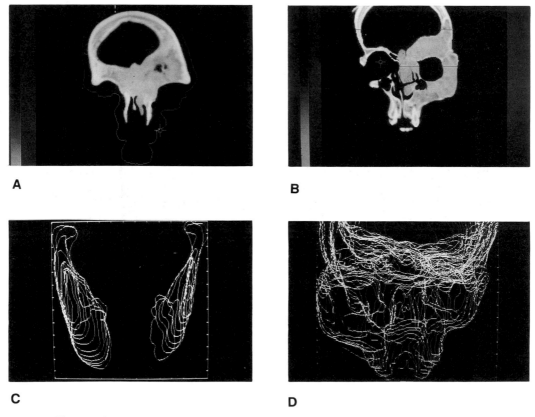

A

B

C

D

Fig. 3. Contours of the soft tissue (**A**) and hard tissue (**B**). Sum of defined mandibular contours monitored to control programming failures, dorsal view, frontal part of mandible not featured (**C**) and skull and upper jaw contours monitored, axial view (**D**).

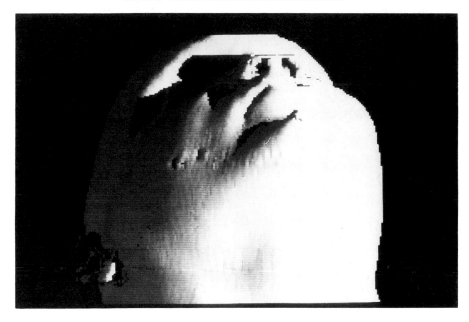

A

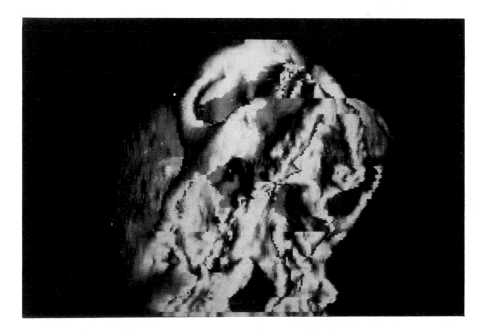

B

Fig. 4.   TV-monitor visualization of the soft tissues (**A**) and the skeletal tissues (**B**), both laterocaudal view.

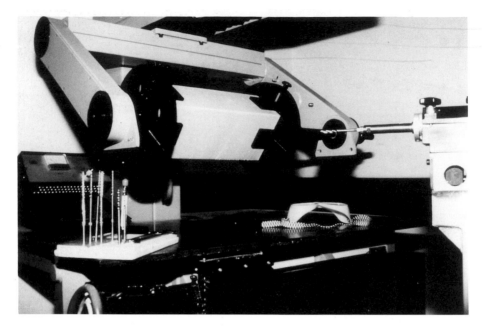

Fig. 5. Milling machine prepared for individual skull model fabrication.

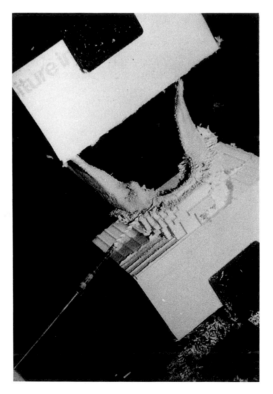

Fig. 6. Milling machine fabricating lower jaw, fine grinding of mandibular structures.

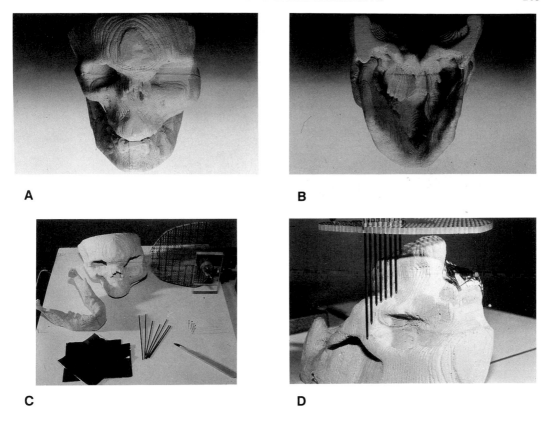

Fig. 7. Three-dimensional individual styrodur model of the skull, frontal (**A**) and dorsal views (**B**); tools for individual skull identification and operation planning (**C**); skull identification per millimeter (**D**).

The user defines the area of interest in the object. Thus, further individualization of skull identification would be possible, especially in asymmetric cases, defects, and problems created through decomposition, since "mirror imaging" allows symmetrical reconstruction of all tissue structures. Furthermore, not only hard tissue but also soft tissue profiles can be made individually.

The individual manufacture of plastic three-dimensional models offers a broad range of possibilities. Since the program permits separate visualization of soft tissues, bones, and air spaces, they can also be constructed and used as composite overlays.

REFERENCES

Brix F, Hebbinghaus D, and Meyer W (1985) Verfahren und Vorrichtung für den Modellbau im Rahmen der orthopädischen und traumatologischen Operationsplanung. Röntgenpraxis 38:290—292.

Gillespie JE, and Isherwood I (1986) Three-dimensional anatomical images from computed tomographic scans. Br J Radiol 59:289—292.

Gillespie JE, Quayle AA, Barker G, and Isherwood I (1987) Three-dimensional CT reformations in the assessment of congenital and traumatic cranio-facial deformities. Br J Oral Max Fac Surg 25:171—177.

Grüner O, and Reinhard R (1959) Ein photographisches Verfahren zur Schädelidentifizierung. Dtsch Z Gerichtl Med 47:247—256.

Helmer R, and Grüner O (1977) Vereinfachte Schädelidentifizierung nach dem Superprojektionsverfahren mit Hilfe einer Video-Anlage. Z Rechtsmed 80:183—185.

Hemmy DC, David DJ, and Herman GT (1983) Three-dimensional reconstruction of craniofacial deformity using computed tomography. Neurosurgery 13:534—541.

Marsh JL, and Vannier MW (1983) The "third" dimension in craniofacial surgery. Plast Reconstr Surg 71:759—767.

Pesce Delfino V, Colonna M, Vacca E, Potente F, and Introna F (1986) Computer-Aided Skull/Face Superimposition. Am J Forensic Med Pathol 7:201—212.

Vannier MW, Marsh JL, and Warren JO (1984) Three dimensional CT reconstruction images for craniofacial surgical planning and evaluation. Radiology 150:179—184.

Chapter 9
Positioning the Skull for Superimposition

P. Chandra Sekharan

Faculty of Forensic Engineering, Anna University, Madras, India 600 025

One often difficult yet very important problem that is encountered when attempting skull–face superimposition involves setting up the skull and photographing it in the same position as the face appears in the photograph of the individual in question (Krogman and İşcan, 1986). It was Brash who first suggested that photographs of the missing person and the skull could be superimposed as an identification technique (Brash and Glaister, 1937). Since then various scientists have utilized this technique in many criminal cases. Webster (1955) gives a detailed description of the superimposition technique adopted in the Plumbago Pit case. For the Corn Field case in Peru, Basauri (1967) also used superimposed photographs along with forensic odontology. In all of these cases, the technique generally adopted has been described as follows: From the original photograph, a negative retake is made. Although the original photograph may be a bust, a full-length photo of the individual, or a group photograph, only the face is reproduced on the negative of definite size, i.e., 4 × 5". The skull is then placed on a tripod, and its position adjusted as closely as possible to that of the face in the photograph. It is then focused on a ground glass of the same size. The reproduced negative is placed on the ground glass, then the image of the skull is adjusted to superimpose on the negative and photographed. The adjustment is made by drawing an outline of or marking the prominent anatomical points of the face on the ground glass. Finally, the two negatives are superimposed to give a positive print. The photograph is then enlarged, coinciding points are noted, and an opinion rendered.

The above procedure has been followed by several forensic scientists all over the world in many criminal cases. Nevertheless, two major problems are associated with Brash's method. First, the position of the skull is usually compromised by placing it on a skull rest and simply moving it by trial and error to match the orientation of the face in the photograph. Second, life-sized measurements are not taken into account. To address this issue, the author (1973) has suggested a rigorous scientific method to accurately position the skull for superimposition studies.

A study of the atlanto-axial and atlanto-occipital joints indicated that the range of movements of the head includes flexion, extension, and rotation. Lateral flexion is permitted by the intervertebral joints of the neck. Hence the posture of the face in a photograph depends on the following factors:

1. Flexion or extension (forward to backward tilt) of the head
2. Lateral flexion right or left (sideways bent) of the head
3. Rotation of the head

These factors must be evaluated accurately before positioning of the skull is attempted. Of the above three factors, the first is the most important for the successful application of the superimposition technique.

DETERMINATION OF FLEXION OR EXTENSION

The forward or backward tilt involves the movement of the head around the transverse axis and the degree to which the face is tilted. The position can be determined in the following way: Consider the erect posture of the head viewed from the side (norma lateralis) (Fig. 1). Imagine two horizontal planes, one of which passes through the "lateral" angle of the eye and the other through the center of the external auditory meatus. The distance d between these two planes (represented by two lines, ab and xy), is a variable factor and depends upon the extent to which the head is tilted forward to backward. The value of d will reach its maximum in the extreme extension of the head when the lateral angle of the eye lies vertically above the external auditory meatus. The distance d becomes zero at a certain position of flexion when both the center of the external auditory meatus and the lateral angle of the eye lie in the same horizontal plane (Fig. 2). In this position, lines ab and xy coincide. If the head is bent still further in the forward direction, the horizontal plane passing through the lateral angle of the eye will lie below the horizontal plane passing through the center of the external auditory meatus. Thus, the distance d is a measure of the tilt

of the head around the transverse axis, and if this distance can be measured accurately, the tilt of the head can be determined. This distance can actually be measured in the life-sized enlargement of the face in norma frontalis. It is therefore necessary to have a life-sized enlargement of the face.

In 1971, the author suggested a revised superimposition technique for the preparation of the life-sized facial photograph of the individual in question. If possible, any articles such as the shirt, spectacles, the chair, etc., found in the photograph should also be obtained. If, for example, the shirt worn by the individual is available, the distance between the two buttonholes that appear in the photograph can be measured; from this distance, the magnification required to enlarge the negative retake to make a life-sized photo can be calculated. Sometimes, it may be possible to work out the magnification data from the body measurements of other living individuals found in the same group photograph. When these distances are measured it is

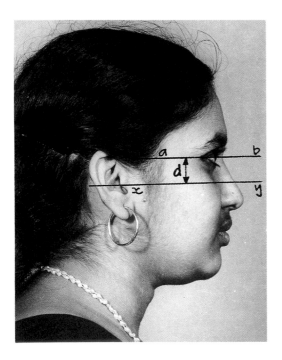

Fig. 1. Lateral view of the erect posture of the head (norma lateralis).

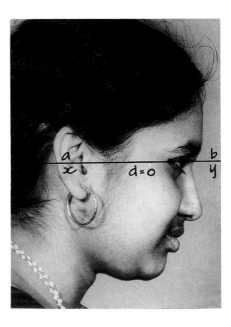

Fig. 2. Position of the head when tilted forward.

essential to select the distances that are involved in linear magnification only. The shirt, the face of the individual, etc., can be considered to be in the same plane, taking into account the distances involved between the camera and the individual when the original photograph was made. Thus a life-sized face can be reproduced.

In the life-sized enlargement of the face in norma frontalis, the two horizontal planes discussed earlier will be represented by AB and XY. The horizontal line AB passing through the lateral angle of a particular eye can be drawn as shown in Figure 3. With reference to the line XY, since the external auditory meatus lies exactly behind the tragus of the ear, it can be fairly assumed that the line drawn through the extreme point of the curved flap of the tragus will represent the desired horizontal plane. The distance between these two lines is then measured as d, and this reading is set between the two horizontal wires of the simple device shown in Figure 4. This device, which was specially designed for positioning the skull, consists of two wooden rings that can be fixed at any position along a vertical rod. Two straight horizontal wires are attached to those wooden rings and a graduated scale is attached to the vertical rod.

This device is kept on the side of the skull, as shown in Figure 5, after setting the distance d between the horizontal wires. Now the skull is adjusted in such a way that the center of the external auditory meatus lies in the horizontal plane passing through the lower horizontal wire of the device, and the point ex (premarked on the outer orbital rim) lies in the horizontal plane passing through the upper horizontal wire of the device. The outer canthus (point ex) can easily be marked on the tubercle of the zygomatic bone, just within the outer orbital margin, as in Figure 6. This tubercle (prominence) marks the attachment of the lateral palpebral ligament.

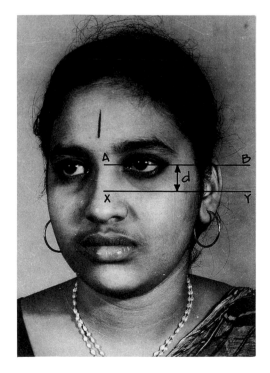

Fig. 3. Oblique view of the face.

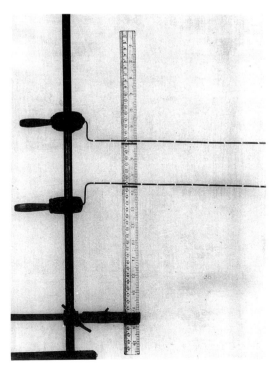

Fig. 4. Tilt-measuring device used in superimposition studies.

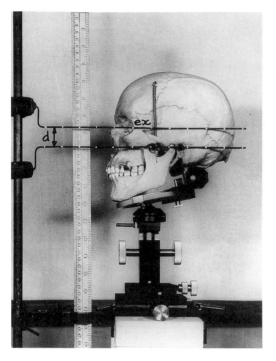

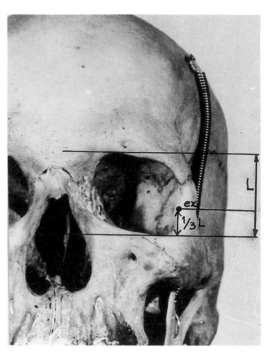

Fig. 5. Skull positioned as per the readings set in the tilt-measuring device.

Fig. 6. Skull showing the position of the outer canthus in the left orbit.

This point corresponds to the lateral angle of the eye and lies exactly in the same horizontal plane in which the lateral angle of the eye is situated. There will, however, be a problem if this tubercle cannot be located. Di Die (1942) placed this tubercle 10 mm below the point where the zygomatico-frontal suture crosses the orbital margin. According to studies by Sakai and Kamijo (1970), the point *ex* lies in the lower third of the outer orbital rim for Japanese skulls. A study carried out by the author (1988a) indicates that in southern Indians, it lies below and at an average of 10.84 mm from the zygomatico-frontal suture in males and 9.96 mm in females.

The skull is fixed on a universal skull rest, a camera stand pan-head, or a universal stage as shown in Figure 5. The advantage of fixing the skull on such a stage is that it can be moved around the transverse and antero-posterior axes, as well as the vertical axis, without disturbing the skull. The skull is then tilted forward or backward accordingly by adjusting the stage,

and its position is set firmly when the point *ex* on the outer orbital rim and the center of the external auditory meatus lie in the corresponding horizontal planes as defined by the two horizontal wires of the device (Fig. 5). After the setting is made, the device is removed, and the camera positioned in front of the skull in the antero-posterior axis for photographing. Now if the skull is enlarged to life size, it will have the same forward or backward tilt as the face in the photograph upon which it will be superimposed. Figures 7 and 8 show the relative positions of the skull set with reference to the tilt of the head seen in Figures 1 and 2. Figures 9 and 10 are the photographs of the skull in norma frontalis for the respective settings shown in Figures 7 and 8. The difference in the structures of the facial skeleton in these two positions may be noted, in particular, the elongation of the features in Figure 10. In the above procedure, two assumptions have been made: (1) The point *ex* in the orbit corresponds to the lateral angle of the eye

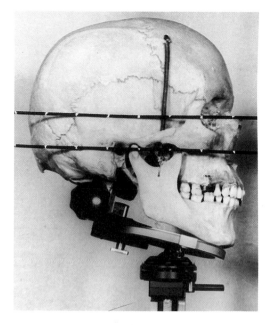 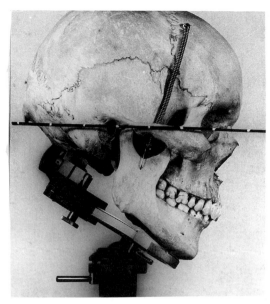

Fig. 7. Lateral view of the skull set in the forward erect posture.

Fig. 8. Lateral view of the skull set in the forward tilt position.

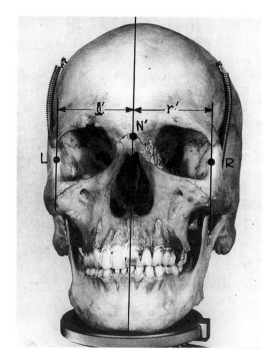 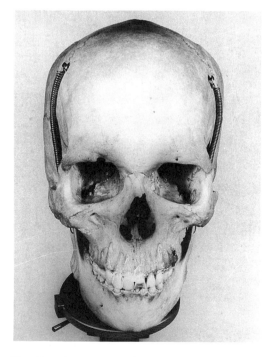

Fig. 9. Frontal view of the skull as per the setting shown in Figure 7.

Fig. 10. Frontal view of the skull as per the setting shown in Figure 8.

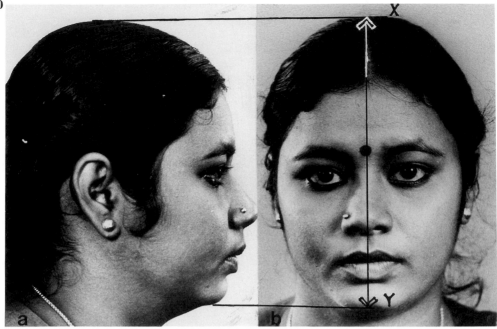

Fig. 11. **a**: Lateral view of the erect posture of the head; **b**: frontal view of the erect posture of the head.

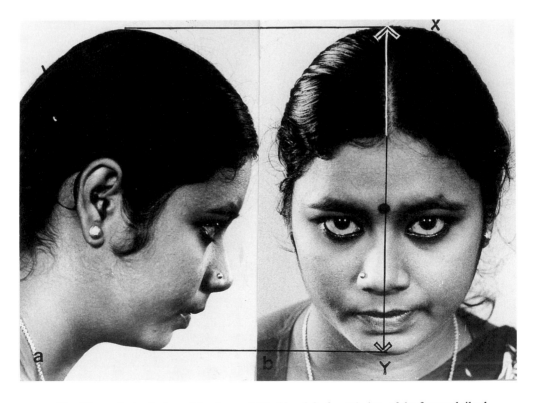

Fig. 12. **a**: Lateral view of the forward tilted head; **b**: frontal view of the forward tilted head.

in the face photograph, and (2) the center of the external auditory meatus will lie in the same horizontal plane as the extreme point of the curved flap of the tragus of the ear. Even though studies have been carried out to establish the accuracy of these two assumptions, some slight deviation is bound to occur in actual cases, and as a result, very slight variations can be noticed in the measurement of the distance *d,* but this variation is negligible.

In cases where the life-sized image of the face cannot be extrapolated, it is still possible to measure the distance between the two horizontal planes as discussed above and establish the exact tilt of the face in the photograph. In such cases, the following procedure is suggested by the author (1988b).

Consider the erect posture of the head (Fig. 11a). Figure 11b shows the frontal view photograph taken in this posture. The vertical median height of the face projected in the photograph can be marked *XY, X* being the highest point in the crown of the head and *Y* being the lowest point in the median plane of chin called the menton. If the head is tilted forward, the facial height in the photograph will appear elongated (Fig. 12). On the other hand, if the head is tilted backward, the facial height will appear shortened, as shown in Figure 13.

For a theoretical consideration, the profile of the face can be approximated to outline *A-M-B-C-D-E-F* shown in Figure 14A The flexion extension movement can be assumed to occur around the transverse axis passing through *D,* which is actually a point at the atlanto-occipital joint, and *M,* the point of intersection of the occlusal line of the lips and the median line.

In the erect profile position of the head, the facial height projected on the photograph—*AB* and *XY*—is the projection of *AB* on the photograph. *XY* in this case will be equal to *AB,* i.e.,

$$(1) \qquad XY = AB.$$

Now XM' and $M'Y$ are the facial heights above and below, respectively, the occlusal line of the lips. The ratio is

$$(2) \qquad XM'/M'Y = AB/MB.$$

If the head is tilted forward by an angle Θ (Fig. 14B), then

$$(3)\ XY = F'B = F'A + AB' = AF\ \mathrm{Sin}\ \Theta + AB\ \mathrm{Cos}\ \Theta$$

and the ratio

$$(4)\quad XM'/M'Y = (AM\ \mathrm{Cos}\ \Theta + AF\ \mathrm{Sin}\ \Theta)/MB\ \mathrm{Cos}\ \Theta.$$

Actually, *AF* represents the cranial length, and *AF'* is the projection of *AF* on the photograph. Thus, in the case of flexion, even though the facial height *AB* is shortened as *AB* Cos Θ, the total facial height projected on the photograph will be more than *AB,* viz.: *AB* Cos Θ + *AF* Sin Θ. This is due to the projection of additional features of the crown of the head on the photograph.

If the head is tilted backward by an angle *O,* the facial height *XY* projected on the photograph will be equal to *AB* Cos Θ, which is less than *AB* (Fig. 14C): '

$$(5) \qquad XY = AB\ \mathrm{Cos}\ \Theta.$$

The XM' = *AM* Cos Θ and $M'Y$ = *MB* Cos Θ and

$$(6)\ XM'/M'Y = AM\ \mathrm{Cos}\ \Theta\ /MB\ \mathrm{Cos}\ \Theta\ \mathrm{or}\ AM/MB.$$

Thus, it can be seen that when the head tilts backward from the erect position, facial height decreases. Similarly, both the heights above and below the occlusal line of the lips decrease uniformly as Θ increases. When the head is tilted forward, the height below the occlusal line of the lips decreases uniformly as Θ increases. But the height above this line increases due to the additional height contributed by the projection of the crown of the head. The shortening or elongation of the facial height will thus depend upon Θ, and the angle through which the head is tilted. Theoretically, *O* can be calculated from the equation:

(7) $\Theta = 2 \tan^{-1} (AF \pm AF^2 - XY^2 + AB^2)/(AB + XY)$.

However, this calculation is not possible, because there are several unknowns in the equation that cannot be evaluated from the photograph. Nevertheless, the facial heights above and below the occlusal line can be evaluated from the face photograph and the ratio of the heights can be calculated. The ratio of these heights is related to the tilt of the head and varies accordingly.

It is therefore suggested that this ratio should first be evaluated from the given photograph (not necessarily life-sized). The skull is then fixed on the stand and its image brought onto the video monitor. The skull is then tilted until the ratio of the measured distances XM and XY equals the same value as that worked out from the photograph. This time point M would, of course, be the point of intersection of the occlusal line of the teeth with the median and the distances XM and XY, which are measured with

help of a divider in the image brought onto the video monitor.

Points X and Y can easily be marked on the skull images. However, there will be some difficulty in marking point X in some photographs if the hairstyle is not simple. But this problem can be overcome by carefully completing the upper outline of the face, ignoring the hair. To decide the angle of rotation and lateral flexion of the head, a life-sized enlargement is not necessary and the method advised by the author (1973) can be used. Once the skull is thus positioned, its 1:1 image is brought onto the video monitor and the image of the face photograph can be zoomed over it with allowance for tissue thicknesses.

This is perhaps the only way to obtain the approximately life-sized image of the face in the absence of magnification data. Nevertheless, this procedure ensures that the skull is oriented scientifically in the same position as the face in the photograph and would obviate

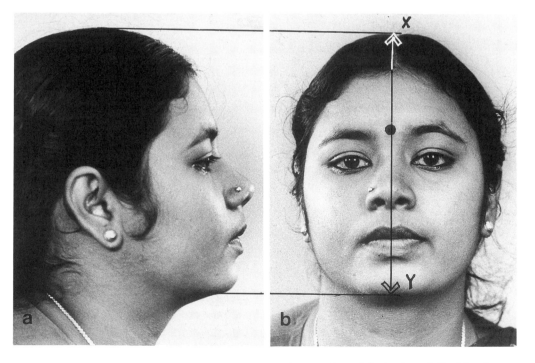

Fig. 13.   a: Lateral view of the backward tilted head; b: frontal view of the backward tilted head.

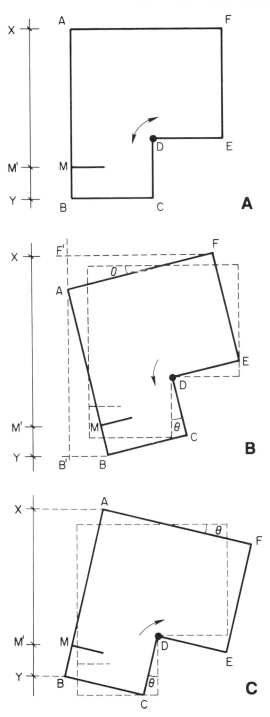

the criticism that there is nothing scientific in manipulating the skull and blindly fitting its image with that of the face.

DETERMINATION OF LATERAL FLEXION

The extent of lateral flexion can simply be calculated from the face in norma frontalis by measuring the angle between the vertical axis of the face in the laterally flexed position and the vertical axis of the face had it been in the erect position (Fig. 15). Line *AB* represents the vertical axis of the face in the erect posture and *XY* represents the vertical axis of the face in the flexed position. The angle between these two lines is measured, and the skull set laterally to this angle by tilting the stage. In fact, this need not be determined precisely; since the lateral

Fig. 14. **A:** Approximated outline of the profile of the face in the erect posture; **B:** approximated outline of the profile of the face in the forward tilted posture; **C:** approximated outline of the profile of the face in the backward tilted posture.

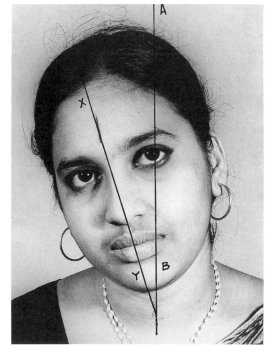

Fig. 15. Frontal view of the laterally tilted head.

flexion is caused by the flexion of the interver-tebral joints and in the coronal plane, the struc-tures on the face and skull in norma frontalis will not be very much altered by slight differ-ences in lateral flexion.

DETERMINATION OF ROTATION

The face in the photograph may appear either straight or rotated toward one side. If it is straight, the breadth of the face on both sides of the median line will be equally recorded in the photograph. If it is rotated toward the left, the breadth of the face on the left side of the median line will be less than that of the face in the right side, and vice versa. The surface of the face is curved postero-laterally on both sides of the median line, and the structures on the face are symmetrically situated. Rotation causes the dif-ferences in breadths.

The photograph of the human face can there-fore be considered as the projection of these curved surfaces on a plane. The length of a line on a plane parallel to it is unaltered by the projection, while the projection of a line on a plane oblique to it is always less than the length, varying directly with the cosine of the angle that the line makes with the plane.

Consider a point in the median line, for ex-ample, nasion (N) in Figure 16. Then consider two other points, each equidistant and sym-metrically placed on the curved surfaces on each side of the face. These represent lateral angles L and R of the left and right eyes, respec-tively. Since L and R are situated postero-later-ally to N, the lines joining these three points, L, N, and R, will be in a plane. Lines LN and RN will subtend an angle w, as shown in Figure 17a. Now consider the projection of the lines LN and NR on the transverse plane TT'. The transverse plane TT' will also represent the plane of the photograph, assuming that the plane determined by L, N, and R is perpendicular to the transverse plane and parallel to the horizontal plane. MN will be the projection of LN, and NO the projec-tion of RN. If Θ_1 and Θ_2 are the angles sub-tended by LN and RN, respectively, to the trans-verse plane TT', then

$$MN = LN \cos \Theta_1 \text{ and } NO = RN \cos \Theta_2.$$

Since L and R are equidistant points, $LN = RN = a$, so that

(8) $$MN/NO = \cos \Theta_1/\cos \Theta_2.$$

When the face is straight,

$$\Theta_1 = \Theta_2 = \Theta, \text{ and } MN = NO.$$

If the face is rotated toward one side, left, for example, by an angle Φ, then $\Theta_1 = \Theta + \Phi$, and $\Theta_2 = \Theta - \Phi$ (Fig. 17b). Therefore, $\Theta_1 > \Theta_2$ or $\cos \Theta_1 < \cos \Theta_2$, since $\cos \Theta$ is a decreasing function of Θ when Θ varies Θ from $0°$ to $90°$, and $MN <$

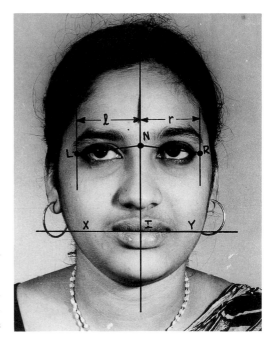

Fig. 16. Frontal view of the face showing the anthropometric points used while calculating the rotation error: N, Nasion; L, left outer canthus; R, right outer canthus; I, point of intersection of the median and occlusal lines; X and Y, intersections of the occlusal line and facial outline.

NO. Also it can be seen from equation 8 that the ratio *MN* to *NO* will depend on Θ_1 and Θ_2 and not on *a,* the distance of the symmetrical points from the median line.

Let us consider these points in the photograph in Figure 16. Point *N* (nasion) can easily be marked in the median line. The respective lateral angles of the eye are marked as *L* and *R*. Let *l* be the length of line *LN* and *r* be the length of line *NR*. Since these distances are measured in the photograph, they are the projections of the actual lengths on the transverse plane. Therefore $l/r = \text{Cos } \Theta_1/\text{Cos } \Theta_2$. Angles Θ_1 and Θ_2 will have definite values for a particular angle of rotation Φ of the face. If Θ_1 and Θ_2 are known, Φ can be calculated. The values of *l* and *r* can be accurately measured from the photograph and the ratio *l/r* can be determined.

As can be observed in Figure 17a, *w* is the angle formed by the lines joining *N* (nasion) and the lateral angles of the left (*L*) and right (*R*) eyes. Let us assume that this angle is 120° for all normal individuals. When the face is straight without any rotation, $\Theta_1 = \Theta_2 = 30°$. If the angle

of rotation Φ of the face takes the values 1°, 2°, 3° . . . , Θ_1 will take the values 31°, 32°, 33° . . . , while Θ_2 assumes the values 29°, 28°, 27° . . . . . Hence the ratio of Cos Θ_1 to Cos Θ_2 for various values of Φ can be worked out and tabulated as in Table 1. Since $l/r = \text{Cos } \Theta_1/\text{Cos } \Theta_2$, the value of *l/r* as worked out from the measurements taken in the photograph will correspond to a particular value of Cos $\Theta_1/\text{Cos } \Theta_2$ in the tabulation, and the corresponding angle of rotation Φ can be determined readily. The skull can then be set in this angle of rotation Φ.

The assumption that *w* is about 120° for all normal individuals is arbitrary. However, there is a means of determining this value for different races through mass studies. From the study undertaken by the author (1973) of 100 normal southern Indian adults, *w* was estimated to be 120° ± 10°. The three points considered in the above discussion do not lie in a horizontal plane, but in a plane slightly inclined to the horizontal plane. Also, the inclination between the plane determined by these three points and the horizontal plane will vary with the rotation of the

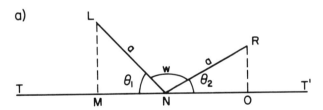

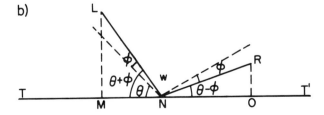

Fig. 17. **a**: Projection of anthropometric points in the photograph where *N* = nasion; *L* = left outer canthus; *R* = right outer canthus; *w* = angle subtended by lines *LN* and *RN*; Θ_1 = angle subtended by line *LN* to transverse plane *TT'*; Θ_2 = angle subtended by line *RN* to *TT'*. **b**: Projection of anthropometric points as above when the face is rotated by angle Θ (angle of rotation).

CHANDRA SEKHARAN

TABLE 1. The Ratios of Left and Right Halves of Facial Projection at Different Angles of Rotation

Φ	Θ_1	Θ_2	$\cos\Theta_1/\cos\Theta_2$
0	30	30	1.0000
1	31	29	0.9802
2	32	28	0.9605
3	33	27	0.9412
4	34	26	0.9223
5	35	25	0.9018
6	36	24	0.8857
7	37	23	0.8676
8	38	22	0.8498
9	39	21	0.8324
10	40	20	0.8153
11	41	19	0.7982
12	42	18	0.7814
13	43	17	0.7647
14	44	16	0.7484
15	45	15	0.7321
16	46	14	0.7160
17	47	13	0.7000
18	48	12	0.6841
19	49	11	0.6683
20	50	10	0.6527
21	51	9	0.6372
22	52	8	0.6216
23	53	7	0.6063
24	54	6	0.5910
25	55	5	0.5758
26	56	4	0.5607
27	57	3	0.5454
28	58	2	0.5303
29	59	1	0.5151
30	60	0	0.5000

face around the transverse axis. Hence, for a particular forward tilt, the plane included by these three points will be horizontal, and in this position points L, N, and R will lie in a straight line in the photograph, while l and r measured in the photograph will give the true values of MN and NO, as discussed earlier. In other positions of forward tilt, these three points will not lie in a straight line, as is the case for Figure 9. In such cases, lines parallel to the median line are drawn through the lateral angles of both the eyes, as shown in Figure 16, and the distances of these two lines from the median line can be measured as l and r, respectively. It is only then that the values of l and r will correspond to the assumed values of Θ_1 and Θ_2.

Studies have also been made by considering

three other points, i.e., the point of intersection of the occlusal line of the lips, the median line, and the two angles of the mouth. The former point can be easily marked in the photograph from the appearance of the philtrum. The angle w will normally be $110° \pm 10°$ when these three points are considered. This value may also vary when a person is smiling. Diseases like facial palsy will also alter the symmetry of the lips. Hence, it is preferable to take nasion and the lateral angles of both eyes into consideration.

Suppose the skull in question is set in the same angle of rotation as the face and is photographed. The corresponding points discussed earlier can also be marked in the skull photograph. Nasion is marked in the median line at the upper end of the internasal suture where it meets the frontal bone. The points ex corresponding to the lateral angle of the eyes are marked on the outer orbital rim of both the orbits, as discussed earlier. The intersection of the occlusal line of the teeth with the median line can also be marked corresponding to the point of intersection of the occlusal line of the lips and the median line. Even if the teeth are not present, prosthion or infradentale can be used. Prosthion is the lowest point of the intermaxillary suture, on the alveolar margin, between the two medial incisors. Infradentale is the highest point on the anterior alveolar margin of the mandible in the median line between the two lower medial incisors. Assuming that the angle of the mouth lies in front of the first premolar, the corresponding points can be marked on the respective teeth or in their respective sockets if teeth are missing.

Now consider nasion and points ex labeled as L, R, and N' in the skull photograph in Figure 9. If l' and r' are the respective lengths of LN' and RN', then the same series of trigonometric formulae hold, with l' and r' replacing l and r. Therefore,

(9) $l'/r = \cos\Theta_1/\cos\Theta_2$ or $l'/r' = l/r$.

From this equation, it is seen that if l' and r' bear the same ratio as l and r, the skull could have been set in the same angle of rotation as the face. Thus, it is possible to place the skull in the same angle of rotation as the face without actually calculating Φ. In actual cases, l and r can be determined from the life-sized enlargement of the face. The skull is set on the stage and rotated in such a way that the values l' and r' measured in the ground-glass image of the skull have the same ratio as l and r. If a large-format camera is used and the image of the skull is focused on the ground glass, the lengths l' and r' can be measured using dividers and their ratio verified. The same procedure is used for the monitor in video superimposition.

In the above procedure, the angle of rotation can be estimated accurately only when the three points chosen for consideration are clearly seen in the photograph. In the first set of points discussed, theoretically, all three points should be visible in the photograph up to a rotation of about 60° of the face, since w is about 120°. But beyond 30° to 35° of rotation, one of the lateral angles of the eye is completely masked by the eyeball, and likewise when the angles of the mouth are considered, one of the angles is masked. Therefore, in photographs in which the face is seen rotated beyond 35°, the following procedure for approximation can be adopted.

After drawing the median line, a line perpendicular to it is drawn through I, the point of intersection of the median line and the occlusal line of the lips. This line will cut the outline of the face at two points X and Y (Fig. 16). The lengths l and r can be measured between these two points and I. The ratio of l and r can be verified in the ground-glass image of the skull by taking corresponding points, as discussed earlier. This perpendicular line can be drawn through any point in the median line in the lower half of the face. In the upper half of the face, placement of the points X and Y will be subject to error due to an asymmetrical hairstyle. In this approximation it cannot be said that points X and Y lie equidistant from I in the face of the individual. Thus, although the theoretical concept discussed earlier does not always hold, setting the skull according to this procedure still offers a fairly close approximation.

As stated earlier, the tilt of the face around the transverse axis is the only major problem in setting up the skull. The determination of the other two factors offers little difficulty, since in a majority of cases lateral flexion and rotation are very slight. The adjustment of the skull according to the above-evaluated factors can be achieved manually. Since manual adjustment may pose certain problems, the remote-operated positioning device, made by Kumari and the author, is suggested for positioning the skull. This device consists of a tripod, a pan and tilt unit (such as the type normally used to operate surveillance cameras), and two control units (one to rotate the pan around the vertical axis, and the other to tilt the pan plate up and down). The pan-head is rotated by the AC servo-motor (M_1), both clockwise and counterclockwise, the angle of rotation being up to 360° (Fig. 18). For superimposition studies, a rotation up to 90°, both clockwise and counterclockwise, will suffice to rotate the skull from right profile to left profile. The pan can be tilted up and down by operating the threaded bolt (S), which runs through the upper plate of the pan. This bolt is rotated by the motor (M_2) both clockwise and counterclockwise so that the pan plate can be tilted up and down. The motor (M_2) is operated by another remote control. The motors (M_1 and M_2) are AC servo-motors, which have quick reversibility and dynamic breaking characteristics. The motors are provided with built-in gear reducers and are lubricated for life. The skull is fixed on the specially designed stem (D) mounted on the pan plate, and tilts forward and backward when the pan plate moves up or down. Once the skull is mounted on this device, its movements are controlled by the two separate remote-control units. The movement of the head sideways (lateral flexion) need not be considered, since, as mentioned earlier, the structures on the face and skull are not affected by this lateral tilt when frontal photographs are taken for superimposition. It is sufficient if the skull and face photographs are fixed parallel to the vertical axis.

The fourth factor that must be considered before actually photographing the skull is the distance between the camera lens and the face of the individual when the photograph in question was taken. This is essential to determine the

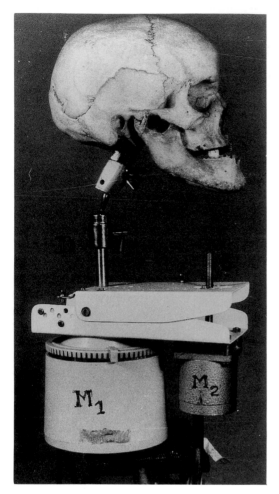

Fig. 18. Remote-controlled skull stand with the "pan and tilt" head run by two AC servo-motors. D, specially designed stem to mount the skull; S, threaded bolt to tilt the pan up and down; M_1, AC servomotor to effect rotation; M_2, AC servomotor to effect the tilt.

perspective. The appearance of a solid object on a plane surface depends on the position of the observer's eye. Obviously, this will vary if viewed from different positions. Therefore, it would be ideal if the skull could be photographed at the same distance as the face was photographed when the individual was alive. It is almost impossible to determine this distance

exactly from the photograph. However, it can be roughly estimated from the camera frame size and nature of the photograph (e.g., bust, full-sized, group, etc.). There is another limitation on this rough estimate because it also depends on whether the photograph is a direct print or an enlargement. A practical suggestion for making this determination is to fix the camera at a distance of 3 feet when a portrait is sent for superimposition studies and at 6 feet when a full-length photograph is supplied.

REFERENCES

Basauri C (1967) A body identified by forensic odontology and superimposed photographs. Int Crimin Pol Rev 204:37–43.

Brash JC, and Glaister J (1937) Medicolegal Aspects of the Ruxton Case. Edinburgh: E & S Livingstone.

Chandra Sekharan P (1971) A revised superimposition technique for identification of the individual from the skull and photograph. J Crimin Law, Criminol Pol Sci 62:107–113.

Chandra Sekharan P (1973) A scientific method for positioning of the skull for photography in superimposition studies. J Pol Sci Admin 1:232–240.

Chandra Sekharan P (1988a) The location of Whitnall Tubercle and its importance in superimposition technique. Indian J Forensic Sci 2:157–162.

Chandra Sekharan P (1988b) Positioning skull for video superimposition. Indian J Forensic Sci 2:166–172.

Di Die LJA (1942) Observacoes Sobre o Tuberculo Orbitario de Whitnall no Osso Zigomatico do Homem (com Pesquisas no Vivo). Anais da Faculdade de Medicinada Universidade de S. Paulo 18:43–63.

Krogman WM, and İşcan MY (1986) The Human Skeleton in Forensic Medicine. Springfield, Ill: Charles C Thomas.

Kumari TR, and Chandra Sekharan P (1992) Remote control positioning device for superimposition studies. Forensic Sci Int 54:127–133.

Sakai and Kamijo (1970) Basic study on superimposition with application of roentgen cephalometry (Report 2): Positional relationship between soft and hard tissues of the human head and face, and study of special camera for superimposition. Rep Nat Res Inst Police Sci 23:10–17.

Webster G (1955) Photography as an aid in identification: The Plumbago Pit Case. Police J 28:185–192.

Chapter 10

Technical Advances in Skull-to-Photo Superimposition

Lan Yuwen and Cai Dongsheng

Tieling 213 Research Institute, Liaoning Province, People's Republic of China 112000

More than 50 years ago, Brash developed a technique for craniofacial superimposition and thus provided an important means of identification from the skull (Glaister and Rentoul, 1962). Along with the development of photographic and video technology, many scientists have significantly upgraded and modified this method. Helmer's success in identifying the remains of Josef Mengele using video superimposition in 1985 is a most convincing example (Helmer, 1987).

In this chapter, we introduce a new technique that uses a microcomputer to accurately obtain the angle of superimposition, an approximation of natural head size, and optimum objective length. There is also a description of the superimposition system constructed for this purpose.

ANGLE OF CRANIOFACIAL SUPERIMPOSITION

One must first adjust the angles of the skull to match the photograph as closely as possible, either by means of photography or television. Accurate superimposition cannot be accomplished without this step. Therefore, it is vital to have a scientific method that is capable of calculating the original angle of the picture, then identically duplicating that position for the skull. The method presented in this chapter can calculate the deflection (rotation) and pitch (upward and downward tilt) angles of the head in the photograph according to the deflection and pitch indices using a photographic test involving 19 angles taken from 100 Chinese Han males ranging in age from 18 to 55 years.

Deflection Index

Set three marking points on the face of the individual to be examined, i.e., taking the left and right ectoconchions as points A and B, respectively, and glabella as point C (positioned on the central line of the nose). Then place an angle marker and scale of measurement on the face, and take photos in 10 angles, with the front position as 0° (0°–90°, 10° change for each angle). Enlarge the photographs to natural head size and measure the distances between points A and C, points B and C, and calculate the deflection index as follows:

Deflection Index = Distance from A to C (mm)/Distance from B to C (mm).

The results, shown in Table 1, indicate an inverse relationship between the deflection index and the deflection angle—the deflection index of the photograph decreases as the deflection angle increases (Fig. 1). We have thus determined that the deflection index can be calculated from the distances between points A and C, and B and C, and then the deflection angle can be measured (Lan and Cai, 1982a).

Pitch Index

For this determination, three points must be marked on the face, i.e., taking glabella as point E, subnasale as point F, and gnathion as point G. Then take the photograph, with point F as the axle point and full frontal orientation at 0°, take photos in nine angles (-20° to 20°, with 5° between angles).

Forensic Analysis of the Skull, pages 119–129 ©1993 Wiley-Liss, Inc.

TABLE 1.   Relation Between Deflection Index and Deflection Angle of Photo[a]

	Deflection Angle of Head									
	0	**10**	**20**	**30**	**40**	**50**	**60**	**70**	**80**	**90**
Deflection index of photo	1.0	0.91	0.80	0.71	0.58	0.49	0.34	0.24	0.13	0
Standard deviation	0	0.01	0.04	0.05	0.02	0.03	0.02	0.02	0.13	

[a]100 persons, 1,000 photographs, and 10 angle groups.

Then enlarge the photos to natural head size, measure the distance from points E to F and G to $F,$ and calculate as follows:

Pitch index = Distance from E to F (mm)/ Distance from G to F (mm).

The results (Table 2) indicate that the pitch index decreases as the pitch angle of the head increases (Fig. 2).

Thus, the pitch index can be calculated using the distances measured from points E to F and G to F in the photo, and the pitch angle can be obtained by measuring the angle formed at the junction of these lines. However, because of the relatively large difference between points E, F, and G for different faces, it is difficult to control the accuracy of the calculation of the pitch

angle using the mean value. Therefore, it is necessary to make some corrections of the values measured from the skull in the following manner. Determine the distances from glabella to subnasale, and from subnasale to gnathion on the skull, and use in the formula below:

$$X = W - A'/B' + A/B$$

where X is the practical pitch index of the tested photo, W is the mean value of the pitch index of the photo, A'/B' is the practically measured pitch index of the skull, and A/B is the pitch index of the photo.

Next, calculate the practical pitch angle (Y) of the photo using this formula: $Y = 94.54 - 98.70X$ as illustrated in Figure 2.

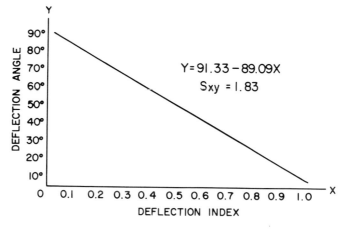

Fig. 1. X, deflection index; Y, definition angle.

TABLE 2.   Relation Between Pitch Index and Pitch Angle[a]

| | Pitch Angle of the Head | | | | | | | | |
	-20	-15	-10	-5	0	5	10	15	20
Pitch index of the photo	1.16	1.11	1.06	1.01	0.96	0.91	0.84	0.81	0.76
Standard deviation	0.01	0.01	0.03	0.01	0.03	0.01	0.05	0.01	0.01

[a]100 persons, 900 photos, and 9 angle groups.

DETERMINATION OF NATURAL HEAD SIZE

Taking measurements over the superimposed image plane geometrically and then developing a reliable scientific evaluation of the results are the essential characteristics of our research system (Lan and Cai, 1988). Only on the condition that the image in the tested photo is restored to its exact or at least extremely close to the natural head size can the above-mentioned data or indices be of value for identification. In this chapter we introduce excerpts of our research on more than 120 Chinese Han females (Lan et al., 1987).

Begin by placing an angle marker and a scale on the face of the (live) person to be examined, take photos at specified angles, and enlarge them to natural head size. Determine the distance between the ectoconchion on both sides in the photo. If the ectoconchion on one side disappears due to an increase in the deflection angle, the remaining length should be used as the total measurement.

The results show that the length of the line segment between the two ectoconchions in the photo shortens gradually as the deflection angle increases (Table 3). The change in length is not linear if it is relatively small for deflection angles below 40°. However, if there is a substantial change (with an angle greater than 40°), the relationship is linear. At 90°, the length of the line segment is 15.02 mm and is the distance between the bridge of the nose and the ectoconchion opposite the one that is turned away from the camera (Fig. 3). The change of length is relatively small if the deflection angle is below 40° and presents in a curve state. The change presents a linear state if the angle is above 40°.

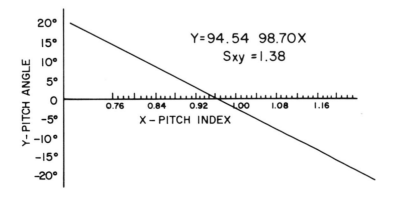

Fig. 2.   *Y*, pitch angle; *X*, pitch index.

TABLE 3. Length (mm) of Line Segment Between the Two Ectoconchions[a]

| | Deflection Angle | | | | | | | | | |
	0°	10°	20°	30°	40°	50°	60°	70°	80°	90°
Mean	89.11	85.53	80.75	75.78	66.25	55.20	45.06	32.61	22.65	15.02
Standard deviation	3.66	3.73	3.59	4.40	3.58	3.80	4.17	3.09	2.47	2.12

[a]120 persons, 1,200 photos, and 10 angle groups.

Using the above-mentioned results, one can calculate a measurement that is extremely close to the actual length of the line segment between the right and left ectoconchions. Based on the deflection angle of the test photo, this length will allow the investigator to extrapolate the natural head size from the photo. However, one must give full consideration to the deviation between individual length and mean value. In other words, one must also use the actual value of the distance between the two junctures of the external orbits of the skull to make some corrections for the mean value. This can be accomplished with the following formula:

$$S = T + (L - L' - S')\text{Cos } X$$

where S is the length of the line segment between ectoconchions in the photo that has already been enlarged to actual head size; T is the distance between the two ectoconchions in the tested photo; L is the distance between the two junctures of the external orbits of the tested skull; L' is the difference between the mean value of the length between the two junctures of the external orbits of the skull minus the distance between the two ectoconchions in the photo; S' is the mean value of the length of the line segment between ectoconchions in the photograph taken at an angle of 0°; and X is the deflection angle.

OPTIMUM OBJECTIVE LENGTH

Successful superimposition must leave the central perspective difference of the skull as close as possible to that of the photo. Yet it seems that there is no way to determine the

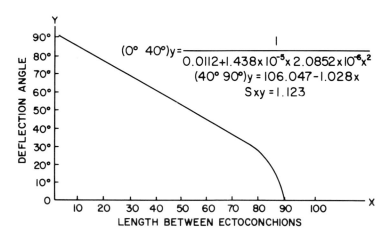

Fig. 3. *Y*, deflection angle of photograph; *X*, length between ectoconchions on photograph.

original photographic length of the test photo. Through research on the central perspective difference, we have established a new concept of "relative parallel" and found that the optimum objective length for photographic superimposition is 1 m (Lan and Cai, 1982a–c).

Relative Parallel Zone

Using a sample of 10 male skulls, we made five vertical and horizontal lines, respectively, on specified positions on the face, and added a scale as shown in Figure 4. Photos were then taken at distances of 0.7, 1, 2, and 3 m, enlarged to half of actual head size, and then measured. These measurements, which appear in Table 4, demonstrate that the values for the breadth and length of the skull and bigonial breadth increase as the objective length increases and, at the same time, increased the length and breadth of the face. In contrast, four other figures, including the trichion line (which forms a part of the breadth of skull), the length between the two junctures of the external orbits, the cheilion breadth, and the lower jawline, show no change as the photographic length increases. The length from trichion to gnathion, which constitutes a part of the length of the skull, also shows no change.

From this, we deduced that when photos are taken within a range of from 0.7 to 3.0 m or even farther, there will be a relatively unchanged zone on the head and face, as can be seen in the white part of Figure 5. This area is a plane, perpendicular to the main axis of the camera lens, formed by connecting lines between trichion, the juncture of orbits, cheilion, and gnathion. This zone can be referred to as the "relative parallel zone" because it does not change in a limited range despite variation in the photographic lengths.

Change Zone

The areas shaded in oblique lines in Figure 5 represent the "change zone," because the size of this part of the image changes with variations in the photographic length. In order to delineate the range of this zone, measurements of the head and face were taken from over 100 (living) male adults of Chinese Han nationality (Table 5). One can calculate the range of each part of the change zone based on the values in this table using the following formulae:

Upper head height = maximum head height -
distance from trichion to gnathion
= 233.6 - 204.1 = 29.5 mm

TABLE 4. Measurements (mm) From 10 Skull Photographs (Mean ± Standard Deviation)

Dimensions	Objective Length (m)			
	0.7	1.0	2.0	3.0
Maximum breadth of skull	65.5 ± 2.55	67.0 ± 2.86	68.5 ± 2.85	69.7 ± 2.80
Maximum length of skull	105.5 ± 4.52	107.4 ± 4.66	108.5 ± 4.52	109.6 ± 4.67
Bigonial breadth	50.8 ± 4.32	52.1 ± 4.55	53.0 ± 4.44	53.7 ± 4.41
Trichion line	49.08 ± 1.95	49.33 ± 1.88	49.06 ± 1.71	49.31 ± 1.64
Length between the two junctures of the external orbits	49.4 ± 1.89	49.4 ± 1.89	49.3 ± 1.89	49.4 ± 1.89
Width of cheilion	25.254 ± 2.01	25.5 ± 2.08	25.5 ± 2.11	25.5 ± 2.17
Lower jawline	25.25 ± 1.99	25.71 ± 1.85	25.52 ± 1.94	25.59 ± 2.03
From trichion to gnathion	96.5 ± 2.72	96.6 ± 2.27	96.6 ± 2.70	96.7 ± 2.64

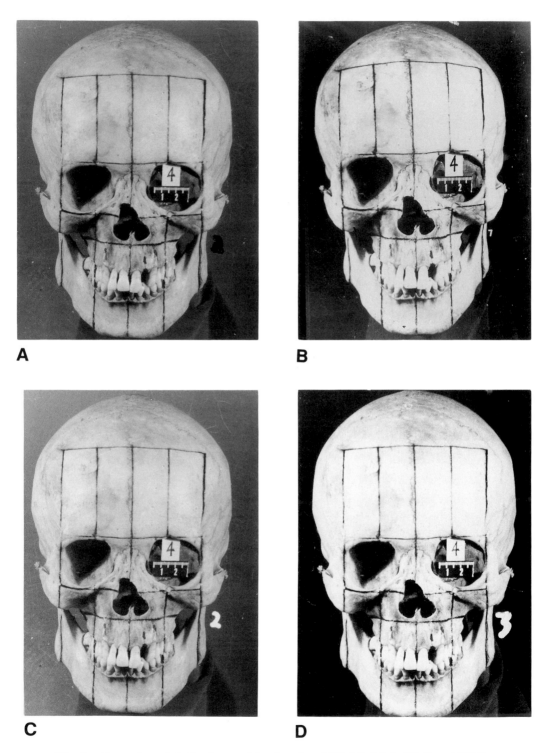

Fig. 4. Front view of skull taken at object lengths of (**A**) 0.7, (**B**) 1, (**C**) 2, and (**D**) 3 m.

Mid-head breadth = maximum head breadth
- length between ectoconchions
= 151.3 - 97.1 = 54.2 mm

Lower head breadth = bigonial breadth -
cheilion (mouth) breadth
= 111.2 - 52.0 = 59.2 mm (rounded to 60
mm).

Differences in Depth of Points

The variation in image size in the change zone of the head and face can be traced to the differences in the depth of points. The maximum cephalic breadth in a frontal photo is the spherical radius of the maximum image of the head and is perpendicular to the center of tragion on both sides. The shaded region in Figure 5A

outside the relative parallel zone represents the area whose maximum breadth corresponds to the distance from ectoconchion to the center of tragion on the same side. The normal value of the difference of the depth of a point is 80 mm.

Relationships between differences in the depth of points, change zone, and changes of image size can be described with the following calculations: The area that exhibits the greatest variation (about 60 mm) in the change zone is the lower part of the head. With a 1 m objective length, its imaging ratio is 1,000/(1,000 + 80) = 0.93, and its real image size is 0.93 × 60 = 55.8 mm, or 4.2 mm smaller due to differences in the depth of points. From this one can deduce the perspective imaging ratio and actual image size at different objective lengths, as shown in Table 6. It is clear that because of the existence of

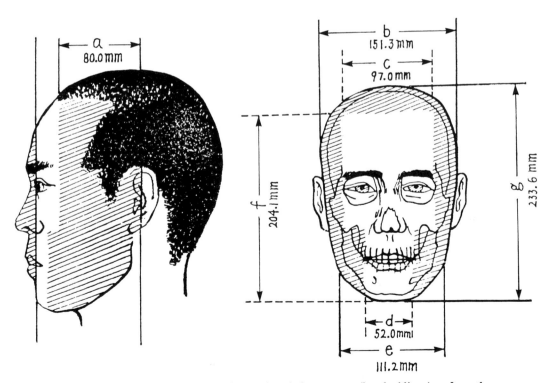

Fig. 5. Relative parallel zone (white area) and change zone (hatched lines). a, Length between ectoconchion and tragion; b, maximum breadth of head; c, length between ectoconchions; d, mouth breadth; e, bigonial breadth; f, length between trichion and gnathion; g, maximum length of head.

TABLE 5. Measurements From Change Zone in Head and Face

	Maximum Head Height	Maximum Head Breadth	Gonial Breadth	Length Between Two Ectoconchions	Breadth of Cheilion	Trichion to Gnathion	Tragion to Ectoconchion
Mean	233.6	151.3	111.2	97.0	52.0	204.1	80.0
Standard deviation	11.0	6.2	6.5	4.5	4.2	10.0	5.0

TABLE 6. Imaging Ratio and Image Size (mm) at Different Objective Length (m) of Photography

	Objective Length (m)											
	0.5	0.6	0.7	0.8	0.9	1.0	1.5	2.0	3.0	4.0	5.0	10.0
Imaging ratio	0.86	0.88	0.89	0.91	0.92	0.93	0.95	0.96	0.97	0.98	0.984	0.992
Image size	51.6	52.8	53.8	54.6	55.2	55.8	57.0	57.2	58.2	58.8	59.0	59.2
Loss in size	8.4	7.2	6.6	5.4	4.8	4.2	3.0	2.4	1.8	1.2	1.0	0.8

variations in the depths of points, the shorter the objective length, the more the image would be reduced. If we take 1 m as the standard photographic distance, image size differs from -2.4 to +2.4 mm as compared to that of the images obtained at photographic lengths ranging from 0.7 to 3.0 m. Because the theoretical deduced value is very close to the actual value, it suggests that the differences in the depth of points is the decisive factor for the variations in image size at different photographic lengths. Furthermore, it also reveals that the influence of this factor is manifest in the change zone of the head and face.

As also can be seen in Table 6, the image taken at the 1 m standard photographic length differs in size within a range of 3 mm as compared to that taken at lengths ranging from 0.6 to 4.0 m, and is in the tolerable range of error for the determination of the thickness of the soft tissue of the gonion. The size difference would be around 3 mm even if the photographic length is further increased. Therefore, we conclude that without knowing the original objective length of photography for a test photo (most probably it was taken with an objective length ranging from 0.6 to 4 m), one should use 1 m as the optimum distance.

SUPERIMPOSITION SYSTEM

The above research has resulted in a theoretical and practical basis for conducting a digitized test using a microcomputer in superimposition. It has paved the way for the creation of the model TLGA-2 skull identification apparatus (Lan and Cai, 1986). This apparatus (Fig. 6) has the following features:

1. An optical system consisting of two groups of objective lenses with specific objective lengths and an optimum imaging ratio capable of simultaneously making the test photo and skull form a superimposed image at half of its actual size on the focusing screen (Fig. 7).

2. An objective lens for the skull that is specially designed to correctly superimpose the skull and photo originally taken at an objective length ranging from 0.7 to 4 m at a photographic distance of 1 m without being influenced by the central perspective difference.

3. Fitted with four groups of objective lenses of different photographic specifications, it is capable of enlarging the test photo from 0.5 to 4 inches to half of actual head size.

4. A skull position-adjusting mechanism designed to simulate the natural movement of human head and capable of automatically adjusting the skull freely in six directions.

5. A mechanism that examines eight lines was designed in accordance with the anatomical proportions of the human face. It is capable of accurately determining the azimuth of superimposition and the object–image proportion. (This is an important achievement of our research.)

6. A testing and measuring mechanism for projection that can enlarge the superimposed image from half to full natural head size and measure the face directly with an accuracy within 0.5 mm.

7. A microcomputer in which the test programs designed according to different types of mathematical models are stored can indicate the azimuth for photographing, provide data corresponding to natural head size, as well as give an accurate scientific conclusion for the superimposition with its present target programs.

8. An automatically exposed photographic mechanism is capable of directly taking the superimposed photo half of natural head size.

9. All controls of this apparatus are located on an easily accessible table. The whole test and examination can be finished by only one operator in 2 hours.

CONCLUSION

The present system was developed on the basis of converting all of the three-dimensional data of the anatomical proportion of the human face into two-dimensional data. Thus one can now proceed with the identification through skull–image superimposition using digitized measurements and calculations based on forensic anthropological and optical theory.

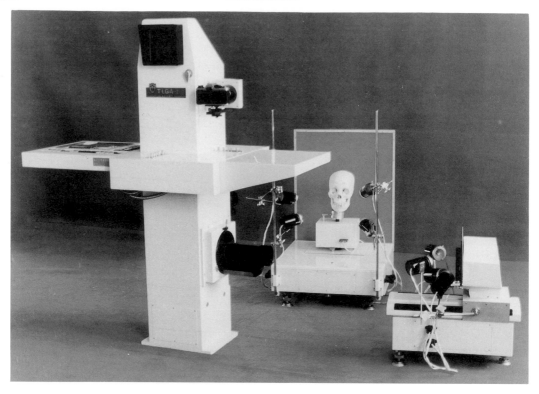

Fig. 6. Model TLGA-2 skull identification apparatus (Lan and Cai, 1986).

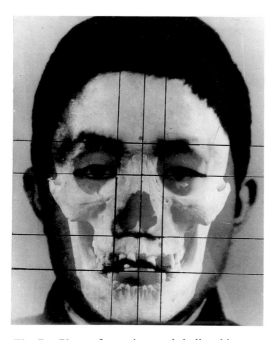

Fig. 7. Photo of superimposed skull and image.

This comprehensive operating system has solved many problems, such as the superimposition angle and distance, and the approximation of natural head size. It works with a precise system for each process and therefore can eliminate blind guessing and strengthen the scientific basis of superimposition.

The use of a microcomputer to make the final judgment for the results of the superimposition allows a more objective analysis, at the same time reducing the subjectivity of the examiner. This makes the conclusions of this test more reliable and convincing.

ACKNOWLEDGMENTS

The editors of this volume are grateful to S.R. Loth for editing this chapter.

REFERENCES

Glaister J, and Rentoul E (1962) Medical Jurisprudence and Toxicology. Baltimore: Williams and Wilkins.

Helmer R (1987) Identification of the cadaver remains of Josef Mengele. J Forensic Sci 32:1622–1644.

Lan Y, and Cai D (1982a) Study on photographic angle of skull–image superimposition. Criminal Technol (Suppl), pp 23–25, Beijing.

Lan Y, and Cai D (1982b) Study on photographic distance in skull–image superimposition. Criminal Technol (Suppl), pp 26–29, Beijing.

Lan Y, and Cai D (1982c) Study on photographic method in skull–image superimposition. Criminal Technol (Suppl), pp 30–33, Beijing.

Lan Y, and Cai D (1986) Technological report on development of Model TLGA-1 skull identification apparatus. Criminal Technol (Suppl), pp 23–35, Beijing.

Lan Y, and Cai D (1988) A new technology in skull identification. Presented at the Advances in Skull Identification via Video Superimposition, Kiel, Book of Abstracts, pp 3–5.

Lan Y, Cai D, Tao C, and Gui Y (1987) Research report of skull–image superimposition on 3 Chinese Han females. Reference Room of 213 Institute, Tieling City, Liaoning Province, China.

Chapter 11

Shape Analytical Morphometry in Computer-Aided Skull Identification via Video Superimposition

Vittorio Pesce Delfino, E. Vacca, F. Potente, T. Lettini, and M. Colonna

Department of Anthropology, Institute of Zoology and Comparative Anatomy (V.P.D., E.V., F.P., T.L.) and Department of Forensic Medicine (M.C.), University of Bari, Bari, Italy 70125

The problem of identifying skeletal remains can be considered in three basic approaches: (1) Observing personal, distinctive characteristics (i.e., morphological variations, pathological signs) within a framework of generic congruence (e.g., sex, age, race, etc.). This approach is obviously limited, both because characteristics uncommon enough to be absolutely individualizing are rare and the antemortem materials necessary for comparison (usually radiographs) are available in very few cases. (2) Plastic reconstruction of physiognomic features from the skeleton. This approach is at present limited by the lack of a complete, self-sufficient theoretical foundation. In fact, these procedures require the forensic expert to make an arbitrary decision for which there are no definite rules, and that have an excessively subjective component. (3) Evaluation of the congruency between skull morphology and photographs taken during life by superimposition of the corresponding images. This procedure may be subjected to rigorous standardization, thus, it is repeatable and quantifiable. Moreover, the reference material is readily available. Therefore, we regard this procedure, in which morphologies of different bony parts are compared, as the one that offers more possibilities for successful application.

There are many considerations. It is necessary to allow for the difficulty of beginning with a scientific principle or procedure and making the transition from an experimental phase to valid application. This is necessary for the results of such techniques to be evaluated and accepted by the legal system.

We can examine the applicability of the procedure for matching a skull and photograph for identification on three levels.

1. Techniques for obtaining superimposed images;

2. Standards to which the procedure must be submitted;

3. Techniques of obtaining definite numerical parameters to be used for statistical evaluation of the results of the match.

As far as point 1 is concerned, the first attempts to use this procedure in forensic anthropology were made by Glaister and Brash (1937) for the Ruxton case. They made a comparison using the photographic technique. However, the difficulties encountered in comparing a tridimensional object with a bidimensional one (Malinowski and Porawski, 1970; Dorion, 1983) made this methodology untenable (even after photographic procedures were successively improved) until the end of the past decade, when superimposition techniques using a closed TV circuit were developed (Helmer and Grüner, 1977; Koelmeyer, 1982).

MATERIALS AND METHODS

There is no doubt that use of video technology offers great advantages over any photographic technique. It allows direct control of the movements of the skull for comparison with the photograph, as well as the recording of any procedural phase, immediate printing of super-imposed images, and improved illumination. The following problem must, however, be resolved.

Transduction of the image from the TV camera into electrical signals and successively the inverse transduction from electrical signals into an image on the observation monitor introduces a geometric distortion effect that must be completely eliminated. This distortion results from different phenomena occurring in various parts of the TV setup (TV camera, control stages, monitor). It is of course possible to eliminate these distortions by setting the monitor to compensate even for distortions introduced by other sections.

However, this is possible only if none of the sections that can introduce distortion are duplicated (except for additional monitors). It is extremely unlikely that two sections, however identically made, could introduce the same effect that could be jointly counterbalanced by the monitor setting. This is particularly true for the TV camera. One must avoid using two separate cameras for recording the skull and photograph and the subsequent electronic mixing of the two corresponding signals.

The solution lies in using only one TV camera with an optical device in front of the lens that can receive both images. This device (SOD-003 by Metamorphosis s.r.l.) is a plane-parallel semireflective glass mounted in a rectangular, parallelepiped-shaped opaque case with one opening on each of three sides (Figs. 1 and 2). The first opening is turned to the TV camera lens, the second is turned to the opposite side on the same optical axis as the lens, and the third at 90° to the other two.

The semireflective glass intersects the optical axis of the lens at a 45° angle, and the semireflective lining side faces the lens. A plane mirror is mounted on the inside wall of the case opposite the opening, situated at 90° to the optical axis. This glass must be made of a material with a refractive index value that can cor-rect the angle of refraction relative to the thickness of the glass itself. For normal use, the device is mounted in front of the lens and can rotate on its axis to lie in a horizontal position; the object (photograph or skull) with the highest average reflectance is framed from the lateral aperture. The paths of the light rays from both objects are of course different. The rays that will form the image of the frontally set object go through the semireflective glass, and get directly to the objective. The rays of light that will form the image of the laterally set object go through the semireflective glass, are reflected by the mirror, and then partially angled at 90° by the glass's semireflective coating, which sends them toward the objective. Obviously, there will be a progressive loss of luminance during this process. This configuration is necessary since the two successive reflections of the photo (or set object) allow the two images to form on the TV camera's sensitive target in a congruent manner.

Naturally, the skull and photograph may be placed independently at different distances from the optical device. Since this distance may be varied, we can easily make the two images dimensionally comparable because they can be enlarged or reduced, independently, by varying their distance from the video camera. The camera contains a lens with a focal length that can reduce the central perspective effects within the depth of the field. This maintains the sharpness of the image while allowing for enlargement or reduction. We know from experience that lenses with a focal length between 16 and 25 mm for ½" video cameras are suitable if the skull is not less than 100 cm from the lens. Moreover, under these conditions, the central perspective distortion effect is absolutely negligible since the procedure involves the successive processing of profiles or curves describing not surfaces but margins detected against a background.

Use of a video camera with a high sensitivity (7 lux minimum) solid state (CCD) will allow the use of diaphragm values that can increase field depth. It is essential for the camera to have a control for excluding the auto-

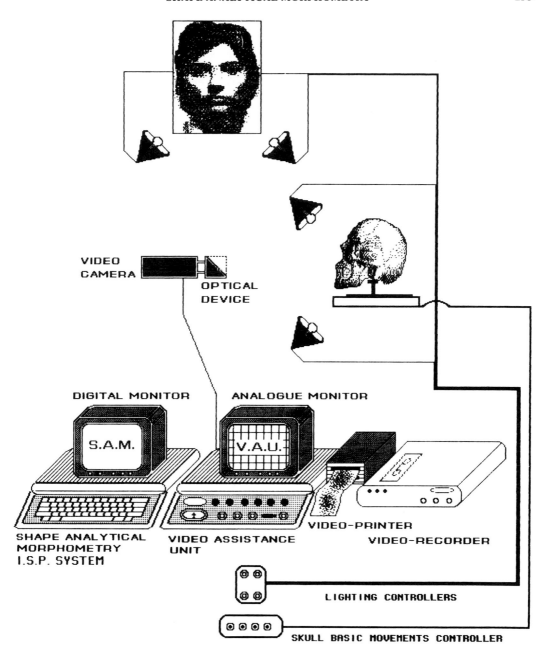

Fig. 1. Diagram of S.A.M. Forensic superimposition work station.

matic gain control (AGC) in order to avoid problems due to the presence of areas of very high or very low reflectance on the skull or in the photograph. Use of a video camera capable of gamma predistortion is also helpful.

The skull and photograph are independently illuminated by adjustable systems using standard spotlights with dimmers so that various

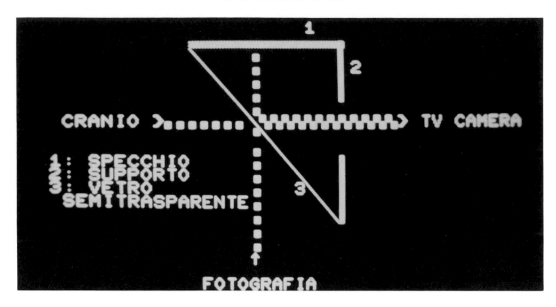

Fig. 2. Scheme of the optical device to be mounted on video camera lens to obtain the optical mixing of skull image and face image from photograph. 1, Mirror; 2, case; and 3, semireflective glass.

mixings of the two images will be possible. The skull and photograph are placed on two separate supports that can allow all necessary movements. The use of motorized and servo-assisted supports, with a telecontrol, facilitates some phases of the superimposition. Movements to roughly position the skull can be easily servo-assisted (see Chapters 9, Chandra Sekharan, and 12, Seta and Yoshino, this volume). The final fine adjustments are generally highly complex, and therefore stands with omnidirectional clutch movement and weight-balancing systems are recommended. The skull placement system represents a particular problem for the stands. The classic clamp at the *foramen magnum* isn't always the best method, because, for one thing, this part may be missing. Furthermore, movements from this anchorage point are not easily verifiable since the foramen magnum is quite far from the geometric center of the skull. The best solution consists of a rod-screwing system in a circular support that can be used on any bony part. The rods can always be oriented toward the geometric center of the skull and positioned so as not to interfere with the bony

parts chosen for the superimposition. We used this method for positioning the skull, and mixed electromechanical and manual manipulations for moving the stand (S.S.D.-100 by Metamorphosis s.r.l.).

The photograph is placed on a stand equipped with a vertical magnetic plane that can rotate both horizontally and vertically. Once the optical TV line has been hooked up, the monitor is geometrically set to return the images without distortion so that the setting deals with images of both the skull and photograph at the same time. The geometric setting of the monitor should be checked at least every 6 months.

The signal from the video camera feeding and control unit (Microconf by Metamorphosis s.r.l.) is not sent directly to the monitor. It first goes to the input gate of a computer ISP (Image Signal Processor by Metamorphosis s.r.l.) (Fig. 2), which uses a software system (S.A.M. Forensic, Shape Analytic Morphometry by Metamorphosis s.r.l.) to control the superimposition and process the images produced to quantify parameters (Pesce Delfino and Ricco, 1983). The computer also controls the various peripherals for printing results, image printing and storage, and recording numerical data, along with files containing series of coordinate values of the processed profiles, supplementary monitors, photographic reproduction set, and video recorder.

This computer can superimpose a net reference system, point array, and vertical or horizontal lines on the video signal. The reference system allows step-by-step continuous regulation. There is a software function for net setting and numbering to guarantee reproducibility. This reference system is visualized on the monitor screen and is therefore completely free of parallax distortion with respect to the image of the superimposition. Moreover, the software can produce luminous pointers (up to six) on the monitor screen where the image of the superimposition is displayed. The pointers can be positioned on the points in the photograph that must match the position of the skull.

The superimposition image looks analog rather than digitized. This way the problems of image degradation related to digitization have been avoided. Furthermore, continuous visual control in real time, even during displacements of the skull and photograph, is possible.

The computer is also equipped with a second monitor, which displays alphanumeric messages and graphics. The computer interacts with the superimposition image only through a very small luminous spot (a pixel in a 255×255 matrix) which can easily be moved in any direction by the operator. It functions both as a pointer to read coordinate values and as a probe in punctiform reading of luminance values encoded in 64 gray levels. Contouring is accomplished with a manual software-assisted tracking system.

The operator can choose software functions from selections listed on the menu. It can be useful, though not necessary, to preprocess the superimposition image to improve and enhance contrast and boundary detection, luminance equalization, filtering (Laplace, Interference), tonal inversion, and false color encoding. This increases the yield of useful details for evaluating congruency between the skull and photograph.

Classical image analysis systems digitally produce an image to be frozen and successively processed. However, this procedure is not recommended when it is necessary to visually control the effect of fine displacements of the skull in relation to the photograph. It is thus better to use an image processor in real time, which also permits elaborations as above on images in motion. For this we use the VAU 101 (Video Assistance Unit by Metamorphosis s.r.l.) wired in the ISP video line-up unit between it and the Microconf unit powering and controlling the video camera (Fig. 1). Figures 3–7 contain examples of these preprocessing procedures. With real-time technology, we can recognize the profile during movements required for fine adjustments of the superimposition by simply turning a switch.

To begin the superimposition, the skull is placed on a stand and suitably illuminated. The image is centered on the monitor at about two-thirds the size of the screen. The photograph is placed vertically on its stand and illuminated separately.

The video camera with the optical device for superimposition fitted in front of it must be set on a horizontal plane determined by an inclinometer. In this phase, the photograph and the skull are viewed separately, alternating the two images by turning the corresponding lighting sets on and off. The reference net system is then superimposed on the images.

The next step is to separately reduce the images of the skull and the face in the photograph to the same scale by positioning the control network so that the selected horizontal lines lie through the detectable craniometric points on the two halves of the face. The points are chosen based on the position of the face, and are set by a specific software function.

Spatially, the face is positioned in a similar manner to that of the head in relation to the camera film plane at the moment the photograph was taken. For this setting, three reference points on the photograph are used: left and right ectocantions, and the infranasal point or the midpoint of the superior contour of the upper lip. These should coincide with the fol-

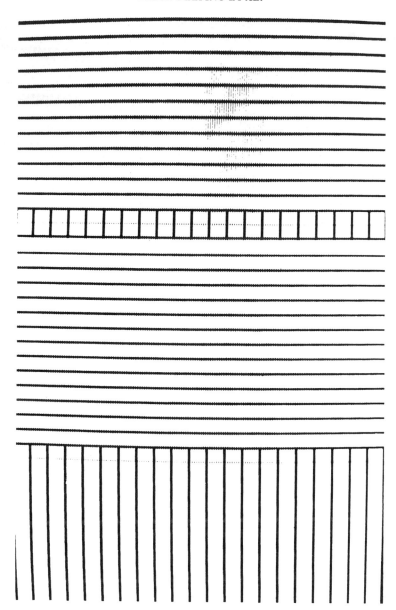

Fig. 3. Pattern to be projected on skull surfaces to point them out and follow the trends aiding visual evaluation of the superimposition. Side with vertical lines downwards, projecting on lower jaw; intermediate vertical lines projecting on upper contour of the orbits.

lowing landmarks on the skull: left and right Whitnall malar tubercles (Stewart, 1983) (or below the ectoconchions if the tubercles are missing), and the nasal spine or prosthion, respectively. This is valid for frontal or oblique views. For a lateral view, the three pairs of points are (1) ectocantion and the point immediately below the ectoconchion, (2) infranasal point and the nasal spine, and (3) tragion and porion.

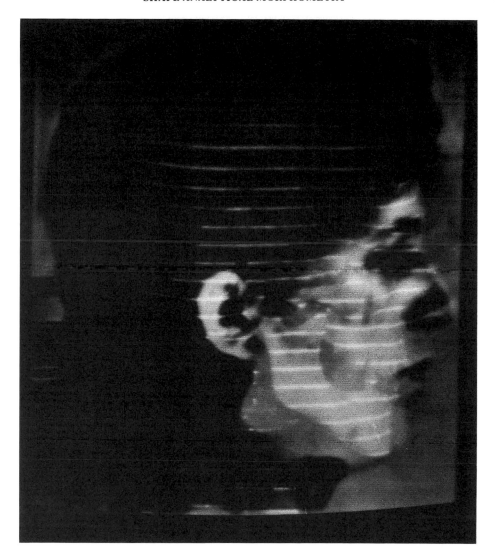

Fig. 4. Video superimposition of case A with its own skull in lateral view. Situation is just before beginning analytical procedures. The profile was worked from the uppermost point of the recognizable frontal profile and the free end of the nasal bone. Reference points adopted for positioning and scaling were the right ectocantion, nasal spine, and right porion.

At this stage, maintaining the visualization of both network and reference points, the two images are mixed by light dimmers. Where previous constraints have been set, they are dimensionally comparable and will superimpose with fairly good correspondence if they belong to the same individual. Then, it will only be necessary to adjust the position of the skull with small complex movements that will not alter the previously fixed and continuously verifiable (by means of luminous reference points on the analog image) dimensions of the skull on the monitor. In this way we will obtain the optimum superimposition whose correspondence can be

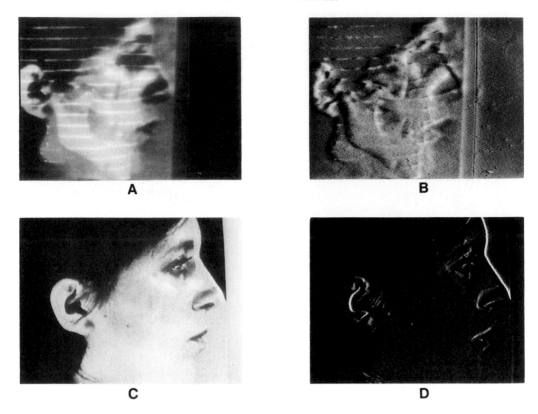

Fig. 5. Superimposed image of case A taken by (**A**) video camera and ready for processing and (**B**) real-time processing by VAU 101 to enhance differences between bony and soft parts of the nasofrontal area (Laplace and Interference filtering). Photograph of case A (not superimposed) taken from (**C**) video camera and (**D**) real time processing by VAU 101, i.e., contrast manipulation, interference filter, and partial tonal inversion to detect the boundary (profile) for the S.A.M. analytical procedures.

visually evaluated. We must allow for various anatomical variations and the following basic parameters: frontal contour, orbit outline, cheekbones, nasal bones and pyriform aperture, upper jaw and alveolar arch corresponding with the upper lip, lower alveolar arch with lower lip, and lower contour of the face and inferior margin of the mandible.

To further verify the fit of the superimposition visually, additional luminous grids can be projected on the skull where curvatures of the bone deform the grid and allow better observation of the correspondence of different parts of the skull and photo. Several patterns are available, but we have found that in most cases, the

pattern (NP 31 by Metamorphosis s.r.l.) composed of white and black lines (Fig. 3) is very useful because the vertical lines project themselves on the superior orbital margins and inferior edge of the jaw, and horizontal lines delineate the surface of the facial bones.

Once the superimposition has been made (Figs. 4–6), it is possible to go on with its parametric evaluation. The aim of these evaluations is to get numerical parameters that can individually describe the shape of corresponding segments on the skull and in the photograph. Indicators of the fit attained by the superimposition come from the comparison of parameters with appropriate statistical evaluators.

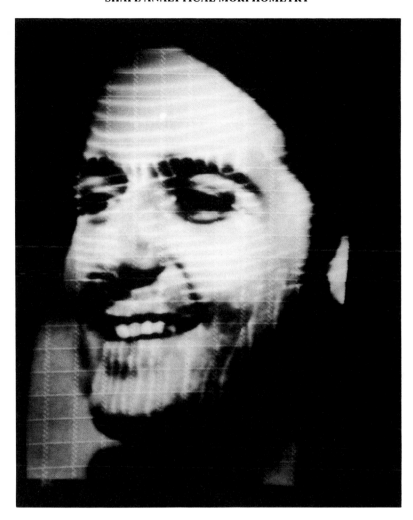

Fig. 6. Video superimposition of case E with its own skull in oblique view. The image shows the face and skull from which the pattern of Figure 3 was projected, and the electronic reference network synthetizable on the monitor screen. The right frontal profile from the uppermost point to the eyebrow was used for the analytical match. Reference points adopted for positioning and scaling were the right and left exocantions and nasal spine.

It is important to stress that the only useful parameters for this are those that can describe the shape, since discrete measurements and their corresponding derived fractions cannot describe small local differences in features that allow individualization. This problem can be addressed by procedures derived from analytical geometry (Lestrel, 1974; Aherne and Dunnil, 1982)(polynomial functions, Fourier harmonic analysis), and are therefore given the generic term "analytical morphometry" (Pesce Delfino and Ricco, 1983). The anatomical parts such as profiles can be processed this way because they are considered as curves, and it is necessary for them to appear in the superimposition images in appropriate projections so that they can be detected (that is why photographs in lateral or oblique positions are usable). Since the same

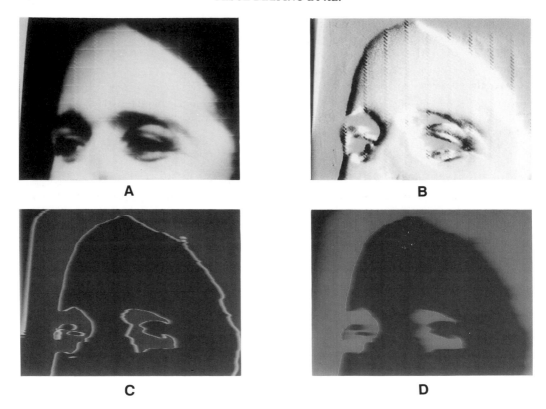

Fig. 7. **A:** Photograph of the face of case E without any treatment: In this case, the profile to be detected is the right frontal one. The shadowing does not make the profile easily recognizable, so that processing is required to digitize the profile. **B:** Real-time processing by VAU 101 of the same image with sharpened boundaries (Laplace and Interference filtering). **C:** The next step in real-time processing: tonal partial inversion added to the image allowing for a contouring effect. **D:** A deeper setting in tonal partial inversion starting from the image thinning the contour track: profile is detected, ready to be digitized by ISP unit in a known coordinate point array to be submitted to S.A.M. analytical procedures.

profiles on the skull and in the photograph must be compared, one must use anatomical areas with defined soft parts exhibiting the same trend that can be followed for some length without interference by the presence of other anatomical components—in particular, the anatomical areas where the soft parts are of limited thickness and run with a trend parallel to the planes of the bone. (It is specifically determined in different regions such as the frontal area, nasal bones and zygomatic district, the superior and lateral orbital contours, and the inferior margin

of the mandible.) The analytical evaluation we propose can be applied only under these conditions.

The morphological characteristics responsible for individual physiognomy contain much information that, if effectively extracted, lets us take a statistical approach to personal identification despite the fact that only a few parts of the face are suitable. Since profiles are represented by a series of (analytically processed) points, the concept of "statistical evaluation" must not be treated as a comparison among various cases, but rather as a comparison of data derived from corresponding parts of a skull and photograph.

We used the S.A.M. Forensic work station (Fig. 1) for the numerical parametrization of the superimposition leading to identification (Colonna et al., 1980, 1982, 1987, 1988a,b; Pesce Delfino and Ricco, 1983; Pesce Delfino et al., 1983, 1986, 1988). The procedures we use yielded an analytical description of the curve profile of the skull and photograph, respectively, and provided numerical parameters with descriptive and consequently comparative meaning. The procedures include (1) upper degree polynomials; (2) Fourier harmonic analysis; and (3) Janus procedure.

Polynomial Functions

Polynomial function coefficients are computed as follows:

$$(1) \qquad f(x) = a + \sum_{k=1}^{D} b_k x^k$$

where $f(x)$ is the dependent variable to be computed, x is independent variable, D is the polynomial degree (order), b represents equation coefficients, and a is the constant indicating the curve position in the coordinate system. Such coefficients are computed by an interpolation/regression algorithm with the least-squares method, where the interpolating curve is characterized by the lowest value of both the deviation square sum and estimated variance. Such polynomials improve the fit of the series of points by decreasing the variance according to the series of points establishing the original curve when the degree of the equation is increased. Therefore, the fit is evaluated by computing the analysis of variance along with the coefficients of polynomials to progressively increasing degrees. A degree can be reached where the variance gets so small and trends decrease so little that it is no longer useful to go on to a higher degree equation. This is how one determines that the best approximation polynomial

equation has been found. Generally, polynomials between the sixth and ninth degrees are most efficient.

The polynomial acts to smooth the curve representing the investigated profile and reduces the effects of local characteristics due to photographic anomalies or irregular soft tissue patterns. The square root of the mean square error is used to calculate the distance in terms of reciprocal point-by-point error between polynomial function curves obtained for the skull and photograph profile, respectively. If comparing a photograph with the same exactly oriented skull, this error quantifies the soft tissue thickness. It is a matter of only a dimensional residual difference. Since, as we have already pointed out, only shape differences are considered significant, the square root of the mean square error is computed under minimization conditions; one of the two profiles is being progressively shifted along the abscissa, and for each position the value is recomputed and the lowest value recorded. If the correspondence is perfect, this value equals zero (the soft tissue effect is, in this way, eliminated). However, this is only possible theoretically and has not been attained in actual practice. If the value is greater than zero, as commonly occurs, it suggests shape differences between the two profiles stemming from the inexact residual positioning of the skull in relation to the photograph. If it exceeds given cut-off values, it may be traced to real differences and indicates that a match has not been made.

Fourier Harmonic Analysis

The sine–cosine coefficients of the Fourier trigonometric series are computed with the following algorithm (Pesce Delfino et al., 1987b):

$$(2) \qquad f(x) = a + \sum_{k=1}^{N/2-1} b_k \sin kx + c_k \cos kx$$

where $f(x)$ is the dependent variable, x is the independent variable (angle value driving the period value of the increasing order harmonic contributors), N is the number of curve points, a is the constant indicating the position of the curve in the coordinate system, $N/2 - 1$ is the maximum order of the harmonics, and b and c are the sine and cosine coefficients, respectively.

The Kth order polynomial smoothes the data through regression/interpolation, while the Fourier analysis considers the profile as an irregular periodic function whose sinusoidal contributors are found and precisely described. Unlike what has been reported (Lestrel, 1974), the S.A.M. system applies the Fourier trigonometric polynominal to an orthogonal coordinate system rather than to a polar coordinate system. The dependent variable is represented by the distance of each point on the curve from a reference line (zero line) whose position is defined by specific standards for different profiles. This is possible in the usual applications of the S.A.M. Forensic system because the investigated profiles are represented by open curves without recursiveness or folding and profile scanning is done in the highly standardized video line set (raster mode).

Calculation of the sine–cosine coefficient allows us to obtain the amplitude and phase values of each harmonic. Most of the information refers to low-order harmonics (the first three or four), which represent the basic profile shape; the exact description of the profile is found by adding the rest of the increasing order harmonics. The maximum number of harmonics is stated by $N/2 - 1$, where N is the number of the points into which the profile was subdivided. The sinusoids of the same-period amplitudes add up perfectly if they are in phase; if in phase opposition, they are completely canceled out. All intermediate relationships due to phase shift are admissible and play their role in shaping different results, by the combination of sinusoids of a regularly increasing period from one to maximum order. Since it is well known that the harmonics are independent of each other, it is possible to use their different combinations in subsets or even the separate harmonics to carry out the phase and amplitude comparisons. The

sum of the amplitude differences of the sinusoidal contributors between profiles of the skull and photograph represents the second independent parameter for numerical comparison.

Janus Procedure

This procedure was implemented to offer comparisons in terms of symmetry. In this way we generated numerical evaluators of isometric and allometric differences that are particularly useful to complete the parameter set used in a numerical evaluation of correspondence in skull–photograph superimposition. This is because allometric differences must reveal the comparison between the photograph and skull, and, moreover, these differences should not be related to the effect of soft tissue thickness. We called this the "Janus" procedure (after the double-headed Latin god Janus, the bifront) because the two profiles are faced (separated by a straight line) after a specular inversion of one profile. Computing the coefficients of the following equation (Colonna et al., 1982):

$$(3) \qquad f(x) = a + bx + cx^2$$

it is possible to obtain an arc–chord complex consisting of the parabola segment corresponding to the computed function (arc) whose ends are joined by a straight line (chord). If the two profiles are identical, the quadratic coefficient will equal zero and a line can be drawn whose intercept and angle coefficient values force it to lie on the vertical line dividing the two domains.

If the two profiles are different, the three coefficients can vary independently, fitting the equation for any given combination of curves, such as the convexity of parabolic curvature, the intercept value, and for the inclination of the corresponding chord, so that an arc–chord complex is formed and simultaneously inclined and shifted. In any case, the surfaces on both sides of the parabola will be equal. This way, an expression of the trend differences between the two profiles can be obtained and considered as a vector. The modulus (magnitude) is expressed by a numerical value (normalized to the circle) of the relationship between the total arc and chord length and the area they delimit (this parameter was called SAE: shape asymmetry evaluator) (Colonna et al., 1987; Pesce Delfino et al., 1989). The direction is expressed by a line perpendicular to the chord, while the orientation is from the convexity of the parabola toward the chord. Actually the parameter represents a whole family of vectors, each of them having the same direction and orientation, but differing in their moduli and application points. Indeed, the application points are arranged in a series along the chord and the single modulus corresponds to the distance between these points and the corresponding points on the parabola. Using this procedure, two other parameters (besides SAE and orientation angle) can be obtained. These parameters are the *allometric percentage,* which corresponds to the area included between the chord and the parabola, and the *isometric difference,* which corresponds to the area defined by the separation line of the same composition and the current chord. The significance of these four parameters must be considered when the results of the Janus procedure are examined. It must be kept in mind that (1) the SAE value is the number that expresses the convexity of the parabolic arc curve defined by the equation. It represents the *modulus* of the vector and increases when the convexity *magnitude* of the profile on the same side of the parabolic convexity points toward the contralateral profile. This parameter is completely independent of the corresponding profile domain.

(2) The arc–chord complex slope indicated by a degree value obtained from the chord angle coefficients is analogously independent of this domain. The slope provides optimal conditions for parabolic "fitting" since a parabola can express the difference between the two profiles and a straight line cannot. The position of the straight-line segment is not exclusively connected to the profile convexity variations; therefore, when the chord slope nears 90°, the differences in the general trend between the two profiles are very small.

The other two parameters, (3) the isometric difference percentage and (4) allometric percentage, divide and compartmentalize the surfaces constituting the two domains, and since the parameters depend on these latter ones, it is better to express them as percentages. The first one shows what can be attributed to the dimensional differences (isometric fraction); the second elucidates the profile shape difference (allometric fraction). In any case, because the four parameters are independent they can be used in different statistical combinations.

In summary, the SAE value defines the global symmetry difference between the two profiles; the isometric difference reflects dimensional discrepancies; the inclination angle of the chord indicates the effects of positional differences, and the allometric fraction manifests differences in shape. The isometric and allometric differences can be numerically merged.

The S.A.M. Forensic system presents a user interface organized as a menu, and each procedure requires, on the average, four or five simple keys to run. These procedures yield the following results that can be saved on a disk: (1) the coordinate value of a series of processed profiles; (2) the coordinate value series of points obtained by interpolation with corresponding polynomial equations; (3) Fourier trigonometric polynomial coefficients; (4) parabolic coefficients in the Janus procedure. Saving this information allows tables and graphs to be made and stored.

Printouts are graphic representations of the (1) processed profiles; (2) polynomial function curves; (3) match between the original profiles and their polynomial functions; and (4) Fourier spectra as bar graphs in normalized scale. The harmonics are represented from left to right in ascending order (corresponding to the period of each sinusoid). The sine coefficients (odd series) are represented in the first bar (striped); the cosine coefficients (even series) are represented in the second bar (solid); the positive values are above and the negative ones, below. The Fourier spectrum pair for each comparison (of skull and photograph) is represented by the same graphic scale for immediate comparison. These include (5) the amplitude and phase values table of Fourier harmonics; (6) graphic representation of the contributors and Fourier synthesis results; (7) graphic representation of the Janus procedure with the arc–chord complex; (8) table of the synthetic parameters obtained by the single procedures with the corresponding final evaluator; and (9) video prints of analog images of the superimposition.

In this study, 10 superimpositions were investigated, four of them from forensic cases that have been positively identified after the superimpositions were performed. Six superimpositions were made by comparing photographs of two subjects (for whom the corresponding skulls were available) with three skulls belonging to other individuals. These skulls were characterized by dimensions and relative indices that were very similar to those in the actual skulls corresponding to the photographs. The dimensions included bi-euryonic breadth; basion–bregma, porion–bregma, prosthion–glabella, and orbital heights; glabella–opisthocranion length; and maximum and minimum frontal and bizygomatic breadths.

RESULTS

The results are reported as typical outputs of the S.A.M. system, primarily in graphic form. The numerical values are listed in tables. This system permits the extraction of more than 100 parameters in 10 independent groups for its use in the parametrization of the skull–photograph match. In superimposition where identification is the only aim, three parameters are used. For matching polynomial curves, we use the square root of the mean square error, i.e., the average of the deviations between the two compared curves weighted for the number of points into which the curves are subdivided. It should be noted that in "true" superimpositions, the values in standard position are higher than those after minimization, with small differences (due to the effect of the soft tissue thickness and residual errors in skull positioning). Differences in the above factors are greater for "false" superimpositions because the actual differences in shape are added (Table 1).

From the Fourier harmonic, we used the sum of amplitude differences of each harmonic of a curve and the corresponding harmonics of the other curve.

From the Janus procedure, the sum of the value of the allometric area (surface delimited by the parabola arc and the straight line joining its ends) is used, with the value of the area delimited between the line of separation of the domains corresponding to the two profiles with the shifted and angled straight line joining the ends of the parabola (isometric difference). The result of this sum is expressed as a percentage of

TABLE 1. Differences of Values of Square Root of Mean Square Error (Morphological Distance)[a]

| | Square Root of Mean Square Error (Polynomials)[b] | | | | | |
| | True | | | False | | |
	S	M	D	S	M	D
1.	1.19	1.16	0.03	4.728	2.73	1.998
2.	1.909	1.36	0.549	4.334	3.7	0.634
3.	1.205	1.19	0.015	6.293	3.34	2.953
4.	1.886	1.56	0.326	13.539	4.62	8.919
5.				7.326	3.29	4.036
6.				10.606	3.59	7.016

[a]Computed from polynomials in standard position and after minimization together with their differences, for true and false comparisons.

[b]S, standard, M, after minimization, D, difference.

the total surface. The numerical value of the three indicators increases as the morphological differences between the two matched profiles increase. The final synthetic evaluator is obtained by multiplying the numerical values of the three parameters. The curves of profiles used each time are derived from the procedure based on upper degree polynomial equations. These can be shown either in standard position or in the one they assume reciprocally after the minimization procedure. Table 2 presents the values for the square root of the mean square error (after minimization) for four cases of "true" and six cases of "false" superimpositions.

The profiles are shown in standard position for cases A and E (Fig. 8A,B). For each case, from left to right, the comparisons reported are those between (1) the original profile and its polynomial function on the photograph, (2) the original profile and its polynomial function for the skull, (3) the original profiles of the photo-

graph and skull, and (4) the polynomial functions of the photograph and skull. It can be seen that correspondence is so high for the first two comparisons in both cases that the two curves are graphically indistinguishable and, in fact, appear as a single curve. In contrast, skull–photograph comparisons of the two curves show obvious differences that can be related to soft tissue thickness and residual errors in skull positioning. However, the differences between the original profiles of the skull and photograph may be greater than the differences in the corresponding function curves because the smoothing effect of the equation eliminates very small irregularities. Comparisons of the photographs of cases A (left) and E (right) with profiles of three skulls from different subjects in "false" comparisons under standard conditions are presented in Figure 8C,D. For each pair of curves, skull profiles appear on the left and the profile of the photograph on the right. The correspond-

TABLE 2. Numerical Values of the Three Main Analytical Parameters (One From Each Procedure) Together With the Synthetic Final Evaluator for Four True and Six False Comparisons

Match[a]	Point Number	Square Root of Mean Square Error Minimized (Polynomials)	First 15 Fourier Harmonics (Sum of Differences)	Allometry and Isometry % Differences (Janus)	Final Evaluator
True					
Case E (OV)	103	1.16	2,384	0.72	1,991[b]
Case A (LV)	76	1.36	3,935	1.55	8,294
Case H (LV)	53	1.19	2,674	1.07	3,404
Case I (LV)	52	1.56	3,402	2.73	14,488[c]
False					
Face E/Skull A (OV)	103	2.73	8,611	1.92	45,135[d]
Face E/Skull F (OV)	103	3.70	13,350	3.30	163,003[e]
Face E/Skull G (OV)	103	3.34	10,251	2.00	68,476
Face A/Skull B (LV)	76	4.62	11,041	3.14	160,169
Face A/Skull C (LV)	76	3.29	7,275	2.21	52,895
Face A/Skull D (LV)	76	3.59	8,487	3.78	115,170

[a]OV, oblique view; LV, lateral view.

[b]Minimum value for true comparison.

[c]Maximum value for true comparison.

[d]Minimum value for false comparison.

[e]Maximum value for false comparison.

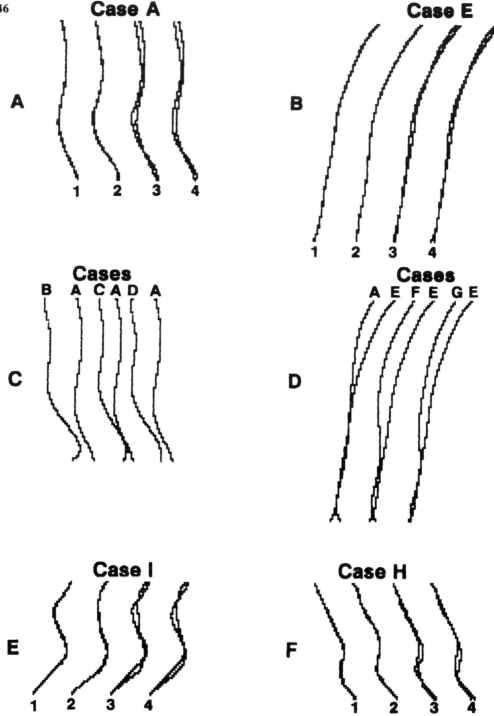

Fig. 8. Profile comparisons of "true" superimpositions for cases A (**A**) and E (**B**). From left to right, the comparisons are between the (1) original profile and its polynomial function on the photograph, (2) original profile and its polynomial function for the skull, (3) original profiles of the photograph and skull, and (4) polynomial functions of the photograph and skull. Profile comparisons of "false" superimpositions of face A (**C**) and face E (**D**) with three skulls from different subjects. For each pair of polynomial curves, profiles from the skull appear on the left and those from the photograph on the right. Comparisons are shown of original profile and polynomial function curves for "true" superimposition for cases I (**E**) and H (**F**).

ing numerical values of the square root of the mean square error are reported in Table 1, together with the values after minimization. Curves C and D in Figure 8 also illustrate the strong morphological differences and the divergency situation of different comparisons. Graphs of cases I and H—"true" superimpositions—are displayed in Figure 8E,F (Table 2). Following the scheme of Figure 8, Figures 9–13 report the Fourier spectra of different profiles in "true" and "false" superimpositions; for each comparison the graphic scale is the same and the sine–cosine coefficients of the first 15 harmonics are represented. Figure 9A,B contains the Fourier spectra of photo A on top and skull A on the bottom ("true" superimposition in lateral view, Fig. 4), while Figures 10 and 11A report

the Fourier spectra of skulls B, C, and D ("false" superimposition with photo A). The comparisons should be made harmonic by harmonic on the same order of amplitude. This is a function of the size (bar height) of sine and cosine coefficients together. All differences in Fourier spectra are related to very subtle (individual characteristics) differences in profile shapes.

The same, previously mentioned, considerations should be made for case E in Figures 11B,C and 12. The Fourier spectrum of photograph E and skull F ("true" superimposition in oblique view, Fig. 6) appear in Figure 11B,C, and Fourier spectrum of skulls A, F, and G (Fig. 12) that were used for "false" superimpositions in oblique view with photo E. The general trend of Fourier spectra was very similar in the same

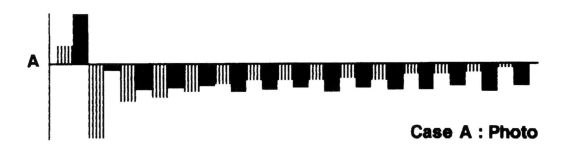

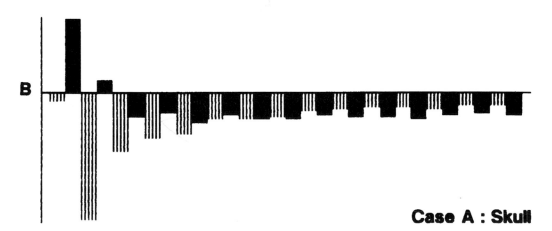

Fig. 9. Fourier spectra for (**A**) photo A and (**B**) skull A. Striped bars, sine coefficients; solid bars, cosine coefficients.

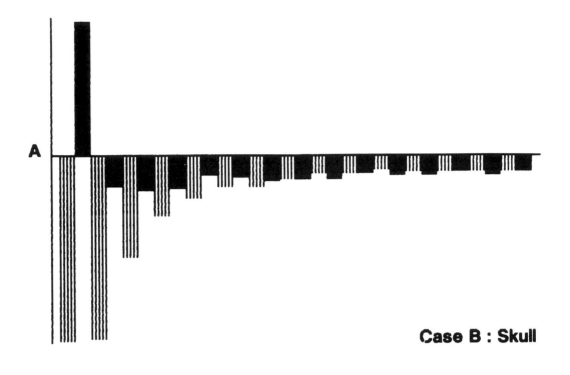

Case B : Skull

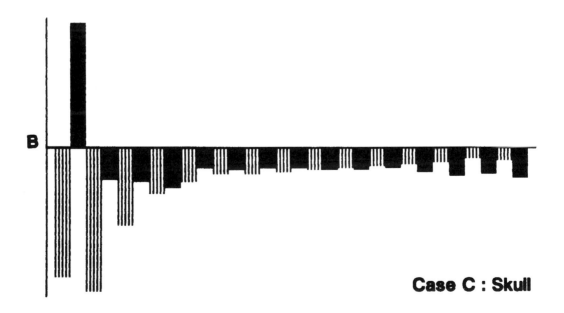

Case C : Skull

Fig. 10. Fourier spectra for skull B (**A**) and skull C (**B**) to be compared with photo A (Fig. 9A). Striped bars, sine coefficients; solid bars, cosine coefficients.

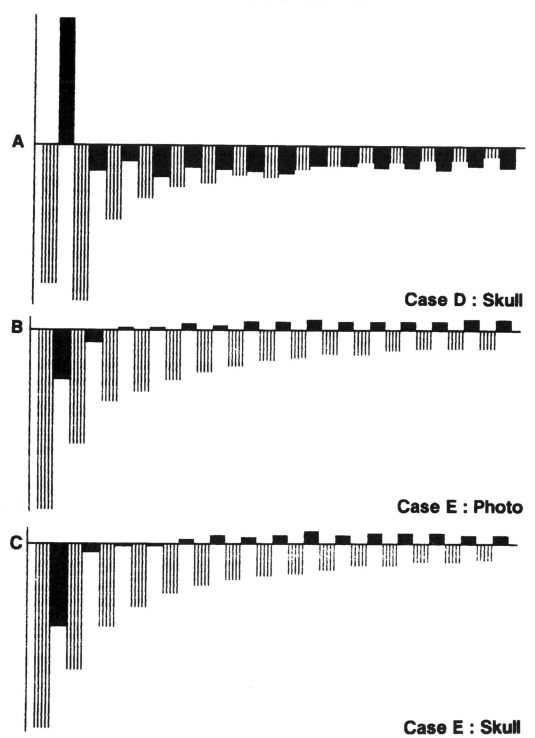

Fig. 11. **A**: Fourier spectrum for skull D to be compared with photo A (Fig. 9A). Fourier spectra for photo E (**B**) and skull E (**C**). Striped bars, sine coefficients; solid bars, cosine coefficients.

views for both "true" and "false" comparisons, apart from amplitude differences in coefficient size (related to truth and falseness). The general trend differs for different views because different anatomical regions have different profile-shape patterns. Figure 13 shows the Fourier spectrum of the profiles from the photo and skull of case I (a "true" superimposition in lateral view of the nose profile). The general trend is similar to the one in photo A (lateral view), but it is completely different from the general trend of the Fourier spectrum comparison of photo F. Table 2 lists numerical values of the Fourier sum of differences for comparisons of all the given spectra, and Figures 14 and 15 present examples of Fourier synthesis. A com-

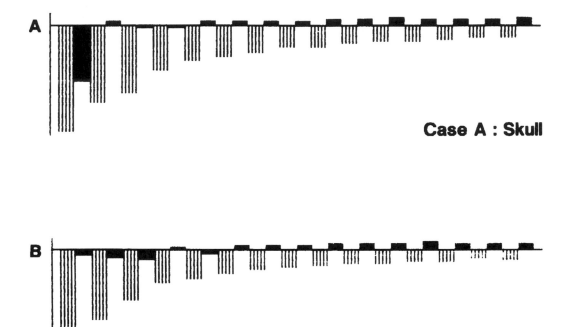

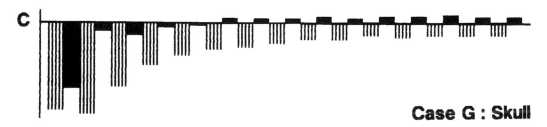

Fig. 12. Fourier spectrum for (**A**) skull A, skull F (**B**) and skull G (**C**) to be compared with photo E (Fig. 11B). Striped bars, sine coefficients; solid bars, cosine coefficients.

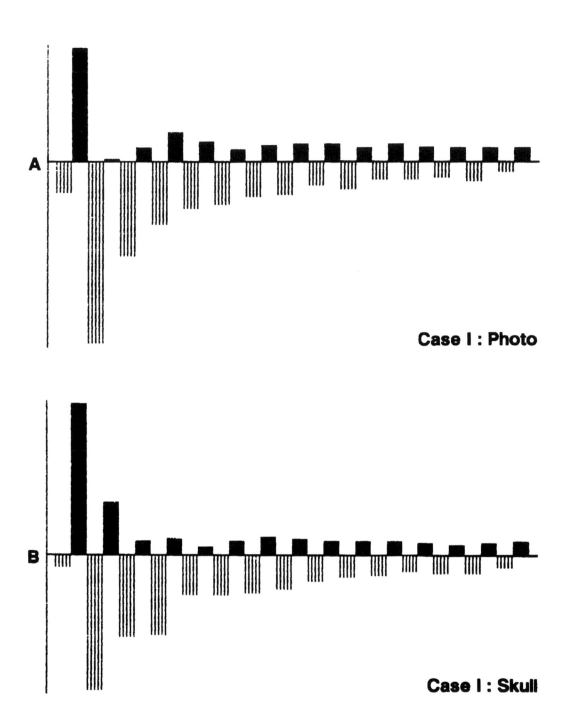

Fig. 13. Fourier spectra for photo I (**A**) and skull I (**B**). Striped bars, sine coefficients; solid bars, cosine coefficients.

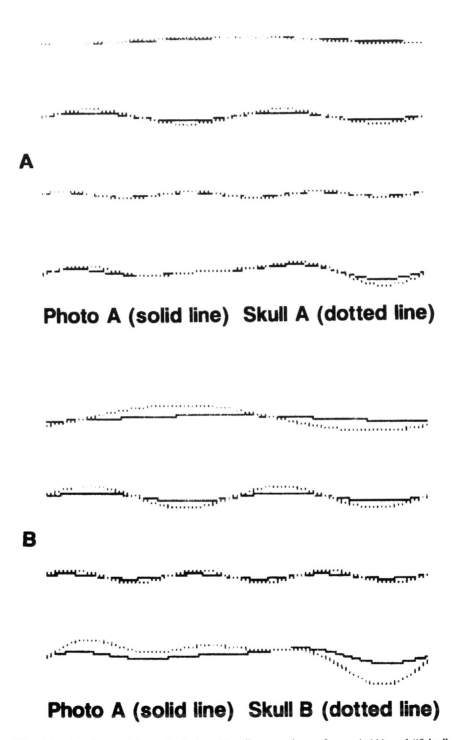

Photo A (solid line) Skull A (dotted line)

Photo A (solid line) Skull B (dotted line)

Fig. 14. Fourier partial synthesis in a "true" comparison of case A (**A**) and "false" comparison of face A with skull B (**B**).

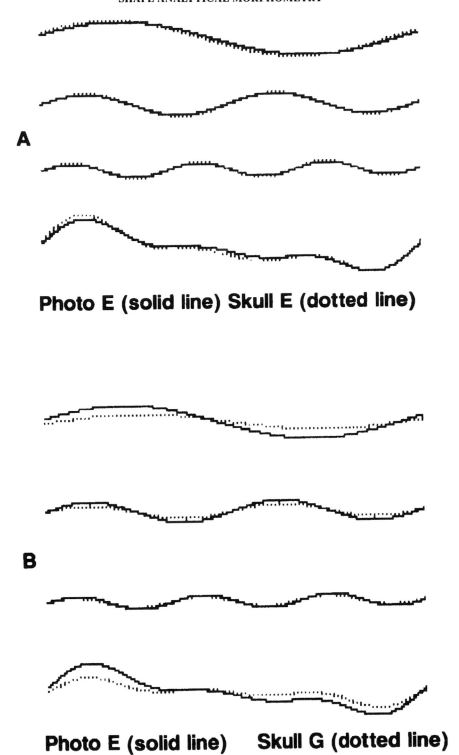

Fig. 15. Fourier partial synthesis in a "true" comparison of case E (**A**) and "false" comparison of face E with skull G (**B**).

parison by direct graphic match of the first three sinusoidal contributors (1, 2, 3) and the result of their sum (4) for face A and skull A appear at the top of Figure 14 and represent a true superimposition in lateral view (refer to Fourier spectra in Fig. 9). The same analysis for face A and skull B appears at the bottom of Figure 14 and shows a false superimposition in lateral view (refer to Fourier spectra in Fig. 10). Note the slight discrepancies in the match of sinusoids and results in the true comparison in contrast to the strong ones in the false match.

The same considerations should be stressed for Figure 15 regarding the comparison of face E and skull E at the top, a true superimposition in oblique view (refer to Fourier spectrum in Fig. 11B,C), and for face E and skull G at the bottom of Figure 15, a false superimposition in oblique view (refer to Fourier spectrum in Fig. 12B,C).

The numerical values of parameters adopted from the Janus procedure can be found in Table 2. The graphic results of the Janus procedure are as shown in Figure 16. The three degrees of freedom of the arc–chord complex should be considered; in "true" comparisons (Fig. 16A,E,I,J) the parabola is almost completely flattened and with no inclination, but only a slight shift in respect to the separation line. In all the other (false) comparisons, the arc–chord complex is shifted, but it is also inclined, and the convexity of the parabola is more pronounced until maximum allometric differences are detected in the comparison of face A–skull D (Fig. 16D) and face E–skull F (Fig. 16G). This last figure may be used for a more detailed discussion. The profile of photo E (on the left in the Janus composition) shows a more convex trend than the corresponding profile of skull F (right), and its domain (between the profile and separation line) is larger. The arc–chord complex (parabola and straight line joining its ends) shifts toward the left to evaluate isometric difference related to domain-size differentials. This complex then tilts to point in the direction of the allometry vector whose modulus is related to the increasing convexity of the parabola. This evaluates the allometry in terms of a more pro-

nounced convexity in the left profile compared with the right one.

The minimum and maximum values of the analytical parameters used as the final evaluator to determine the veracity of a superimposition appear in Table 2. For true comparisons, these values are much lower than for false ones and no overlaps occur except for the parameter from the Janus procedure. This is explained by the fact that the Janus procedure deals with symmetry of profiles of corresponding anatomical regions. "False" superimpositions exhibit the same symmetry arrangement; but the square root of the mean square error from polynomials and the Fourier sum of the differences reveal distinctly separated values because the first one is a "total morphological distance" evaluator and the second can detect very subtle (individual) differences due to "local" features of the profiles. However, we also use the parameter from the Janus procedure as the final evaluator because when allometric differences are detectable, they are to be considered very significant.

DISCUSSION

To successfully match skeletal remains to a particular individual using this approach, one must evaluate all shapes in the processed images. The procedure presented in this chapter can be effective for this purpose. This approach approximates the natural logic with which we usually identify a person known to us. We base recognition on the physiognomy of this person—his or her dimensions, color, and, above all, the shape of constituent elements (nose, forehead, or any other profile, narrow areas or wide regions). The trend of an anatomical profile (its shape) undoubtedly contains more information than any other evaluation made in the same region. For example, any dimension measurable between glabella, the nasal spine, and the extremity of the nasal bones will not tell us anything about the shape of the nose. However, the profile between those points represents the characteristic with physiognomic value—this forms the basis for any identification operation.

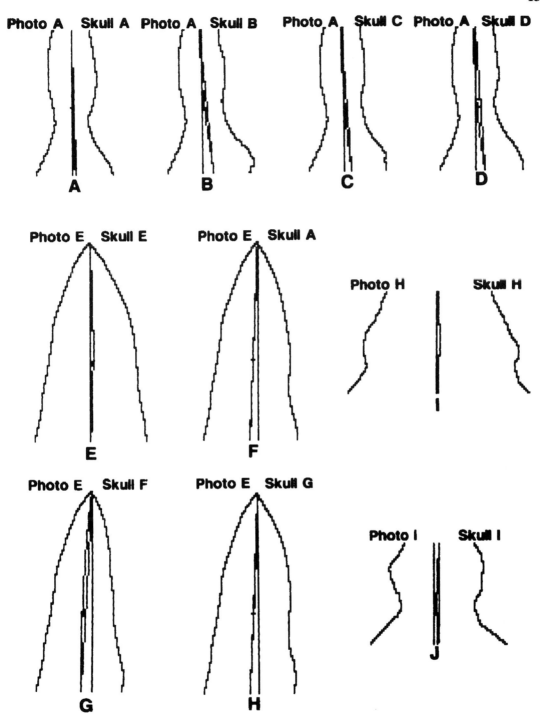

Fig. 16. A: Janus procedure for "true" comparison of case A; **B**: "false" comparison of face A with skull B; **C**: "false" comparison of face A with skull C; **D**: "false" comparison of face A with skull D; **E**: "true" comparison of case E; **F**: "false" comparison of face E with skull A; **G**: "false" comparison of face E with skull F; **H**: "false" comparison of face E with skull G; **I**: "true" comparison of case H; **J**: "true" comparison of case I.

It is a case of the classic morphological problem of the relationship between "size" and "shape." Actually, our visual perception is very effective in understanding and using the information of "shape." Yet, in contrast, methods that quantify morphology have already produced relatively simple and effective procedures for dimensional evaluations by calling for specific solutions for numerical descriptions of the "shape" in order to make them good parameters for discriminating statistics. This is exactly what is required in a comparison between a skull and photograph. Since the "shape" of an anatomical region must be reduced to the characteristics of the profiles that compose it and since these profiles can be fully considered as curves, the solutions that can describe them must revert to analytical geometry.

It is, however, necessary to include the algorithms in a strictly defined logical architecture. The logical architecture of the S.A.M. system, originally developed to address the anthropological problems of evolutionary morphology, and subsequently expanded to numerous domains of morphological diagnosis, assumes that each irregular shape contains elements of two distinct logical domains: gross distortions that interest the profile as a whole, and relatively minor local variations. In fact, any irregular object in an image can be subjected to this logic, either when the morphological differences are very pronounced, as in a large number of paleoanthropological applications (Pesce Delfino et al., 1987a,b, 1989), or when these differences are subtle, as in monitoring modifications made during corrective orthodontic procedures (Ricco et al., 1988, 1989a,b).

The information is processed separately by appropriate procedures so as to acquire independent parameters both on the logical level and the numerical one. The following strategy is applied in personal identification by comparing the skull and face: Once the superimposition has been achieved, the corresponding profiles in the photograph and on the skull are described separately by analytical procedures and a parameterized description is secured. The parameters will be compared to obtain numerical evaluators of "morphological distance." The smaller these indicators are, the better the congruence between the examined skull and photograph will be. Since it is a matter of numerically and logically independent parameters, the final evaluation will be based on their suitable combination.

The parameters from the three procedures are mutually independent, either from a logical or a computational point of view, and are multiplied between them to obtain a single final synthetic evaluator that expresses the degree of coincidence between the compared profiles of the superimposed skull and photograph. In false (noncorresponding) superimpositions, the final evaluator implies a variation of the magnitude order. We must stress that, from the quantitative point of view, the final evaluator values in lateral standard positions are not comparable to and must be considered separately from those obtained from oblique projections.

The use of superimposition between a skull and photographs of the living subject face is a technique of great importance in the identification of skeletal remains. Although this technique has been improved by using video systems, some questions about the validity of the method have been expressed. Difficulties have been reported in normalizing the dimensions and position of the photo and skull. There are also questions about whether a photograph could correspond to more than one skull and vice versa. Some experts have stated that the skull–photograph superimposition methods are probably more reliable for excluding rather than securing a positive identification (İşcan, 1988).

Thus, a major problem in superimposition is the search for the exact factors in the photograph that are related to the skull. This point remains critical even if closed-circuit TV systems are used. In fact, we have already pointed out in our previous works that it must be precisely controlled and standardized (Colonna et al., 1980, 1987).

The second critical problem concerns the control systems used to coordinate the fit of the superimposition. Obviously, the accuracy of the evaluation depends on the quality of the materials available for the investigation. The best results will be obtained if frontal, oblique, and lateral photographs of the head are available.

The quantitative evaluation of the degree of image correspondence represents the next step to eliminate the limitations associated with subjective assessment. In fact, the superimposition can only be performed by controlling the correspondence of clearly definable single points. In this phase of the procedure, a stable and perfectly repeatable reference system should be guaranteed. Within the limits of this system, individual points of correspondence are determined. These points are joined by curves constituting the profile to be investigated; but a visual evaluation of the correspondence of irregular curved lines with similar trends is extremely difficult.

The comparison of two similar curves depends on the fact that the architectural scheme of the anatomic areas is the same. It does not mean that differences cannot exist—recognizing an individualizing characteristic is the aim of any identification procedure. In other words, it is necessary to clearly distinguish between the coincidence of the discontinuous reference points and that of curves constituting the profile that develops between these points. In the first case, coincidence can be verified for many skull–photograph pairs if restrictive controls are not in place. In the second case, however, the coincidence can occur only if the skull is compared with the photograph of the subject to whom it belongs.

Hence, the coincidence of previously determined points (e.g., canonical craniometric points) does not represent the end of the superimposition investigation, but rather the starting point for matching the curves constituting the profiles by describing them through analytical procedures (Fig. 7C). Once we have progressed from the anatomical term "profile" to the analytical term "curve," many descriptive quantifications are possible.

These procedures consider the analytical description of the curve profile by polynomials: Kth order polynomials or Fourier trigonometrical polynomials; in the first case the curve is resolved in a series of coefficients describing its different parts; in the second, the curve is considered as the result of a set of sinusoids of given period whose sine–cosine coefficients are found as well as their amplitude and phase values. In both cases it is easy to obtain synthetic indicators, expressed by a single value, that characterize each curve and, above all, convey the degree of coincidence between the two matched curves.

Not all of the different components of the facial profile can be used in quantitative evaluations. This can be traced to the presence of thin soft tissues that are parallel to the planes of the bone and to the lack of other anatomic structures crossing the profile, which stands out on the background of the image.

The analysis is done by interpolating the empirical values in a series of the profile points with an upper degree polynomial by means of the least squares method. The comparison is carried out by verifying the divergence between the two series through reciprocal error evaluation (mean quadratic error under minimization conditions). This procedure considers the curves in their entirety and evaluates their corresponding morphological distance.

The second algorithm used is the Fourier harmonic analysis, which visualizes a sufficiently large number of harmonics (at least the first 15). The two algorithms we used are very different. The first one smoothes data by regression/interpolation, while the second considers the profile as an irregular periodic function whose sinusoidal contributors it computes. This approach evaluates the difference between the two curves by pinpointing their local variations. Although these are very effective analytical procedures to describe biological structures, there remains an important consideration: One of the two profiles (e.g., the profile of a certain anatomical part on the photograph) can be considered as an allometric transformation of the corresponding profile (e.g., on the skull) with which it is being compared. Therefore, a procedure that can distinguish the allometric differences from the isometric ones should be quite useful to complete the parameter set that will be used for a numerical evaluation of correspondence in a skull–photograph superimposition. Because the allometric differences have to characterize the comparison between the photograph and the skull of a different subject, these differences should be further separated from the effect of soft tissue thickness. This procedure guides the matching by pointing out the "rough distortions" or asymmetries.

The proposed quantitative procedures are the continuous analytical type, and are not represented by discrete measurements between the pairs of points. As the profile is subdivided into many points, it yields a great deal of extractable information. In the end, this does affect the value of the final numerical evaluators, which, if less than 20,000, as is the case for comparisons between the skull and photograph of the same individual (true), ensure a positive identification by differentiating them from false comparisons.

The latter ones show the values of synthetic evaluator differences, even in magnitude order, related to the corresponding comparisons. Investigations of new cases, besides those presented here, continue to confirm the conclusions reached in this chapter. One of these included a recent true comparison for the Court in Rome that yielded the lowest final evaluator (1,562) yet recorded (minimized square root of mean square error = 0.967; sum of differences of Fourier harmonics = 2,448; and allometry and isometry differences = 0.66%).

ACKNOWLEDGMENTS

This work was performed in cooperation with the University of Bari and the DIGAMMA Research Center, Bari, Italy. The authors thank Drs. E. Ferrara and C. Villasmunta, and Mr. D. Vinci for their valuable help. The editors of this volume are grateful to S.R. Loth for editing this chapter.

REFERENCES

Aherne WA, and Dunnil MS (1982) Morphometry. London: Edward Arnold.

Colonna M, Pesce Delfino V, and Introna F Jr (1980) Identificazione mediante sovrapposizione cranio-foto del viso a mezzo di circuito televisivo: Applicazione di una nuova metodica. Boll Soc Ital Biol 56:2271–2276.

Colonna M, Pesce Delfino V, and Introna F Jr (1982) Consideration sur cinq cas d'identification par superposition televisée entre photo du visage et crane. Proceedings of the XII Congress of the International Academy of the Forensic Society of Medicine, Vienna, May 17–22.

Colonna M, Lettini T, Potente F, Vacca E, and Pesce Delfino V (1987) Valutazione computerizzata della sovrapposizione cranio-foto del viso: Utilizzazione di un nuovo parametro. Rassegna Medico-Forense, December, No 1–2.

Colonna M, Lettini T, Potente F, Vacca E, and Pesce Delfino V (1988a) A case of identification by skull–face computer aided superimposition. 12th International Congress of Anthropol Ethnol Sci, Zagreb, July 24–31.

Colonna M, Potente F, Vacca E, Lettini T, and Pesce Delfino V (1988b) S.A.M. (Shape Analytical Morphometry) strategy in some actual cases of identification by skull–face matching. Paper presented at the International Symposium "Advances in Skull Identification via Video Superimposition," 3–5 August, Kiel.

Dorion RBJ (1983) Photographic superimposition. J Forensic Sci 28:724–732.

Glaister J, and Brash JC (1937) Medico-Legal Aspects of the Ruxton Case. Edinburgh: Livingstone.

Helmer R, and Grüner O (1977) Schädelidentifizierung durch Superprojection nach dem Verfahren der electronischen Bildmischung, modifiziert zum Trickbild. Differenz-Verfahren Z Rechtsmed 80:183–187.

İşcan MY (1988) Rise of forensic anthropology. Yrbk Phys Anthropol 31:203–230.

Koelmeyer TD (1982) Videocamera superimposition and facial reconstruction as an aid to identification. Am J Forensic Med Pathol 3:45–48.

Lestrel PE (1974) Some problems in the assessment of morphological size and shape differences. Yrbk Phys Anthropol 18:140–162.

Malinowski A, and Porawski R (1970) L'utilité de l'expertise anthropometrique pour les essais d'identification des crânes humains par la methode de la superprojection photographique. Zacchia 45:77–97.

Pesce Delfino V, and Ricco R (1983) Remarks on

analytic morphometry in biology: Procedure and software illustration. Acta Stereologica 2:459–464.

Pesce Delfino V, Colonna M, Introna F Jr, Potente F, and Vacca E (1983) Identification by computer aided skull face superimposition. XI International Congress of Anthropol Ethnol Sci, Vancouver, August 20–25.

Pesce Delfino V, Colonna M, Vacca E, Potente F, and Introna F Jr (1986) Computer-aided skull/face superimposition. Am J Forensic Med Pathol 7(3):201–212.

Pesce Delfino V, Vacca E, Lettini T, and Potente F (1987a) Analytical description of cranial profiles by means of Kth order polynomial equations, procedure and application on *Plesianthropus transvaalensis* (STS5). Anthropologie 25–26:47–55.

Pesce Delfino V, Potente F, Vacca E, Lettini T, and Lenoci R (1987b) Analytical morphometry in fronto-facial profile comparison of Taung1, *Plesianthropus transvaalensis*, *Homo sapiens* infant and *Homo sapiens* adult. In V Pesce Delfino (ed): Biological Evolution. Bari: Adriatica, pp 151–188.

Pesce Delfino V, Vacca E, Potente F, Lettini T, and Colonna M (1988) Analytical methods by S.A.M. (Shape Analytical Morphometry) work station in computer aided skull identification via video superimposition. Paper presented at the International Symposium "Advances in Skull Identification via Video Superimposition," 3–5 August, Kiel.

Pesce Delfino V, Vacca E, Potente F, and Lettini T (1989) Analytical morphometry on S. Sergi's craniograms: Morphological distances and allometry detection. In G Giacobini (ed): Hominidae: Proceedings of the 2nd International Congress of Human Paleontology. Milan: Jaca Book, pp 363–367.

Ricco R, Di Gioia E, Potente F, Vacca E, Ditolve P, and Pesce Delfino V (1988) L'analisi di Fourier nello studio delle forme di profili fronto-facciali nelle cheilogniatopalatoschisi. Atti del Convegno Biennale S.I.D.O., Florence, October 13–16.

Ricco R, Di Gioia E, Potente F, Vacca E, Ditolve P, and Pesce Delfino V (1989a) Applicazione di morfometria analitica in ortodonzia. Atti del X Congresso Nazionale S.I.D.O., Turin, October 26–29.

Ricco R, Di Gioia E, Ditolve P, Vacca E, Potente F, and Pesce Delfino V (1989b) Proposta di un valutatore analitico (SAE: Shape Asymmetry Evaluator) nello studio delle asimmetrie cranio mandibolari. Atti del X Congresso Nazionale S.I.D.O., Turin, October 26–29.

Stewart TD (1983) The points of attachment of the palpebral ligaments: Their use in facial reconstructions on the skull. J Forensic Sci 28:859–863.

Chapter 12

A Combined Apparatus for Photographic and Video Superimposition

Sueshige Seta and Mineo Yoshino

First Forensic Science Division (S.S.) and First Medico-Legal Section (M.Y.), National Research Institute of Police Science, Chiyoda-Ku, Tokyo 102, Japan

For more than 20 years, the authors have been concerned with the identification of skulls by photographic superimposition. In the last 10 years, video superimposition has proven to be a very successful craniofacial identification (Helmer and Grüner, 1977; Koelmeyer, 1982; Dorion, 1983; Krogman and İşcan, 1986; Iten, 1987). As suggested by several authors, this technique presents enormous advantages over photographic superimposition. This stems mainly from the fact that it is much easier to orient the skull to correspond with a photograph of the face to which it will be compared. Despite this advantage, it should be noted that photographic superimposition yields finer images for an identification report. With this in mind, the authors have attempted to build a combined system for both photographic and video superimposition.

EQUIPMENT

This apparatus is composed of the skull-positioning box, two video cameras, electronic and picture-mixing units, a TV monitor, and a photography stand to hold the photograph for comparison. As can be seen in Figures 1 and 2, the equipment was set up as a compact working system.

Positioning Box for the Skull

This unit constitutes the most essential part in the present system because it was specifically devised to allow movement of the skull. Careful attention was paid to the mode of skull movement, which is one of the most critical factors in achieving successful superimposition. For this purpose, a skull rest with variable positioning was devised (Fig. 3). It was equipped with a slightly modified Martin-type craniophore. The movement of the skull rest is controlled by a motor-driven mechanism, which can be operated with an easily accessible joystick lever that was incorporated into the control panel with other function buttons (Fig. 4). The range of motion of the skull on this unit is upward and downward (± 20 mm), left and right (± 40 mm), forward and backward (± 20 mm), rotation around the axis ($\pm 100°$), flexion and extension ($\pm 30°$), and tilt to the left and right ($\pm 15°$) (Fig. 5). The combination of the variable movement functions was sufficient to duplicate the normal movements of the neck. Skull size determination, which is a crucial problem in obtaining a reasonable correspondence to the compared face, was made by adjusting the zoom lens of a color video camera recording the skull. This operation is controlled by pushing a button located on the right upper side of the control panel (Fig. 4). The combined use of each movement function while monitoring the skull and picture (a front or lateral/semilateral view), can sufficiently lead to the establishment of precise and easy-to-obtain skull orientation and size corresponding to the face to which it is compared. The skull in the box was illuminated by a total of 34 10-watt white fluorescent lamps. They were arranged so as to almost surround the skull in the box with 11 lamps above, nine lamps on each side, and five lamps below. Depending on the color of the

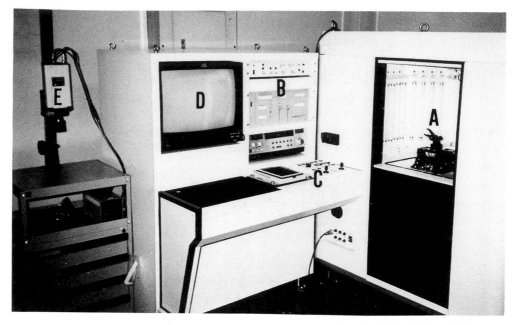

Fig. 1. General view of the apparatus. A, Skull box equipped with a skull rest. B, Electronic and mixer units. C, Control panel. D, TV monitor. E, Photographing unit with a video camera for the comparison face. The window of the skull box can be shut with a black metal curtain during the superimposition process.

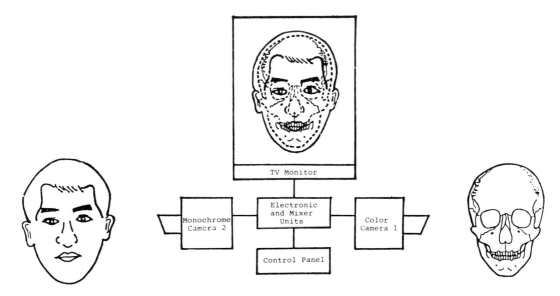

Fig. 2. Illustration of the apparatus. The apparatus is composed of two video cameras (color camera 1 and monochrome camera 2), electronic and mixer units, and one TV monitor. Variable mixing of skull and comparison face images can be made on a single TV monitor, taking into account the thickness of soft tissues. All operations are run from a control panel.

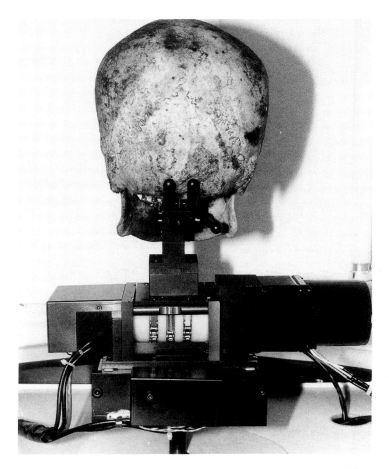

Fig. 3. View of the skull rest with a craniophore. The rest can be moved by a motor-driven mechanism. The craniophore is devised to prevent any movement.

skull in question, the intensity of the lighting can be adjusted by varying the number of lamps.

Optical Pathway of the Apparatus

For reproducing the skull and comparison face photograph together in one monitor, the apparatus is equipped with two video cameras, electronic and mixer units, and a TV monitor. Video camera 1 (10–100 mm, 200 mm lens, f1.6, metal oxide semiconductor color tube) and video camera 2 (50 mm lens, f1.5, monochrome tube) are used for reproducing the skull and comparison face photograph, respectively. In the present apparatus, special technical care was focused on providing the simultaneous reproduction of the skull image both on the TV monitor and the photographic ground-glass plate. This is because the skull image photographed on this plate is finer than if it were directly photographed from the TV monitor. For this purpose, two optical pathways were formed by differentially combining the reflection mirrors. The reflection efficiency of the system was specially enhanced with an aluminum coating. As shown in Figure 6, four reflection mirrors (mirrors 1–4) were used to reproduce the skull image on the TV monitor. Each mirror was aligned

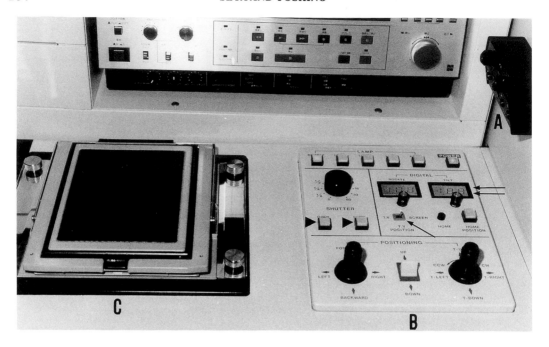

Fig. 4. View of the control panel. A, Zoom operation of video camera 1 for determining the skull size. B, Operation of skull movement, lighting selection, and choice of photographic or video superimposition (arrow). C, Ground glass for photographic superimposition. The skull is photographed at half original size on cabinet-sized film with the shutter button (arrowheads). For tilt and rotation movements, a digital readout supplies the values or deviation from the median–sagittal plane on which the skull is set at the beginning of superimposition (double arrows).

so that it would transmit the ray of light at a 45° angle. Video camera 1 was set in front of mirror 4 to reproduce the skull image on the TV monitor. To focus the skull image on the ground glass, mirror 4 was made to slide out of the optical pathway by a motor-driven mechanism. Instead of mirror 4, a projection lens (Fujinon 600 mm, f11.5) was inserted in the optical pathway to focus the skull image on the ground-glass plate through mirror 5 (Fig. 6). The projection lens was designed to focus the skull on the film plate at just half the original skull size.

Picture-Mixing Unit

During video superimposition, the skull in question and the photograph in question are reproduced on a single screen; thus, both images can be moved. The picture-mixing unit for superimposing both images allows not only an infinitely variable mixing of the two pictures but also the creation of horizontal and vertical image sections at any desired positions on the TV monitor (Fig. 7). "Fade-out" facilitates the comparison of two pictures as a whole, especially the comparison of the contour of skull and face. For documentation, the entire superimposition procedure can be recorded on videotape from the monitor.

PHOTOGRAPHIC AND VIDEO SUPERIMPOSITION

The skull is first recorded with video camera 1 and displayed on the TV monitor in the Frankfort horizontal plane (Ohraugen-Ebene). To

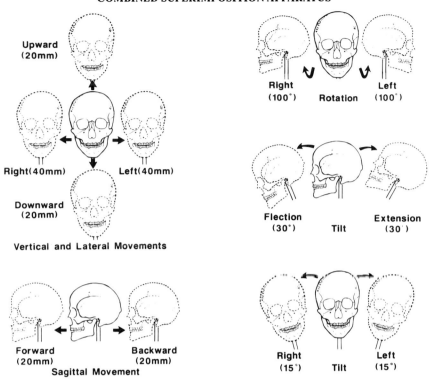

Fig. 5. Illustration of skull movement. Combining use of each movement attains motion almost similar to that of the neck. These movements can be made from outside the skull box by the appropriate button on the control panel.

make the comparison, the photograph of the face is then reproduced on the TV monitor using video camera 2. The skull is then oriented to correspond to the angulation of the face. To account for soft tissue thickness, skull size is determined using the zoom mechanism of camera 1. In the process of video superimposition, special care has been paid to the problem of image distortion. In order to determine the degree of image distortion, a cross scale was experimentally reproduced on the TV monitor using both video cameras 1 and 2. Ratios of the vertical to horizontal axis distances were estimated from the images. The ratio of both original axes was 1.00. The ratios from video cameras 1 and 2 were 1.004 and 0.994, respectively (Fig. 8). This result suggests that the distortion of the object image reproduced on the TV monitor with both cameras is negligible. The picture-mixing unit allows the variable mixing of two

pictures. The horizontal and vertical sectioning of images at desired points can be efficiently used for comparing all of the anatomical and morphological characteristics, and taking into account the thickness of the soft tissue (Fig. 7). The photographic superimposition was combined with the video superimposition, primarily to obtain a finer matched photograph to be presented in an official report. Though the superimposed result can be photographed directly from the monitor, it is not recommended because of the unsatisfactory quality of the image. In the routine practice of photographic superimposition, after the skull has been correctly oriented on the TV monitor, the skull in question is then focused on the ground glass at half the original skull size and photographed on cabinet size (6.5 × 4.75") film. The picture of the face used for this purpose is enlarged from the original photograph to correspond to the

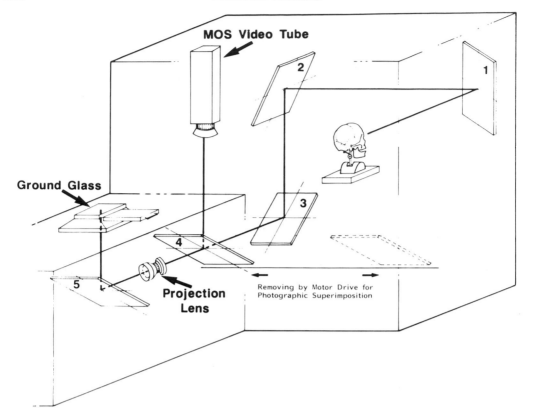

Fig. 6.   Illustration of optical pathway devised for the apparatus. The optical pathway is produced by the combination of four reflection mirrors. Each mirror is arranged to meet at a 45° angle to a ray of incident light. For video superimposition, four mirrors (mirrors 1–4) are used as shown in the figure, and for photographic superimposition the fourth mirror plate is designed to slide out of the optical pathway in order to focus the skull on the ground glass via a projection lens and mirror 5.

size of the skull, with enough space to account for the thickness of soft tissue at the anatomical landmarks. Basically, the frontal view of the photograph is enlarged based on bizygomatic width and soft tissue thickness at zygion. In the lateral view, the facial photograph is enlarged based on glabella–gnathion distance and soft tissue thickness at gnathion. Figure 9 shows the photographic superimposition made in an actual investigation. The skull transparencies were made after the skull was correctly oriented in a frontal and a slightly lateral view, respectively. In normal practice, a blue transparency is used in order to enhance the contrast of the skull image with the transparency of the face.

DISCUSSION

It has been suggested by several authors (Helmer and Grüner, 1977; Koelmeyer, 1982; Dorion, 1983; Krogman and İşcan, 1986; Iten, 1987) that video superimposition provides enormous advantages over the usual photographic superimposition, so that comparisons can be made rapidly and in greater detail than is possible with static photographs. Helmer and Grüner (1977) pioneered the development of video superimposition and promoted its use in the investigation of a skull in question. They reproduced images of skull and photograph on two monitors using two separate video cameras, and elec-

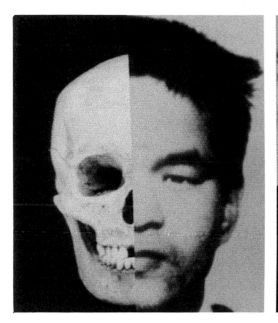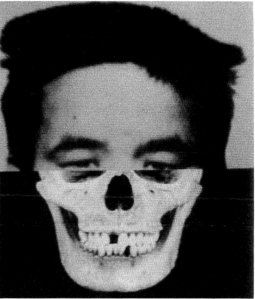

Fig. 7. Mixing and producing picture sections, vertical or horizontal, at the desired points, one is able to compare all the anatomical and morphological characteristics, taking soft tissue thickness into account. The stills are directly photographed from the TV monitor.

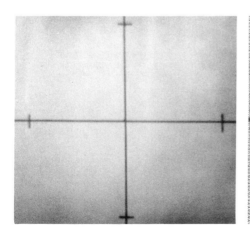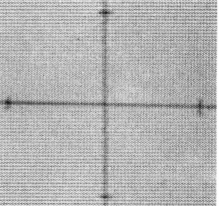

Fig. 8. Examination of the degree of optical distortion in reproducing the image on the TV monitor from video camera 1 (**left**) and 2 (**right**). An experimentally depicted cross (vertical 1:horizontal 1) was reproduced on the TV monitor using cameras 1 and 2. The ratios of the vertical axis distance to the horizontal calculated on the monitor was 1.004 in camera 1 and 0.994 in camera 2, suggesting that the image distortion is almost negligible.

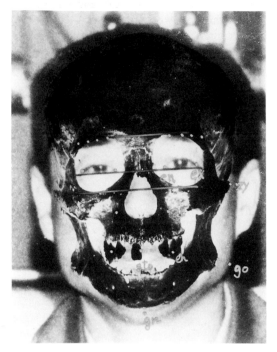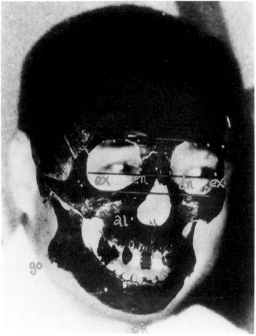

Fig. 9. The result of photographic superimposition. After the skull was correctly oriented during the process of video superimposition, it was focused on the ground glass to make the transparency for the photographic superimposition. The comparison photograph is enlarged corresponding to skull size, based on anatomical landmarks of the skull. The purpose of photographic superimposition is to get finer matching images for submitting a case report.

tronically mixed them in overall and partial views. Dorion (1983) also employed video cameras for superimposition. He used a transparency of the photograph of the face set just in front of the skull, and displayed the skull and the transparency on a single monitor. İşcan briefly described his experience with video superimposition using two studio cameras, a special-effects mixing and dissolving switch, and a 19" monitor (Krogman and İşcan, 1986). Iten (1987) recently recommended the following equipment for video superimposition: two video tubes (1 and 2), electronic mixer units, and three monitors. The skull was photographed using tube 1 and the image was reproduced on monitor 1. The facial photograph was then reproduced with tube 2 on monitor 2. The mixed picture and horizontal and vertical sections were

displayed on monitor 3 by means of the electronic mixer units.

Among many investigators of superimposition, it has been a matter of primary concern to obtain a quick, precise orientation of the skull that corresponds with the comparison photograph. In fact, it would be very difficult to obtain the technical specifications used to take the antemortem photograph. Therefore, a number of devices have been designed to position the skull so that it will match the orientation of the face in the picture. In the present apparatus, the skull and face were both reproduced in movable images on a single monitor to rapidly obtain an accurate skull orientation. The movement of the skull can be made efficiently (taking soft tissue thickness into account) through the control panel arranged outside the skull box, which includes the zoom lens for determining skull size, tilting to the left and right, as well as conventional movements (flexion, extension, left and right lateral, upward and downward, and rotation). This was, in fact, found to be the best method of orienting the image of the skull to correspond with that of the face. The entire video superimposition process can be easily accomplished by one person, without direct manipulation of the skull.

The photographic superimposition aspect of this apparatus is used solely for preparation of the forensic report. Under the optical pathway devised in the present apparatus, the optical distortion of the reproduced skull and facial photograph is negligible. The quality of the superimposed image is superior to the image directly photographed from the monitor, which is an advantage over equipment currently used in forensic practice.

It is worth noting that although a match was obtained with the photograph of the suspected missing person, a good match was also obtained with another photograph of a person known to be alive. Superimposition should be able to prove whether or not the skull and photograph belong to the same individual. As a general rule, it can be stated that superimposition is of greater value in ruling out a match, because it can be definitely stated that the skull and photograph are not those of the same person. However, if they do align, it can only be stated that the skull might possibly be that of the person in the photograph, because of the chance that another skull of that size and contour may also line up with the photograph (see İşcan, 1988). The recognition of individualizing features such as acquired or congenital anomalies reinforces the probability that the skull and face are those of the same individual.

REFERENCES

Dorion RBJ (1983) Photographic superimposition. J Forensic Sci 28:724–734.

Helmer R, and Grüner O (1977) Vereinfachte Schädelidentifizierung nach dem Superprojektions-verfahren mit Hilfe einer Video-Anlage. Z Rechts-med 80:183–187.

İşcan MY (1988) Rise of forensic anthropology. Yrbk Phys Anthropol 31:203–230.

Iten PX (1987) Identification of skulls by video superimposition. J Forensic Sci 32:173–188.

Koelmeyer TD (1982) Videocamera superimposition and facial reconstruction as an aid to identification. Am J Forensic Med Pathol 3:45–48.

Krogman WM, and İşcan MY (1986) The Human Skeleton in Forensic Medicine. Springfield, Ill: Charles C Thomas.

Chapter 13

Standards for Skull-to-Photo Superimposition

Cai Dongsheng and Lan Yuwen

Tieling 213 Research Institute, Liaoning Province, People's Republic of China 112000

The success of craniofacial superimposition as a method of establishing identity in the Ruxton case by Brash in 1935 attracted much attention from medico-legal experts in many countries (Brash and Glaister, 1937; Krogman and İşcan, 1986). The interest thus generated spurred more research that has led to numerous improvements and modifications of the standards of identification and methods of superimposition. However, many felt that it was difficult to make an accurate, scientific evaluation from the results of this procedure due to inevitable photographic variations, the basic similarity of human skull morphology, and the lack of anthropological data on two-dimensional projections of the face.

The present research has revealed the intrinsic characteristics of the face and skull and their interrelationship from an anthropological perspective. Through radiographic examination of 224 individuals (100 male and 124 female) of Chinese Han nationality ranging in age from 18 to 55 years, the authors found that there is an obvious uniqueness and exclusivity for the landmarks of the face and corresponding locations on the skull in a two-dimensional relationship. This provided a solid foundation for the identification of a skull by means of superimposition (Cai and Lan, 1982a). The purpose of this chapter is to introduce a series of objective standards to evaluate the results of superimposition.

RELATIONSHIPS BETWEEN LANDMARKS IN THE FACE AND SKULL

This method of superimposition begins with the radiographic recognition and labeling of landmarks on the face and skull. First, place a drop of lead (2 mm in diameter) on each of 28 landmarks on face of the person to be examined. The positions of these points are illustrated in Figure 1. Then have the subject sit facing the radiographic film box and take X-rays in seven pitch angles (from -15° to +15°, with 5° between angles) and 10 deflection (rotation) angles (from 0° to 90°, with 10° between angles), respectively, using the two ectoconchions in the skull as objective points with a subject-to-film box distance of $d = 45$ mm and an X-ray unit-to-film plate distance of $D = 2$ m (Figs. 2, 3). This will reveal the superimposition relationship of the skull and face (Cai and Lan, 1982b; see also Lan and Cai, Chapter 10, this volume).

After the radiographs have been developed, take measurements and calculate the distances between related landmarks on the skull and face, as well as indices, and make corrections for radiographic distortion of the measurements to make them conform to their actual values. Corrections should be made using the following formula:

$$R = (D - d) \times I/D$$

where R is the value after correction and I is the actual value measured from the X-rays.

From the above test, we obtained projectional plane data and index relationships between landmarks in related parts of the skull image and soft tissue of the face. We also calculated the displacement formulae and projectional data of different superimposed marking points at different angles. A standard identification system consisting of 58 targets in four

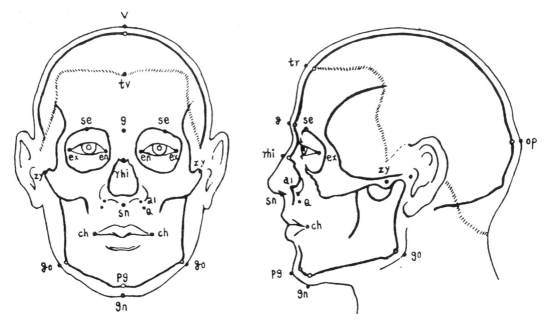

Fig. 1. Landmarks on the skull and face.

groups was thus established for superimposition.

Group 1 is composed of superimposed landmarks that include 28 targets, some of which appear in Table 1. The distance targets, or measure of space between two points, of the landmarks in Table 1 were calculated from the two-dimensional distance between corresponding points in related parts of the soft tissue of the face and the skull images. The index targets were calculated from the anatomical projection proportion of the related parts of the face and skull images. For example, to calculate the endocanthion index, use the formula $a = d/h$, where a is the endocanthion index, d is the length between endocanthion in the face image to the tangent of the upper orbit of the skull, and h is the height of the orbit of the skull.

Group 2 features eight examining lines in related positions on the face and skull images as targets to determine the proportional positions of the five sense organs accurately and to calculate the azimuth for the superimposition photograph (Fig. 4, Table 2). The related indices of the eight examining lines change along with the

change of the deflection angle. The three vertical lines will be displaced as the image deflects. For instance, the central line of the face superimposes completely with that of the skull, whereas if the image is deflected, the two lines will separate. This separation will further increase as the deflection angle increases. This relationship is defined by the following equation:

$$Y = X/9 \text{ (mm)}.$$

The five horizontal lines would be displaced if the image is pitched. For instance, the subnasale line is 3.63 mm lower than the lower tangent of the piriform aperture in norma frontalis. This line will move upward if the face in the image is pitched upward, and downward if it is tilted down. This change can be calculated with the following formula (Table 4, line 4):

$$Y = -2.9186 + 0.4696X.$$

Group 3 includes 13 targets to gauge soft tissue

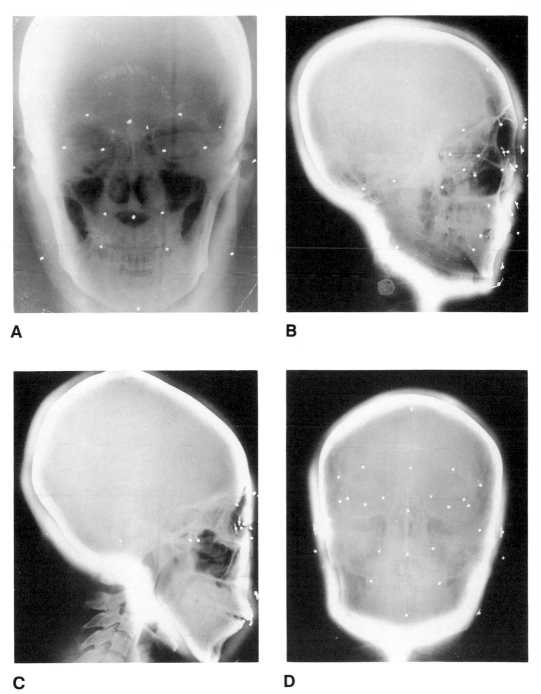

Fig. 2. Landmarks and position variations in radiographs. **A**: Front position, 0° both in pitch and deflection; **B**: 45° deflected; **C**: 90° deflected; **D**: 15° up pitch.

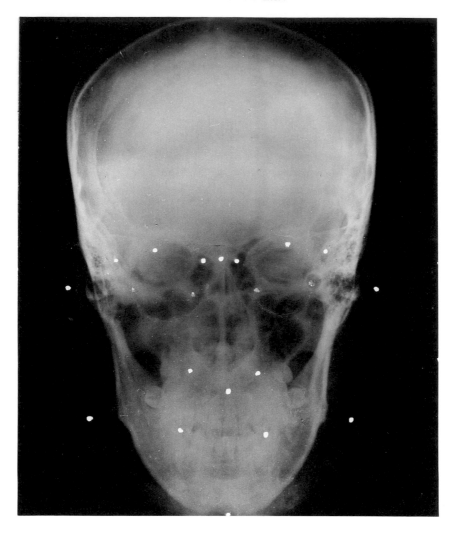

Fig. 3.   Radiograph of a skull with a 15° down pitch.

thickness. Thickness is calculated by measuring the distance between the external edge of the soft tissue of the face and that of the skull at the target points (Table 3). This table shows that the change of angle does not influence the thickness of soft tissue but relates directly to the appearance of different target points. For example, points below opisthocranion can be seen only at 90°.

Group 4 contains nine contour targets based on the anatomical relationships and morphology of the face (Fig. 5). Table 4 lists the names

of each contour and its appearance at different angles, as well as illustrating that the appearance of the contours is directly related to the deflection angle. For example, the head vault, eyebrow, and gonion curves are hidden behind the projection plane at angles greater than 45°, 60°, and 90°, respectively, and the back of the head, forehead, and pogonion curves are seen only at 90°. These targets exhibit a high degree of exclusivity and are thus important factors in individualization that can lead to identification.

TABLE 1. Changes in the Relationships of Group 1 Landmarks in the Face and Skull During Projection

Variables	Front Position (0°) $X \pm$	Formulae for Change Based on Facial Angle in Photo
Distance between glabella and upper orbit tangent	-9.69 ± 1.74 mm	Pitch: $y = -0.298X$ mm
Ectocanthion index	0.61 ± 0.050	Pitch: $y = 1/(-1.732 \times 10^{-5} - 1.564 \times 10^{-5} \cdot X + 0.0268X^{-2})$
Endocanthion index	0.67 ± 0.047 mm	Pitch: $y = 0/6586 - 5.714 \times 10^{-3}X$
Subnasale to apertura piriformis lower tangent	-3.63 ± 1.769 mm	Pitch: $y = -2.9186 + 0.4696X$
Distance from 1st molar line to lower edge of piriform aperture	29.1 ± 3.07	Pitch: $y = 1/(4.441.908 \times 10^{-5} \cdot X + 0.345X^{-2})$
Distance between ectocanthions	90.78 ± 4.233 mm	Deflection: $y = 2.9633 \times 10^{-2} - 1.1659 \times 10^{-2}X + 9.078X^{-2}$
Distance between junctures of orbit	96.28 ± 4.272 mm	Deflection: $y = 1/(-1.943 \times 10^{-3} - 7.5545 \times 10^{-5}X + 0.5451X^{-2})$
Index of distance between ectocanthions	0.94 ± 0.02	Deflection: $y = (X - 0.94)(-6.1035 \times 10^{-5} - 100X)$
Distance between endocanthions	35.36 ± 2.669 mm	Deflection: $y = 1/(-4.0149 \times 10^{-5} + 6.9779 \times 10^{-6}X + 2.0281 \times 10^{-2}X^{-2})$
Distance index between endocanthions	0.37 ± 0.03	Deflection: $y = 0.37$
Vertical line through endocanthion to upper teeth	Third tooth (left, right)	Deflection: $y = 3$
Distance between ectocanthion and external orbit tangent (left, right)	2.18 ± 0.457 mm	Deflection side: $y = (X - 2.41)(5.2165 + 0.0878X)$ Opposite side: $y + (X - 5.13)/(1.0314 + 4.603 \times 10^{-2}X)$
Index of cheilion line	1.183 ± 0.2355	Less change in pitching
Index of distance between gonions	0.799 ± 0.04	Deflection: $y = \sqrt{7519} \times 10^{-4} + 1.9318 \times 10^{-6}X + 0.638X^{-2}$
Index of distance between cheilions	0.489 ± 0.06	Deflection: $y = 0.00035 - 4.5556 \times 10^{-5}X + 0.489X^{-2}$
Vertical line through center of tragion to gonion	20.60 ± 1.71	Deflection: $y = 2.5641 \times 10^{-2} - 1.3801 \times 10^{-3}X + 12.607X^{-2}$

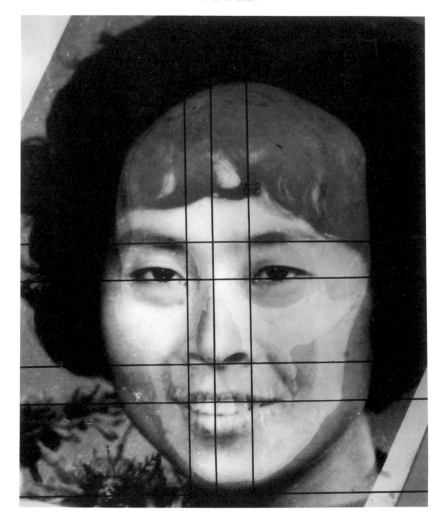

Fig. 4. The eight examining lines.

TABLE 2.   Group 2 Examining Lines on the Face and Skull Images

Face Image	Skull Image
Glabella line	Upper orbit tangent
Central line	Central line
Gnathion line	Gnathion tangent
Ectocanthion line	Line between junctures of external orbit
Subnasale line	Piriform aperture lower tangent
Cheilion line	Mouth line
Vertical line through left endocanthion	Left canine
Vertical line through right endocanthion	Right canine

TABLE 3. Group 3 Targets of Soft Tissue Thickness (mm)

Target of Marking Point	Mean and Standard Deviation of Deflection Angle					
	0°	15°	30°	45°	60°	90°
Vertex	6.08 ± 0.84	6.12 ± 0.82	6.12 ± 0.96	6.04 ± 0.76	6.10 ± 0.74	6.22 ± 0.94
Gnathion	7.37 ± 1.87	7.61 ± 1.57	7.50 ± 1.42	7.38 ± 1.31	7.41 ± 1.31	7.41 ± 1.31
Euryon (left)	7.34 ± 1.28	8.20 ± 1.27				
Euryon (right)	7.27 ± 1.23	7.30 ± 1.14				
Zygion (left)	6.95 ± 1.61	8.53 ± 1.79	9.69 ± 1.66			
Zygion (right)	6.95 ± 1.61	5.96 ± 1.54				
Center of tragion (left)	8.34 ± 1.79	8.90 ± 1.79				
Center of tragion (right)	8.34 ± 1.79	6.11 ± 1.25				
Gonion (left)	10.80 ± 2.46	14.50 ± 3.11	15.82 ± 2.7	14.80 ± 2.13		
Gonion (right)	10.80 ± 2.46	10.10 ± 2.55				
Cheekbone		9.22 ± 1.57	10.30 ± 1.58	10.90 ± 1.57	11.3 ± 1.56	
Opisthocranion						6.95 ± 1.38
Trichion						5.03 ± 1.64
Glabella						5.71 ± 0.94
Dorsonasale						3.13 ± 2.20
Subnasale						10.60 ± 2.57
Pogonion						11.30 ± 2.48

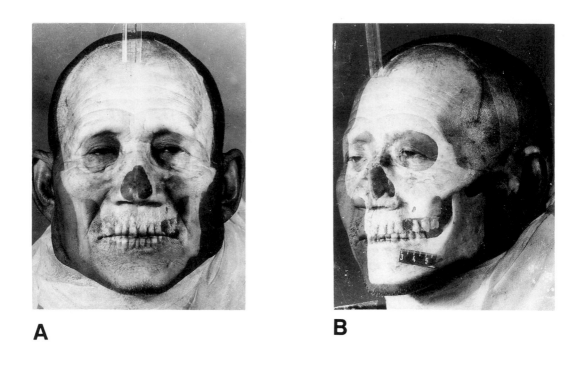

A   B

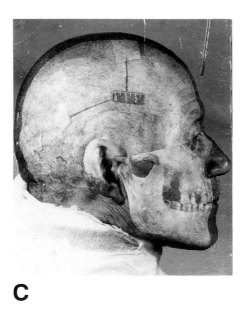

C

Fig. 5. Contours of the face in (**A**) full frontal position, (**B**) half-profile, and (**C**) full profile.

TABLE 4.   Appearance of Group 4 Contours in Deflection Photography (Deflected Toward Left)[a]

Number	Contour	Deflection Angle					
		0°	15°	30°	45°	60°	90°
1	Head vault curve	+	+	+	+	-	-
2	Eyebrow curve (left)	+	+	+	+	+	-
	Eyebrow curve (right)	+	+	+	+	+	+
3	Nose curve	+	+	+	+	+	+
4	Gonion curve (left)	+	+	+	-	-	-
	Gonion curve (right)	+	+	+	+	+	+
5	Lower jaw curve	+	+	+	+	+	+
6	Rear head curve	-	-	-	-	-	+
7	Forehead curve	-	-	-	-	-	+
8	Pogonion curve			-	-	-	+
9	Cheekbone curve (left)	+	+	+	-	-	-
	Cheekbone curve (right)	+	-	-	-	-	-

[a]+ indicates that the related contours can be seen and - cannot be seen.

REPLICABILITY OF STANDARDS

Using the examination standards established for male and female adults of Chinese Han nationality, superimposition tests were conducted on each known skull and its corresponding photo from 166 (100 male and 66 female) individuals. The resulting data for all targets were within a permissible range of the mean and standard deviation. This demonstrates that our standards for the examination for superimposing the skull and photo of the same individual are repeatable.

EXCLUSIVITY OF STANDARDS

In order to confirm and verify the exclusivity and reliability of the examination standards, we have run 10,000 tests of the probability of incorrect superimposition using 1,000 randomly selected pictures of Chinese Han adult females. The photos ranged in size from 2 to 4 inches and were superimposed on 10 skulls from different females. These were tested using the eight examining lines and contour curve systems from the female standards.

The results of the test in Table 5 show that only the central and ectocanthion lines superimposed with 100% probability. The superimposition probabilities of the cheilion and subnasale lines are relatively high at 36.75% and 33.11%, respectively. It is notable that the contour line exhibits the minimum superimposition probability, with only 832 cases of superimposition (8.32%). This indicates that the contour curve

TABLE 5.   Conditions of Superimposed Examining Lines

Examining Line	Number of Superimposed Cases	Probability of Superimposition (%)
Central line	10,000	100
Ectocanthion line	10,000	100
Glabella line	2,400	24
Subnasale line	3,311	33.11
Cheilion line	3,675	36.75
Gnathion line	2,980	29.80
Vertical line through endocanthion (left)	2,081	20.81
Vertical line through endocanthion (right)	1,446	14.46
Contour curve	832	8.32

has the highest degree of individual eccentricity of the examining lines tested and is thus a reliable target.

To make additional observations of the superimposition rate of the examining lines, we divided them into groups for the simultaneous superimposition of more than one line and conducted a statistical analysis. The results, listed in Table 6, show that the superimposition rate for three lines (including the two specified baselines, which must be superimposed) is 100%; for four lines it drops to 55.48%. For more than five lines, the rate decreases sharply as the number of lines increases—using eight lines it is only 0.05% and in no cases could nine lines be simultaneously superimposed. The tests indicate that the eight examining lines plus the contour curve adopted in this research possess very high exclusivity and thus are of great value in eliminating problems stemming from the basic similarities of the human face. This is very helpful in screening out invalid superimpositions.

DISCUSSION AND CONCLUSIONS

This chapter presents an analysis of the relationship between the landmarks on the face and corresponding locations on radiography of the skull. Four groups of standards using a total of 58 examining targets have been established for identifying a skull by superimposition. These include 8 targets for the examining lines, 9 for the contour curve, 13 for soft tissue thickness, and 28 for the relevant relationships of the landmarks. The 58 targets may not be totally visible at the same time in any single examination angle, but may be partly manifested at different deflection and pitch angles. In order to estimate the morphological variation, each target has a mean value and standard deviation. Relevant relationships of landmarks in the face and skull can be assessed with a relatively high degree of accuracy because they are determined by forming indices and deduced from mathematical formulae that calculate their variations.

The reliability of the standards developed from this research have been demonstrated using 166 cases of known skull and photo pairs to conduct 10,000 tests of superimposition probability. If all visible targets are completely superimposed using our system of standards, it can be considered a positive identification. On the other hand, a match is ruled out if two or more targets cannot be superimposed. Finally, when only one target does not fit, the possibility of identification exists. In this case, the test must be repeated on another photo taken at a different angle in the hope of obtaining a more definitive result. With these standards, the authors have identified 108 unknown skulls in the last five years. All were verified when the criminal cases were solved.

The present chapter deals only with the results of skull–photo superimposition tests on male and female adults of Chinese Han nationality. Of course, further study of race- and age-related variation is still needed.

ACKNOWLEDGMENTS

The editors of this volume are grateful to S.R. Loth for editing this chapter.

TABLE 6.   Superimposition Rate for Examining Line Groups

	Number of Simultaneously Superimposed Lines						
	3	4	5	6	7	8	9
Number of cases superimposed in 10,000 tests	10,000	5,548	1,310	275	45	5	0
Rate of superimposition (%)	100	55.48	13.10	2.75	0.45	0.05	0

REFERENCES

Brash JC, and Glaister J (1937) Medicolegal Aspects of the Ruxton Case. Edinburgh: E & S Livingstone.

Cai D, and Lan Y (1982a) Research on standards for skull to photo superimposition. Criminal Technol (Suppl), pp 34–40, Beijing.

Cai D, and Lan Y (1982b) Research on landmarks on face in skull–image superimposition using X-ray photographing. Criminal Technol (Suppl), pp 17–22, Beijing.

Krogman WM, and İşcan MY (1986) The Human Skeleton in Forensic Medicine. Springfield, Ill: Charles C Thomas.

Chapter 14
Principles of Facial Reconstruction

G.V. Lebedinskaya, T.S. Balueva, and E.V. Veselovskaya

Institute of Ethnography, 117334 Moscow, Russia

Discussions of the advantages and disadvantages of methods for facial reconstruction from the skull and their significance for anthropology and forensic medicine suffer from the fact that two major problems remain unresolved. These are: the study of the interrelationships between the soft tissues of the face and their bony support, and development of criteria for establishing similarity.

Although this field has attracted attention for nearly a century, and its history features such prominent scientists as Virchow, Kollmann, His, von Eickstedt, Gerasimov, and others, our knowledge in this area is far from complete (Krogman and İşcan 1986). This situation can be traced to the fact that anatomical and X-ray methods have thus far failed to produce sufficient data on various population groups for statistical analysis. The results of controlled studies and the application of the reconstruction methods for craniofacial identification reveal the existence of multiple connections between the morphological features of the face and skull (Balueva et al., 1988). However, reliable standards can be established only on the basis of statistically valid data.

ULTRASONIC ECHO LOCATION

In the last few years, governed by the above assumptions, we undertook studies of various ethno-racial population groups from the former USSR to add to our data bank. The program included research into correlations between the thickness of soft tissues from different parts of the face, as well as verification of the connections between morphological features of the face and their bony support.

This research resulted in a new method of ultrasonic echo location for measuring soft tissue (Lebedinskaya et al., 1979). Unlike previous methods (measurements of corpses and X-ray analysis of profiles), ultrasonic probing has a number of significant advantages. It allows studies of very large populations without endangering health, and thus provides a massive amount of information. Also, the ultrasonic apparatus (Echophthalmoscope EOS-21) is easy to use and readily transportable. The investigation covers 17–20 anthropometric points of the face from five morphological zones, where the thickness of the soft tissues is measured (Fig. 1).

At present, a total of 1,695 individuals, including groups of Koreans, Buryats, Kazakhs, Bashkirs, Uzbeks, Armenians, Abkhazians, Russians, and Lithuanians, have been studied. Because age-related changes affect the thickness of soft tissues at the surface of the face (Veselovskaya, 1989), the sample was limited to persons between the ages of 20 and 50 years.

Table 1 includes the means and standard deviations for the thickness of soft tissue features in the groups studied. Calculations of asymmetry and excess coefficients reveal that the distribution of the features under discussion fit within a normal range of variation. The standards presented for the thickness of soft tissues at different parts of the face can be recommended for specialists in craniofacial identification.

To study the correlative variability of these features, correlation matrices were produced for each of the groups. X^2 statistics with transformed Z-scores were then used to test the significance of differences in the correlation coefficients for each pair of features in all groups. In the majority of cases, the differences turned out to be insignificant. The correlation matrix struc-

TABLE 1. Variation of Soft Tissue Thickness (mm) in Males and Females of Different Ethnic Groups

Landmarks	Sex	Koreans Mean	S.D.	Buryats Mean	S.D.	Kazakhs Mean	S.D.	Bashkirs Mean	S.D.	Uzbeks Mean	S.D.	Armenians Mean	S.D.	Abkhazians Mean	S.D.	Russians Mean	S.D.	Lithuanians Mean	S.D.
N	M	91		95		84		155		55		55		50		72		188	
	F	91		167		99		—		71		74		59		101		188	
Metopion	M	4.5	0.98	4.5	0.88	4.5	0.87	5.1	0.85	5.1	0.71	4.7	0.81	4.5	0.72	5.3	0.86	4.7	0.83
	F	4.5	0.89	4.7	0.95	4.9	0.90	—	—	5.0	0.71	4.9	0.91	4.6	0.77	5.3	0.77	4.6	0.67
Superciliary	M	5.2	0.81	5.4	0.79	5.2	0.82	5.6	0.89	5.4	0.76	5.2	0.83	5.2	0.72	5.8	0.98	5.1	0.72
	F	5.2	0.86	5.7	1.00	5.6	0.87	—	—	5.5	0.77	5.8	1.09	5.4	0.63	5.9	0.95	5.3	0.70
Glabella	M	5.1	0.80	5.4	0.75	5.3	0.79	5.6	0.84	5.4	0.75	5.3	0.90	5.2	0.74	5.8	0.79	5.5	0.75
	F	5.4	0.89	5.6	0.88	5.6	0.86	—	—	5.5	0.77	5.7	0.98	5.4	0.75	6.0	0.89	5.5	0.78
Nasion	M	4.5	0.79	4.8	0.85	4.8	0.91	5.8	0.85	5.7	0.87	5.8	0.89	5.8	1.15	5.6	0.94	5.4	0.96
	F	4.4	0.86	4.5	0.89	4.6	0.70	—	—	5.3	0.77	5.7	0.84	5.4	0.84	5.5	0.90	5.0	0.77
Rhinion	M	2.8	0.31	2.8	0.43	3.0	0.38	3.8	0.56	4.1	0.68	3.2	0.47	3.0	0.41	3.8	0.81	3.1	0.20
	F	2.9	0.35	2.8	0.30	2.9	0.38	—	—	4.0	0.56	3.4	0.62	3.0	0.61	3.7	0.70	3.1	0.25
Lateral point of the nose	M	2.9	0.31	2.9	0.33	3.0	0.36	4.0	0.75	3.9	0.66	3.3	0.51	—	—	3.9	0.83	3.1	0.27
	F	2.9	0.28	2.9	0.33	3.0	0.33	—	—	3.9	0.58	3.5	0.51	—	—	3.8	0.75	3.2	0.22
Maxillary	M	13.2	1.86	14.5	1.96	13.2	1.63	11.6	2.36	14.1	1.88	13.2	2.58	—	—	12.4	2.36	12.4	1.83
	F	13.9	1.65	15.8	1.79	14.5	1.90	—	—	15.5	2.14	15.2	1.84	—	—	14.2	2.49	13.5	1.39
Malare	M	9.8	1.85	10.6	1.77	9.8	2.02	9.3	1.47	9.3	2.04	9.3	1.31	—	—	9.8	1.60	9.3	1.64
	F	12.2	2.02	13.6	1.78	12.6	2.09	—	—	11.7	1.93	12.3	2.09	—	—	12.4	1.97	11.7	1.77
Zygion	M	4.7	0.80	4.5	0.89	4.5	0.78	5.0	0.93	4.5	0.58	4.8	0.66	—	—	5.1	0.87	4.7	0.64
	F	5.6	0.90	5.0	0.77	5.3	0.88	—	—	5.0	0.70	5.3	0.96	—	—	5.4	0.92	4.9	0.65

Measurement	Sex	1	SD	2	SD	3	SD	4	SD	5	SD	6	SD	7	SD	8	SD	9	SD
Supracanine	M	10.4	1.33	10.8	1.21	10.7	1.34	10.1	1.34	10.2	1.66	10.5	1.41	10.7	1.34	10.5	1.30	11.2	1.32
	F	9.3	0.95	9.8	1.04	9.9	1.01	—	—	9.8	1.04	9.6	0.93	9.7	1.24	9.7	1.14	9.6	1.15
Philtrum	M	11.1	1.44	11.8	1.52	11.7	1.40	11.6	1.64	11.9	1.63	12.0	1.53	—	—	11.5	1.59	12.5	1.45
	F	9.6	1.13	10.2	1.23	10.3	1.30	—	—	11.0	1.27	10.1	1.06	9.7	1.04	10.6	1.49	10.6	1.49
Upper lip	M	12.6	1.73	13.5	1.90	12.4	1.70	13.0	1.90	13.1	2.02	12.8	1.75	12.0	1.80	12.4	1.91	13.2	1.83
	F	10.6	1.57	11.7	1.81	11.1	1.53	—	—	12.1	1.51	10.8	1.52	10.0	1.47	10.9	1.77	11.0	1.79
Lower lip	M	13.8	1.51	14.5	1.63	13.7	1.61	14.5	1.72	14.0	1.98	14.3	1.51	13.3	1.77	13.8	1.75	14.1	1.60
	F	12.3	1.49	13.1	1.73	12.4	1.42	—	—	13.1	1.52	12.2	1.45	11.9	1.51	12.3	1.70	12.2	1.57
Upper point of the chin	M	11.3	1.34	11.7	1.53	11.2	1.07	11.3	1.47	11.2	1.46	11.2	1.19	11.7	1.50	11.5	1.40	11.1	1.26
	F	11.1	1.16	11.2	1.37	11.1	1.20	—	—	10.8	1.40	10.4	1.21	11.5	1.78	11.1	1.21	10.5	1.40
Chin	M	10.6	1.85	11.4	1.93	10.9	1.66	10.9	1.88	11.2	1.90	11.2	1.89	11.7	1.89	11.6	1.83	11.5	1.76
	F	11.1	1.71	11.9	1.82	11.4	1.53	—	—	10.6	1.52	10.8	1.57	11.3	1.87	11.8	1.74	11.1	1.53
Gnathion	M	6.3	1.17	6.8	1.18	6.4	1.25	—	—	6.4	0.97	6.8	0.88	—	—	—	—	6.7	0.94
	F	6.5	1.12	6.9	1.28	6.6	1.21	—	—	6.3	1.00	6.3	0.90	—	—	—	—	6.2	0.98
Mandibular body	M	12.8	3.43	13.1	3.12	12.6	2.80	10.1	2.26	11.4	2.94	13.3	2.51	—	—	12.0	3.07	13.2	3.15
	F	14.6	2.83	14.8	2.54	14.6	2.72	—	—	13.1	2.40	14.3	2.77	—	—	13.8	2.65	14.6	2.55
Lower margin of mandible	M	6.1	1.62	6.2	1.43	5.6	1.22	—	—	6.0	1.46	6.8	1.24	—	—	—	—	6.0	1.07
	F	6.9	1.53	7.2	1.57	7.0	1.58	—	—	6.5	1.09	7.1	1.38	—	—	—	—	6.0	1.15
Mandibular branch	M	17.0	2.26	17.2	2.02	17.0	2.06	—	—	16.8	2.02	—	—	—	—	—	—	18.0	2.08
	F	17.0	2.18	17.5	1.67	16.9	2.13	—	—	16.9	1.95	—	—	—	—	—	—	17.5	2.10
Gonion	M	4.6	0.96	4.5	0.94	4.6	0.79	5.4	1.07	5.1	0.72	5.2	0.82	—	—	5.2	1.05	4.7	0.76
	F	5.4	1.22	5.1	1.01	5.2	1.24	—	—	5.3	0.99	5.5	1.00	—	—	5.3	0.98	4.7	0.85

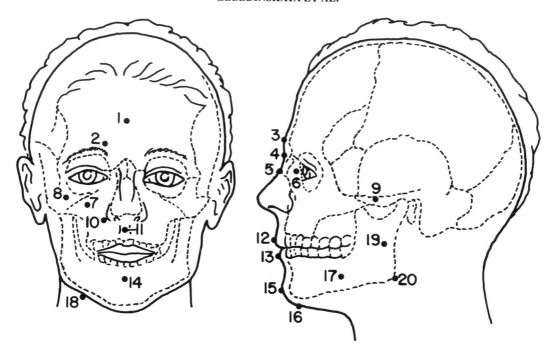

Fig. 1. Points where soft tissue thickness are measured. **Forehead**: 1, Metopion; 2, superciliary; 3, glabella. **Nose**: 4, Nasion; 5, rhinion; 6, lateral point of the nose. **Cheekbones**: 7, Maxillary; 8, malare; 9, zygion. **Mouth**: 10, Supracanine; 11, philtrum; 12, upper lip; 13, lower lip. **Lower jaw**: 14, Chin fissure (upper point of the chin); 15, chin; 16, gnathion; 17, middle of the mandibular body; 18, lower margin of the mandible; 19, mandibular branch; 20, gonion.

ture reflects uniform variability within groups, and all of the groups displayed considerable similarity of matrices with no significant differences in correlation coefficients. This similarity allowed us to produce average matrices—one for males, another for females (Fig. 2). (The data on Abkhazian groups were not considered due to a lack of information on a number of features. The average matrices included 17 features, present in all remaining groups. The initial number of features was left unchanged.)

An analysis of the diagrams (Fig. 2) discloses that high positive correlations exist between features within each of the five morphological zones of the face (forehead, nose, cheekbones, mouth, and lower jaw). The analysis of the relative variability of features, reflecting the distribution of soft tissues at different zones of the face, reveals high values for correlations

between points of the forehead, cheekbones, and mandibular regions, as well as at nasion. Lack of significant correlation coefficients for points in oral and nasal areas (except nasion) with those from other facial zones indicates the independent variability of soft tissue thickness in these zones.

In the next step, cluster analysis was carried out on the basis of the average correlation matrices. Dendrograms (Fig. 3) illustrating the process of clusterization were built, and clearly show three clusters. The first includes all points of the forehead, cheekbones, and mandibular zones, along with nasion. The second cluster is composed of points in the oral region, and the third, situated farther away from the rest, includes rhinion and the lateral point of the nose. In this way, the entire system of features was subdivided into three independent complexes,

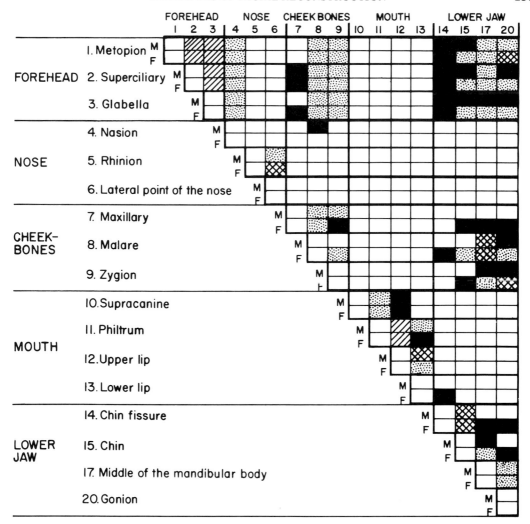

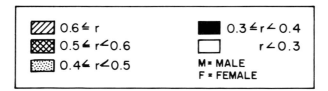

Fig. 2. A system of feature correlations for soft tissue for the face in males and females.

each one demonstrating a high degree of positive correlation of the features in the complex. This analysis also revealed a slight difference in correlative variability between the sexes. In females, the soft tissue at nasion varies more independently from other points of the face than in males.

Canonical analysis was chosen to assess differentiation between groups on the basis of distribution within groups. This method, applied to

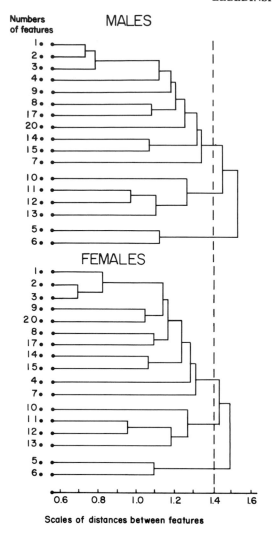

Numbers
of features

MALES

FEMALES

0.6   0.8   1.0   1.2   1.4   1.6

Scales of distances between features

Fig. 3. Graphic representation of cluster analysis of soft tissue thickness (based on intragroup average correlation matrices).

intergroup covariance matrix was calculated that reflects the intergroup variability of the whole set of features. The average intragroup covariance matrix—an indicator of variability of the features within groups—was also computed.

The application of canonical analysis results in a set of discriminators (Y_1, Y_2, . . .) and corresponding vectors. Personal or private number is the special mathematical term for this vector and is symbolized by the letter **L**. The value of this vector is determined by the total diversity and intragroup dispersion.

Canonical analysis chooses features that provide maximum discrimination between individuals. These are the features that differ most distinctly among the groups studied. Each feature is weighted by a discriminator component whose value reflects its usefulness in separating groups. For example, if the value corresponding to a certain feature is nearly zero, it does not contribute much to this process, whereas a high figure for the vector Y component makes the feature a valuable indicator of intergroup diversity.

An important property of canonical analysis is that it can generate a convenient graphic presentation of the relative location of the groups in question in the plane of the first two discriminators, which describe the most important variables of intergroup variability. First, the specific values of the discriminators are established for each group. These present a sum of discriminator components corresponding to particular features multiplied by the average absolute value of all the features in the given group. The resulting group means of the first and second discriminators serve as coordinates (Y_1 and Y_2) pinpointing the location of each group in the plane.

In the present study, intragroup dispersion was estimated from average covariance matrices of all the male and female groups studied. Intragroup covariance matrices were calculated to estimate the intergroup dispersion of features involving zonal distribution of soft tissue thickness.

Table 2 illustrates the means for components

a multitude of groups, results in a few discriminators that subdivide them into naturally existing sets. Among the latter, differences in the discussed complexes of features are considerable, while there is no significant difference within groups (Deryabin, 1983).

The mean values of features form the basis for canonical analysis and the covariance matrices calculated for each of the groups. Next, an

TABLE 2. Results of Canonical Analysis Applied to Features of Soft Tissue Thickness[a]

Features	Males			Females		
	Y_1	Y_2	Y_3	Y_1	Y_2	Y_3
Metopion	0.234	-0.070	0.468	0.198	-0.092	0.311
Superciliary	0.306	-1.017	-0.056	-0.357	0.791	-0.274
Glabella	-0.649	0.901	-0.750	0.087	-0.522	0.261
Nasion	0.368	0.462	0.291	0.501	-0.195	0.208
Rhinion	0.932	-0.064	1.527	1.073	0.179	-0.500
Lateral point of the nose	0.779	0.010	0.323	0.973	0.582	0.333
Maxillary	-0.107	-0.084	0.220	-0.035	0.397	-0.020
Malare	0.019	-0.381	-0.097	-0.118	0.138	0.123
Zygion	0.069	0.035	-0.334	-0.005	-0.438	-0.806
Supracanine	-0.149	0.271	-0.081	-0.119	0.127	0.053
Philtrum	0.040	0.330	0.103	0.240	-0.281	0.342
Upper lip	-0.030	-0.106	0.036	-0.815	0.177	-0.037
Lower lip	0.075	-0.050	-0.106	-0.007	0.155	0.040
Chin fissure	-0.074	-0.250	-0.052	-0.158	0.058	-0.178
Chin	0.028	0.150	0.028	-0.027	-0.047	0.138
Middle of the mandibular body	-0.154	0.170	-0.005	-0.029	-0.163	0.124
Gonion	0.446	-0.009	0.226	-0.124	0.056	-0.564
Personal No. L	199.33	54.60	22.17	174.36	69.16	24.14

[a]Discriminator components, Y_1, Y_2, and Y_3, and personal numbers, L.

of the first three discriminators, Y_1, Y_2, and Y_3, and the corresponding means of personal numbers. It can be seen that the contribution of the third discriminator is already eight to nine times smaller than the contribution of the first: $L_{Y3} =$ 22 and $L_{Y1} = 199$ in men, $L_{Y3} = 24$ and $L_{Y1} = 174$ in women. Thus, the addition of other vectors will not significantly improve the results.

In both sexes, the superciliary point and glabella from the forehead zone, all the points of the nasal zone (nasion, rhinion, lateral of the nose), and gonion from the mandibular zone contributed significantly to intergroup diversity according to the three directions outlined. In males, metopion and malare points, and in females, maxillary, zygion, and supralabial points are also important discriminators (Table 2).

Discriminant scores for each ethnic group were calculated by multiplication of the average mean of the feature and corresponding element of the vector. The sum of the former results provides the first two discriminators (Y_1

and Y_2) in each of the groups (Table 3). The following tabulation demonstrates how these values are obtained in Russian females:

Site of Soft Tissue Thickness	Mean	Discriminators	
		Y_1	Y_2
Glabella	5.0	0.30	0.08
Nasion	3.0	-0.21	0.10

using this data and the following discriminant formulae:

$$Y_1 = 5.0 \times 0.30 + 3.0 \times (-0.21) = 0.87$$
$$Y_2 = 5.0 \times 0.08 + 3.0 \times 0.10 = 0.70.$$

Figure 4 illustrates the relative locations of the groups in the plane of the first two discriminators. Each point defined by coordinates Y_1, Y_2 forms the center of the intragroup distribution. The circles constructed from these centers (with $r = t$) include the areas of individual means in each of the groups. If this area in-

TABLE 3. Sums of Values of the First and the Second Discriminators of Canonical Analysis (Y_1, Y_2) in the Ethnic Groups Studied

Groups	Y_1 Men	Y_1 Women	Y_2 Men	Y_2 Women
Koreans	4.665	-3.429	1.645	7.371
Buryats	3.756	-4.775	1.671	8.900
Kazakhs	4.293	-3.622	2.246	7.879
Bashkirs	7.229	—	2.088	—
Uzbeks	6.857	-1.657	2.284	9.182
Armenians	5.397	-1.815	3.135	8.326
Russians	6.590	-1.210	2.199	8.006
Lithuanians	4.613	-2.634	3.517	7.149

cludes 95% of the observations, then according to the properties of normal distribution, its radius equals 1.96 units of discriminator; for 99% of cases, 2.58; and at 99.9% it increases to 3.30 units.

In order not to overload the picture, the circles in Figure 4 were constructed from the centers of intragroup distributions belonging to the most distant groups. For males, these turned out to be Buryats and Bashkirs, and for females, Buryats and Russians.

As can be seen from the diagrams, there is considerable overlapping of individual means in the terminal (most distant) groups, where $t = 3.30$. It includes the majority of other group centers. The areas covering 95% of observations ($t = 1.96$) for the most distant groups show much less overlap and include only the closest center. It is, however, easy to presume that if all of the circles are constructed from these centers, then all significant gaps between populations will disappear.

The above information presents evidence of minor differences in zonal distribution of soft tissue thickness in the face, which are most clearly expressed between those group clusters that are farthest apart on the drawing. In both sexes there is some overlap of Mongoloid and Europoid groups. It is interesting to note that one group of mixed origin—Kazakhs—approaches the Mongoloids, while another—Bashkirs—approaches the Europoids.

The male groups of Bashkirs, Uzbeks, and Russians, when compared to Buryats, Koreans, and Kazakhs, exhibit somewhat thicker soft tissues in the nasal region (at all three points) and gonion, while thickness decreases at glabella. Armenians and Lithuanians are about average

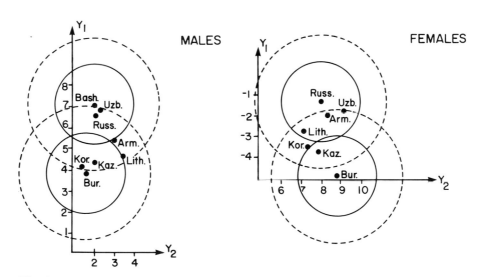

Fig. 4. Graphic representation of the canonical analysis results. Relative positions of the ethnic groups in the plane of the first two discriminators Y_1 and Y_2. The radii of circles correspond to $t = 1.96$ (———) and $t = 3.30$ (– – –).

in these areas. The second discriminator did not contribute to further separation (Fig. 4, Table 3).

Among females, the representatives of the Russian, Uzbek, and Armenian groups display a tendency for greater soft tissue thickness in the nasal region and insignificant thickness in the superciliary and supralabial points when compared to Buryats. The same is true to a slightly lesser degree when they are compared to Kazakhs and Koreans. Lithuanians display average means of informative features. For the second vector, the means of the discriminators were close for all groups.

Thus, canonical analysis demonstrated considerable uniformity of the groups, as far as zonal distribution of soft tissues is concerned. A tendency for some increase in the thickness of soft tissues in the nasal region was noted in both sexes of Europoids as compared to Mongoloids.

Thus, analysis of intergroup variability of the feature complexes revealed a certain gradient of variability, along which the studied groups are regularly distributed. Areas of individual means of all groups overlap significantly. However, in males, and to a slightly lesser extent in females, there are concentrations of groups in the regions of the opposing poles of the revealed direction of variability. One of these poles features predominantly Mongoloid groups, the other predominantly Europoid groups.

Like any independent system of features (morphological, odontological, dermatoglyphic), the parameter complex of zonal distribution of tissue thickness displays its own regularities in intergroup differentiation. These do not strictly follow the morphological race classifications. Each is particular to and significant for the feature system studied.

RADIOGRAPHIC APPROACH

Far more complicated is the approach to the study of physiognomy and the corresponding morphological features of the cranium. In the first place, the correlative dependences can be revealed only on a great deal of data. The ana-

tomical method does not provide such quantities, not to mention the inevitable posthumous changes in soft tissues that seriously alter the actual correlations.

The dissection of corpses provided us with a single result—a rather more accurate location of the origin of the ligamentum palpebrale mediale, locating the position of the medial corner of the eye (Lebedinskaya, 1957). Unfortunately, such functional relationships are scarce among features of interest to us.

The radiographic method also has serious faults. Radiographs are suitable for measurements only if special conditions are followed (distance from tube focus: 1.5–2 m fixed position of the head, etc.). For that reason, the archives of clinics cannot provide reliable material for our studies. This makes it impossible to obtain material on different population groups.

In the early 1950s we collected a considerable number of X-rays (415) of Russians that met the standards necessary for measuring. The bone contour and face profile were readily discernible. This collection provided the basis for the study of correlations between the parameter of the external nose and the cranial nasal notch. The highest correlations were found between the height of the bony nose and general length of the nasal ridge ($r = 0.8$) and the height of piriform aperture and length of the cartilaginous nose ($r = 0.7$). Dependence between protrusion of the cartilaginous nose, general length of its ridge, and height of the nose on the skull was slightly weaker ($r = 0.5$–0.6). This refers also to the relationship between the nasal notch (incisura nasalis) and the form of the cartilaginous nasal ridge ($r = 0.6$ after Spearman). A low positive correlation was found for the position of the nasal tip and direction of the anterior nasal spine. Dependence was found to be very low for the direction of the anterior nasal spine and the angle of the nasal base. There was practically no relationship between the width of the nose and width of the piriform aperture (Lebedinskaya, 1973).

The most difficult object in reconstruction of the face from the skull is the form of the vertical profile of the nasal ridge. On the basis of the X-ray series mentioned above, a method of nasal profile reconstruction, somewhat different from Gerasimov's (1949), was developed (Lebedinskaya, 1976). The construction of the profile on the lateral craniogram is based on the vertical line connecting two craniometric points (nasion and prosthion). A parallel line passing through the most protruding point of the nasal bones (the latter is established in relation to nasion–rhinion) presents the "axis of symmetry" for the outlines of the nasal notch in the skull (incisura nasalis) and of the cartilaginous parts of the external nose.

The method was tested by comparison of the actual profile and the profile reconstructed from the same radiograph. When the results were verified, it was found that 83.1% of the cases corresponded accurately, 4.6% showed a definite similarity, and 13.3% were in error.

To check a new method of nasal reconstruction, the investigator constructs the external nose, based on the outline of the nasal notch drawn from a radiograph of the cadaveral head. Then, the somatological program (Bunak, 1941) was used to compare the reconstruction of the nasal ridge (points 1–4) made by the investigator with the actual nasal profile of the individual in the X-ray. It is important that the investigator did not see the actual radiographs or cadavera (i.e., he did not know the real shape of the external nose). A comparison of these results gave 63% full correspondence, with 28% exhibiting deviations of one point, and 9% deviating at two points (in all of the cases, mistakes concerned the second and third points of the vertical profile of the nasal ridge).

It was also important to learn if this method, developed on Russians, could be applied to other groups. Therefore, it was used for the comparison of data acquired during somatological studies of the morphological features of profiles in contemporary populations that were reconstructed from a recent cranial series taken from the same region. This study involved Buryats, Eskimos, Tchuktches, and Highlanders of Pamier, and the results revealed that the method can also be used for these groups (Zolotarieva et al., 1984).

The material in forensic departments, i.e., the skull and photographic image of the living person, is an unreliable source for verification of correlations between the skull and soft tissue. These are random assemblages not systematically related to any particular population, or territory. Furthermore, the number of usable photographs in this group is severely limited by their generally poor quality—most of them were not taken by professionals and do not meet the standards needed for photographic anthropometry.

PALPATORY MARKING

Another method—palpatory marking—suggested and tested by the authors turned out to be much more effective. For convenience and measurement accuracy, the palpated points on the face were marked by grease paint with a thin makeup stick. Studies carried out on living people yielded a great deal of data that revealed the interrelationships between separate physiognomic features and correlations between the latter and a number of morphological features in the skull.

Since the 1987 investigations, complete data has been collected from only two contrasting populations: Lithuanians (Europoid group, $N = 468$) and Buryats (Mongoloid group, $N = 237$). A comparison of the respective intragroup correlation matrices revealed a number of complexes of correspondingly varying features. Among them, we used only those that have significance for reconstruction and can be found in all the populations without exception, because they reflect stable biological regularities. In this way chance resemblances can be excluded.

Current studies, based on the radiographic material of the Russian group, revealed that there is practically no dependence between the width of piriform aperture and the width of the nose. Still, our familiarity with forensic material on photographic matching allowed us to observe a correlation between the width of the nose and the distance between alveolar protrusions of the canines (juga alveolaria). The validity of these observations was tested. The alveolar prominences of canines were palpated, marked on the face with grease paint, and measured at the level of subnasale (Table 4).

The correlation matrices revealed a definite interrelated feature complex, including nose width, height of nasal ala, width of divergence of nasolabial folds, and distance between canine alveolar protrusions at the level of subnasale. Multiple regression analysis confirmed the validity of this complex of interrelated features: The coefficients of multiple correlation and regression were highly significant at the $P < 0.001$ level (Table 5).

To test this method, studies were carried out in an abbreviated program, so the correspond-

ing data could not have been included into the tables. It is, however, noteworthy that these data confirm the interrelations between nose width and the distance between canine alveolar prominences at the level of subnasale. Thus, in Russians, the mean of the pair correlation factor is 0.64 (74 males), in Bashkirs 0.45 (277 males), and in Evenks 0.77 (94 males).

In order to account for age-related changes in the facial morphological features, and bearing in mind that nothing is known about the intensity of changes in the supporting bony structures, the material was subdivided by decade. Unfortunately, the male Buryat group in the 18–20-year range turned out to be too small. Therefore, the data presented is only from mature individuals (Fig. 5).

The complex of features from the nasal region also includes, in a certain sense, the width of the oral slit. At the same time, correlation

TABLE 4. Correlation Coefficients Between Facial Dimensions in Lithuanians (191 Males, 227 Females) and Buryats (131 Males, 186 Females)

Facial Dimensions	Lithuanians Males	Females	Buryats Males	Females
Nasal width and distance between canine alveolar protrusions on the level of subnasale	0.52	0.55	0.71	0.61
Nasal width and height of nasal ala	0.50	0.44	0.30	0.37
Distance of divergence of nasolabial folds and distance between canine alveolar protrusions on the level of subnasale	0.62	0.62	0.51	0.68
Nasal width and distance of diversion of nasolabial folds on the level of subnasale	0.50	0.47	0.40	0.61
Oral slit width and distance between canine alveolar prominences on the level of subnasale	0.41	0.37	0.40	0.44
Oral slit width and nasal width	0.52	0.43	0.40	0.47
Oral slit width and divergence of nasolabial folds on the level of subnasale	0.57	0.44	0.41	0.47
Oral slit width and width of the dental arcade at the level of canines	0.37	0.26	0.07	0.25
Oral slit width and width of the dental arcade at the level of 1st premolars	0.24	0.26	0.05	0.25
Oral slit width and widthof the dental arcade at the level of 2nd premolars	0.24	0.26	0.08	0.31
Upper lip height and height from subnasale to the cutting edge of the crown of the upper medial incisor	0.45	0.49	0.77	0.39
Cutaneous part of the upper lip and height from subnasale to the upper point of the crown of the upper medial incisor	0.43	0.46	0.40	0.32

TABLE 5. Results of Multiple Regression Analysis

Dependent Features	Males				Females			
Independent Features	R	R^2	Reg. Coef.	Const.	R	R^2	Reg. Coef.	Const.
Nasal width				Lithuanians				
1. Height of nasal alae	0.65	0.43	0.61	6.14	0.63	0.40	0.48	
2. Distance between canine alveolar prominences	0.71	0.51	0.25		0.56	0.31	0.28	3.63
				Buryats				
1. Distance between canine alveolar prominences	0.70	0.50	0.58	12.11	0.61	0.38	0.28	1.58
2. Height of nasal alae	0.72	0.51	0.14		0.68	0.46	0.44	
Distance between alveolar prominences of canines				Lithuanians				
1. Divergence of nasolabial folds	0.63	0.40	0.35	10.50	0.63	0.40	0.35	7.79
2. Nose width	0.68	0.46	0.52		0.69	0.48	0.38	
				Buryats				
1. Nose width	0.70	0.50	0.65	4.94	0.74	0.55	0.43	
2. Divergence of nasolabial folds	0.75	0.58	0.23		0.68	0.47	0.36	5.70
Width of the oral slit				Lithuanians				
1. Distance between canine alveolar prominences	0.43	0.19	0.50	15.22	0.38	0.14	0.51	19.86
2. Distance between canines	0.49	0.24	0.47		0.43	0.18	0.37	
				Buryats				
1. Distance between canine alveolar prominences	0.42	0.17	0.67	25.61	0.44	0.19	0.54	12.92
2. Distance between second premolars	—	—	—		0.50	0.25	0.31	
Height from subnasale to the cutting edge of the upper media incisor				Lithuanians				
1. General upper lip height	0.47	0.22	0.51	14.25	0.49	0.24	0.56	11.09
				Buryats				
1. General upper lip height	0.47	0.22	0.46	14.25	0.42	0.18	0.21	
2. Height of cutaneous part of upper lip	0.47	0.22	0.29	13.07				
Height from subnasale to the upper point of the crown of the upper medial incisor				Lithuanians				
1. General upper lip height	0.41	0.17	0.29	4.41	0.48	0.22	0.36	2.56
2. Height of cutaneous part	0.44	0.20	0.29		0.50	0.24	0.29	
				Buryats				
1. General upper lip height	0.43	0.19	0.44	5.16				
1. Height of cutaneous part of upper lip					0.32	0.10	0.41	6.60
2. Height of upper lip mucosa					0.34	0.12	0.13	

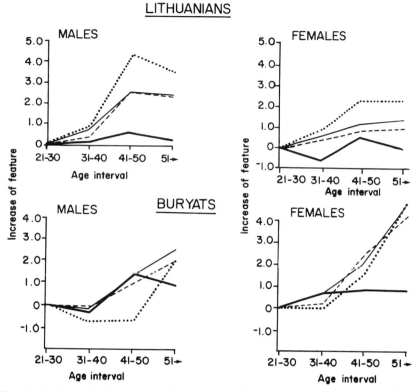

Fig. 5. Relationship between midfacial morphology and age in Lithuanian and Buryat males and females. Nose width (——), distance of diversion of nasolabial folds on the level of subnasale (....), distances between canine alveolar protrusions on the level of subnasale (– – –), and height of nasal alae (——).

between the width of the oral slit and the width of the dental arcade at different levels is low, and practically nonexistent in male Buryats (Table 4). Using multiple correlation and regression, all of the coefficients of these variables are highly significant at the $P < 0.001$ level (Table 5). Thus, in all groups tested, the highest correlation occurs with the alveolar prominences of canines at the level of subnasale.

Age-dependent changes in the width of the oral slit and dental arcade on the levels of canines, first premolars, and second premolars are reflected in Figure 6. To establish the position of the oral slit in relation to the underlying bony structures, measurements were taken of the general height of the upper lip from subnasale and

the distance between that point and the level of the cutting edge of the upper medial incisor. Statistical analysis produced the correlation coefficients shown in Table 4.

Other areas studied included the height of cutaneous part of the upper lip, height from subnasale to the highest point of the crown of the upper medial incisor, height of the mucosa of the upper lip, and crown height of the upper medial incisor. There was no correlation between the cutaneous part of the upper lip and its mucosa, as well as for the height of the mucosa of the upper lip and crown height of the upper medial incisor (Tables 4 and 5).

Figure 7 illustrates age-dependent changes of the general height of the upper medial incisor

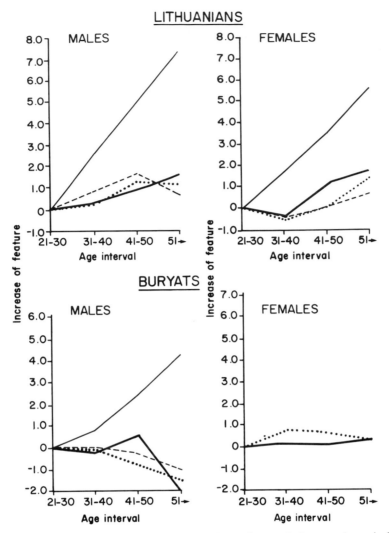

Fig. 6. Relationship between oral slit, dental arcade morphology, and age in Lithuanian and Buryat males and females. Oral slit width (——), width of the dental arcade on the level of canines (– – –), width of the dental arcade on the level of first premolars (.....), and width of the dental arcade on the level of second premolars (——).

and also (separately from the cutaneous part of the lip) its mucosa. It is interesting to note that an increase in the size of the cutaneous part of the upper lip in all groups and both sexes is accompanied by a decrease in the mucosa. The general height of the upper lip and the height from subnasale to the cutting edge of the upper medial incisor display slight age-related changes. The sudden increase in the latter feature in male Lithuanians and female Buryats is probably con-

nected to higher rates of periodontal disease.

THE FUTURE

The continuation of these investigations will help create a data bank from which a reliable basis for methods of facial reconstruction from the skull can be developed. It is only after having that data in our possession that we can

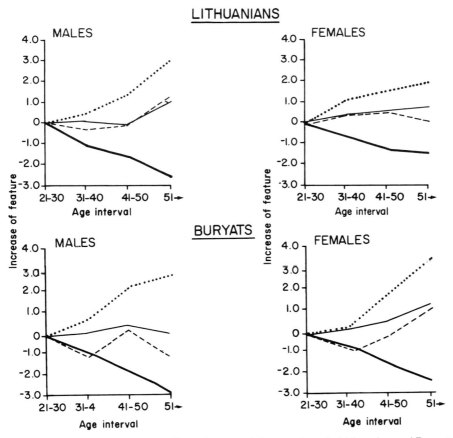

Fig. 7. Relationship between lip region morphology and age in Lithuanian and Buryat males and females. General upper lip height (——), height from subnasale to the cutting edge of the upper medial incisor (– – –), height of cutaneous part of the upper lip (.....), and height of upper lip mucosa (——).

begin to tackle other problems.

It's puzzling that there is only the most general correspondence between racial or ethnic features and the skull. Also, even if all of the points are not precisely matched, it is still possible for the reconstructed image to resemble the original. It seems that ideal precision may not be so important after all. In all likelihood, the human eye does not perceive deviations of a feature within certain limits and permits some leeway. What are those limits? This problem must be studied next.

ACKNOWLEDGMENTS

The editors of this volume and the authors of this chapter are grateful to S.R. Loth for her editing.

REFERENCES

Balueva S, Veselovskaya EV, Lebedinskaya GV, and Pestryakov AP (1988) Anthropological types in the ancient population on the USSR territory. In AA Zubov (ed): Anthropological Reconstructions. Moscow: Nauka (in Russian).

Bunack VV (1941) Anthropometry. Moscow: Uchpedguiz (in Russian).

Deryabin VE (1983) Multidimensional Biometry for Anthropologists. Moscow: Moscow State University Publishers (in Russian).

Gerasimov MM (1949) Principles of Reconstructions of the Face on the Skull. Moscow: Nauka (in Russian).

Krogman WM, and İşcan MY (1986) The Human Skeleton in Forensic Medicine. Springfield, Ill: Charles C Thomas.

Lebedinskaya GV (1957) On the problem of reproduction of the actual shape of the eyes in reconstructions of the face on the skull. Short communications of the Ethnographic Institute of USSR Academy of Sciences, Issue 27, Moscow (in Russian).

Lebedinskaya GV (1973) Correlations between the upper part of the facial skull and the tissues, covering it. In GV Lebedinskaya and GV Rabinovich (eds): Anthropological Reconstructions and Problems in Palaeoethnography. Moscow: Nauka, pp 38–57 (in Russian).

Lebedinskaya GV (1976) Plastic reconstruction of the face on the skull and its developmental trends. Sov Ethnogr 4:63–70 (in Russian).

Lebedinskaya GV, Stepin VS, Surnina TS, Fedosyutkin BA, and Tscherbin LA (1979) The first experience of application of ultrasound for the studies of the thickness of soft facial tissues. Sov Ethnogr 4:121–131 (in Russian).

Veselovskaya EV (1989) Age-dependence of changes in the facial soft tissues in Bashkirs. In VV Koroteyeva (ed): Ethnography, Anthropology and Related Disciplines: Interrelations Between Objects and Methods. Moscow: Institute of Ethnography, pp 78–84 (in Russian).

Zolotarieva IM, Lebedinskaya GF, and Morozova NK (1984) Results of comparison of ancient and recent populations in respect of some racio-diagnostic features. Sov Ethnogr 5:59–69 (in Russian).

Chapter 15

The Relationship of Skull Morphology to Facial Features

Boris A. Fedosyutkin and Jonas V. Nainys*

Scientific Research Laboratory of the Criminalistics Center of the Ministry of Internal Affairs, Moscow 123060, Russia (B.A.F.); Department of Anatomy and Forensic Medicine, Kaunas Medical Institute, Kaunas, Lithuania (J.V.N.)

Identifying the remains of missing persons is often a challenge for law enforcement and investigative bodies. The absence of documents and witnesses, and injury and decomposition often render the body, and especially the face, unrecognizable. High migration rates in large territories with different climatic zones and relatively low population density compound the problem of finding and identifying the skeletal remains of persons whose death ensued under questionable or unknown conditions.

There is no register of population attributes, especially for identification purposes (in contrast to, for example, the fact that many countries maintain dental records), so in any case when remains are detected, identification depends on the availability of objective data on an allegedly missing individual. These may consist of cranial and dental roentgenographs, evidence of blood group, and most importantly, photographs of the face. All available information, including age, stature, dates and conditions surrounding the disappearance of the missing person, and the discovery of an unknown corpse, etc., is considered during the investigation. Analogous materials are used for identification of the victims of accidents and natural disasters.

Paul Broca is considered by many to be the first researcher to study the congruences between the structure of the skull and the overlying soft tissues that define appearance. He noted the complexity of this concept and how it was exacerbated by the great variation in soft tissue thickness from one person to the next. He thus was the first to scientifically consider the concept of individuality in the human face.

Also in the 19th century, Schaaffhausen (1884) reconstructed a woman's head by covering the skull with materials to imitate the soft tissue. In this case, thickness was chosen arbitrarily by the author. At the end of the last century, heightened interest in facial reconstruction from the skull was associated with the identification of skeletal remains belonging to a number of distinguished people, including Kant (Kupffer and Bessel-Hagen, 1881), Bach (His, 1895), Schiller and Raphael (Welcker, 1883, 1896), and Haydn (Tandler, 1909). In turn, this activity led to the search for more accurate methods to assess the correspondence between the skull and soft tissue. Different aspects of this problem were considered in many works, such as those of Stieda (1888) and Weisbach (1889). There were reports of attempts to utilize new methods to establish objective criteria—roentgenography (Welcker, 1896), plaster casts (masks), portraits, and sectional data—to detail the structure of separate parts of the face. Reconstructions were attempted by Merkel (1890) and Kollmann (1910) on the skulls of ancient people, in which information about some characteristics was already consciously used. In particular, these authors pointed out correlations between the structure of the soft tissue formations of the nose with the configuration of the piriform aperture of the skull.

The results of scientific research on this problem that had been published around the turn of the century drew the interest of criminalists. It

---

Professor Nainys died on September 18, 1989.

prompted them to conduct controlled studies, including their comparison with photographs taken during life (Gross, 1899). During the collection of data on correlations of the structure of the face and head, many different, and sometimes diametrically opposing, possibilities arose, meaning that several varied faces could be compatible with any given skull.

Tandler (1909) discovered that the configuration of the soft tissues was not correlated with the contour of the bones near the root of the nose, neither was there a connection between the degree of chin protrusion and the thickness of soft tissues on this part of the face. Correlation of the nature and the degree of pronouncement of the nasal spine with nose protrusion was addressed by Virchow (1912). His (1895) and Birkner (1907) noted variations of the thickness of soft tissues based on racial origin. His considered it impossible to predict individual features of the face and, consequently, for only a generalized reproduction to be obtained by reconstruction.

In Russia, Bogdanov (1882) is credited with the first attempt to extrapolate appearance during life from the skull of fossil man (Gerasimov, 1971). Gerasimov made a reconstruction of neolithic Ladoga and other facial reconstruction of fossil man, and reproduced a number of documented portraits by purely empirical means (Gerasimov, 1971).

Practical experience accumulated in this way formed the basis for the application of this method in forensic cases. Gerasimov's monograph *Principles of Reconstruction of the Face on the Skull* was published in 1949. This was followed by a second monograph, *Reconstruction of the Face on the Skull* (1955), that included the results of his continued systematic studies. In this second edition, he described the basic stages of the method, and added copious information on different problems of skull diagnostics. It should be stressed that because of the extreme variability of characteristics, stemming from a variety of causes, the description of the method did not contain a definitive statement of specifics. Many times, Gerasimov emphasized the fact that reconstruction is one method of

identification through which bone is built upon to resemble a living person. Because reconstruction is a problem with many unknowns, it would be an unrealistic goal to expect an exact likeness; thus, our purpose is to approach it as skillfully as possible to minimize error. To this end he emphasized the necessity of collecting additional data on a number of correlations for separate facial and skeletal elements (Fedosyutkin et al., 1984).

Systematic research on the thickness of the integument of the face of living people was carried out in the former USSR in 1979 by means of ultrasound echo ranging (Lebedinskaya et al., 1979). Statistical data on thicknesses in different parts of the face of males and females at various ages were analyzed to assess their correlation with the shape of the face (see Chapter 14, Lebedinskaya et al., this volume).

In 1981, Yordanov published a monograph entitled *Face Reconstruction from the Skull* that made a definite contribution to the development of this methodology. The author initiated a detailed investigation of the degree of symmetry and asymmetry of the facial skeleton, and characteristics of the structure of the jaws and teeth associated with sex and racial origin. Yordanov based his work on Gerasimov's methodological elaborations, and stressed the possibility of using Gerasimov's data and methods for establishing the appearance of people of mixed (Slavic and other European) ancestry who lived in Bulgaria. He further revealed that despite general affinities, a number of differences existed requiring further study. In 1984, Djagaryan published a monograph on facial morphology and plastic reconstruction. However, he did not present any new useful data on this subject, but merely repeated Gerasimov's work.

PERSONAL IDENTIFICATION

The problems of personal identification are thoroughly elaborated in many scientific works (e.g., Leopold, 1978; Zvyagin, 1981; Helmer, 1984; Krogman and İşcan, 1986; İşcan, 1988). In summarizing the literature to date, three basic areas should be singled out in this most complicated problem. First, there must be a careful, scientific study of both general (group) and particular (individual) characteristics in the skull and postcranial skeleton. The second task lies in the choice of methodology to analyze the data, and creation of the portrait (that is, reconstruction of appearance from the skull). Finally, the third task consists of furnishing evidence of the fact that the examined skull belongs to a particular individual, i.e., the establishment of identity (Nainys and Fedosyutkin, 1988).

Knowledge of the characteristics of the skull structure, its separate elements, and their interconnections is a basic necessity for the successful evaluation of these tasks and, consequently, the problem as a whole. To date, considerable data has been derived from studies of the skull. This research has led to improved metric accuracy in shape definition, spatial arrangement, age, and pathological changes of anatomical structures (Speransky, 1988). The need to further develop forensic identification techniques made it imperative to analyze the appearance of the face during life and its relation to the skull, and in turn the skull and its correlation with the image on a photograph.

The first priority is the assessment of the characteristics of the skull using osteometric data. To conduct a study, we used the skulls and photographs taken during life of identified individuals in our archives. More than 200 skull–photo pairs were comprehensively analyzed using a specially prepared program.

The authors focused on parts of the cranial anatomy that are the most significant to appearance during life. Most of the material consisted of Caucasoid skulls (rather than mixed race or Mongoloid). Thus, the question of how population variation and interbreeding affects the skeleton still must be addressed. Experience in this field points to the conclusion that there are certain universal traits of the skull that influence appearance, regardless of geographic or racial differences.

The authors found definite correlations in the structure of separate skull elements and their expression on the face of that individual. In a complicated volumetric structure such as the head, it is impossible to simply define every similarity. A more reasonable goal is to elucidate trends in the range of variation. This, in turn, should lead to more accurate individualization.

On this basis, the choice of a method of facial reconstruction from the skull moves to the next phase. Depending on conditions, one can use both the traditional method of plastic and graphic reconstruction or computer graphics. We suggest a combined approach.

Discovery of the crucial morphological and dimensional criteria forms the basis for identification, irrespective of execution and illustration—photo combination and video superimposition of skull and face. In this case it is necessary to factor in all the information about the victim's race, age, sex, and data from anatomical, anthropological, and serological investigations. This system should reduce the risk of coming to erroneous conclusions.

INTERRELATIONSHIP OF THE SKULL AND FACE

Determination of sex, age, race, ethnicity, body length, and individual peculiarities is made by cranioscopic and craniometric studies of the skull and postcranial skeleton using methods generally accepted in anthropology and forensic medicine (Lebedinskaya, 1976; Krogman and İşcan, 1986; see also Novotný et al., Chapter 6, this volume). The skull is then placed in the Frankfurt horizontal position and is photographed on transparency film to the scale of the pictures (the scale is defined by the centers of the orbits: the pupils of the eyes). The negative slide of the skull is fixed on the illuminated demonstration screen of the instrument and every characteristic is controlled by overlapping the picture on the skull image.

To establish uniformity and comparability, the following sections (elements) of the skull were delineated: the upper part of the head, including arc of the skull and forehead; the lower part of the face; the area of the eyes; the bridge of the nose and superciliary region; the bottom of the ear; cheekbones; nose; and mouth. When pronounced asymmetries are present, they are quantified. Drawings of paired elements (eyes, eyebrows, and ears) are made separately to better reflect any asymmetries. The analysis of the characteristics of the face as a whole is carried out in the final stage.

The examination starts by defining the shape of the upper and the lower parts of the face. This is important for the definition of overall face shape and the choice of statistical data on soft tissue thickness. In our experiments, ultrasound echo ranging was used to determine soft tissue thickness on living people. In this way, the most reliable correlation of these indicators with face shape in the majority of investigated points was revealed. The basic characteristics for reconstruction in full-face position (norma frontalis) are as follows:

1. The shape of the upper head influences appearance (during life) more in males than in females, and it often defines the hairstyle. Depending on the width of the forehead, the height of the transverse arc, and the protrusion of the sincipital tubercle, the four shapes of the transverse arc are defined as: semisphere, pentagonoid, oval, and rectangular (Fig. 1A). Different variants of the drawings reflect different correlations of the arc height and its width; it is much simpler to select the necessary drawing from its fit on the image of the skull on the slide.

2. The hairline—the transition of the smooth surface of the forehead bone into small, rough, tubercles above the forehead—can be located by microscopy (4.8 × magnification) of the surface after coating it with glycerin. If the hairline is indistinct, it can be masked by the hairstyle.

3. It is simple to select the drawing of the haircut when a sample of or information about the victim's hair color and form is available. In the absence of such information about a man's hair, it is advisable to choose a short, close-cropped style that follows the contour of the transverse arc shape at the distance of 1.7–2 mm (the thickness of the soft tissues in the

evaluation of the scale of the image). A few variants of this style can be used for women, taking into account fashion, age, and race.

4. The shape of the temporal lines gives an indication of forehead width. The presence of frontal bosses and slope of the forehead, as well as the protrusion of the bridge of the nose and upper part of the browridge, are approximated at the final stage by retouching.

5. In general, the shape of the lower part of the face repeats the contour of the mandible (Fig. 1B). Overall face shape is revealed when the upper and the lower facial drawings are combined.

6. The shape of the mandible on the slide does not always give a clear indication of the shape of the lower part of the face. Therefore, the mandible itself must be examined. If the gonial angle is over 125° and the coronoid process is high, the lower part of the face is likely to be one of the narrow variants (oval or triangular shape). Angles less than 125° (approaching a right angle) and wide, low, coronoid process favor one of the wide variants (rounded or rectangular) (Fig. 1C).

7. The presence of convexities in the lower lateral margin of the mandibular body (e.g., rocker jaw) are incorporated on the reconstruction by projections in these areas during retouching (Fig. 1D).

8. The degree of elevation in the frontal part of the mandible and the width of its base define the width of the chin (Fig. 1E).

9. If the height of the mandibular body decreases from the chin triangle to the side of the rami, this forms a high chin (Fig. 2A).

10. Everted gonial regions of the mandible are associated with the wide variants of the lower face (Fig. 2B).

11. If the frontal edge of the alveolar arc of the mandible is well developed, projection of the lower lip is pronounced (Fig. 2C).

By direct examination of the skull and mandible in norma frontalis, lateralis, verticalis, and basilaris, other individual characteristics can be revealed. However, since it cannot always be reflected on the reconstruction in the full-face

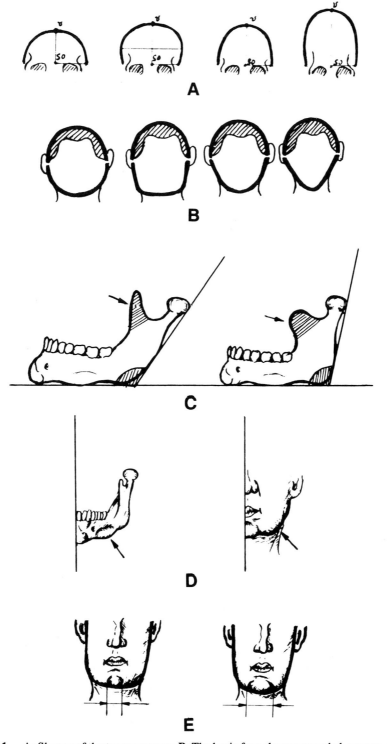

Fig. 1. **A**: Shapes of the transverse arc. **B**: The basic face shapes: rounded, square, oval, and triangular (from **right** to **left**). **C**: The characteristics of the mandibular structure for narrow (**left**) and wide (**right**) variants of the face shape. Arrows indicate differences in the coronoid process. **D**: Convexities in the lower lateral margin of the mandibular body (rocker jaw) and their appearance in the face. **E**: The width of the base of the chin triangle: narrow chin (**left**) and wide chin (**right**).

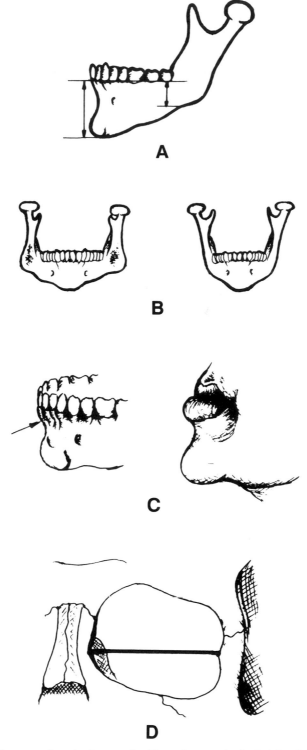

Fig. 2. A: A narrow face is characterized by a decrease in the height of the mandibular body from front to back. **B**: The degree of gonial eversion of the mandible: strong (**left**), absent (**right**). **C**: Pronounced development of the alveolar edge of the mandible. **D**: Location of the eye slit.

projection, we don't dwell on them in detail. When making the drawing of the lower part of the face, it is important to remember that the soft tissue thickness in wide face shapes is about twice that of narrow ones. On our scale, it is 5–6 mm in wide faces, and 2–3 mm in narrow ones. The indices of thickness are relative and can change significantly over one's lifetime. Basic constitution type is more stable, thus we attach great importance to it.

12. The anatomy of the orbit is so complicated and diverse that the characteristics of the eye region on the reconstruction are more often the summary reflection of many attributes. Therefore, we must first investigate all the possible attributes and only then select the optimum drawing. The location of the eye slit is defined by the straight line that connects the tubercle on the lateral border of the orbit (malar tubercle) with the base of the anterior lacrimal crest (Fig. 2D). This tubercle is absent in 15–20% of cases. In these cases, one can use a point on the outer margin of the orbit, 8.4 mm below the fronto-zygomatic suture in males and 9.5 mm below in females.

13. The length of the eye slit is 60–80% of the width of the orbit; its height (the size of the eyelid opening) for Caucasoids is approximately ¼ of the orbit's height for Mongoloids. The pupil of the eye is located in the middle of the orbit (by height).

14. The protrusion of the eyeballs from the orbit is established based on the depth of the orbital cavity, vertical inclination of the orbit, and the thickness and degree of overhang of its upper rim. Deepset eyes are more often found in Caucasoids when the upper rim of the orbit is greatly thickened and protrudes relative to the lower one (in norma lateralis) (Fig. 3A–C).

15. A well-developed (or continuous) browridge and bridge of the nose intensify the impression of deepset eyes because of the shadows cast in the area of the eyelids and the eyes' angles.

16. A wide opening of the eye slit and protruding eyeballs are characteristic of a weak orbital profile, a smooth, thickened outer rim at the transition to the lower part, as it goes to the front of the malar tubercle.

17. In the middle or lateral sections of the upper eyelid, there can be folds that result from characteristics of the structure of the upper rim of the orbit. The fold of the fixed part of the upper eyelid generally traces the direction of the upper rim of the orbit (Fig. 4A). If there is an overhang in the middle part of the superior orbital rim, the fold of the eyelid is located in the middle of it. If the outer rim is thickened and slanted to the back of the upper side of the orbit, the fold is pronounced in this section of the eyelid. When the fold is near the inner angle (epicanthus) of the upper eyelid (which often covers it), it is characteristic of a high orbit, a low- or medium-height nasal bridge, and a long lacrimal fossa. It is most pronounced in Caucasoid and Mongoloid children, but can decrease with increasing age. Both the degree of eyeball protrusion and the folds of the upper eyelid can change as a result of, for example, illness (exophtalmos, edema of the eyelids, etc.), with age, and lid thickness. Information about these conditions must be taken into account from the beginning when planning the eye on the reconstruction.

18. If there is strong development of the supraorbital margin and browridge, the eyebrows are shifted downward, 1–2 mm lower than the upper rim of the orbit, creating the impression of "overhanging" eyebrows (Fig. 4B). This attribute is most pronounced in Caucasoid males and the elderly.

19. The browridge and bridge of the nose define the arrangement and variations of the eyebrows (Fig. 4C). In the case of a weakly developed nasal bridge and browridge, the inner third of the eyebrow (the head) is located in the projection of the orbit, along the supraorbital margin; the middle and outer thirds (the body and tail) of the eyebrows gradually rise to the supraorbital margin and trace its contour.

20. If there is thickening of the outer part of the supraorbital rim and a strong browridge, the eyebrow is arranged over it, forming the angle as shown on the right side of Figure 4D.

21. The mastoid region has morphological attributes that determine some characteristics of

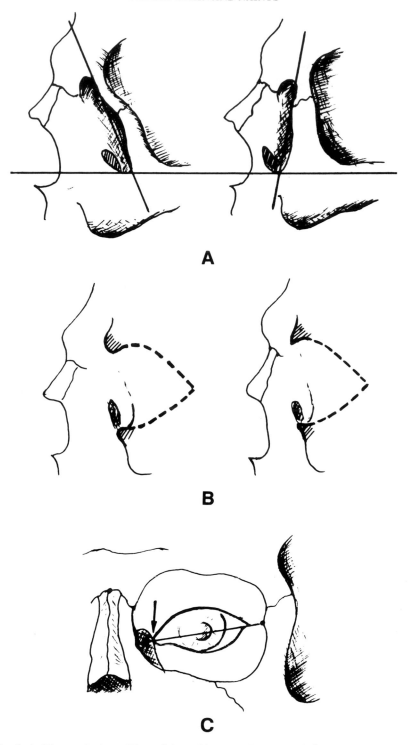

Fig. 3. A: The vertical profiling of the orbit: strongly angled (**left**) and weakly angled (**right**). **B:** Characteristics of the upper margin of the orbit: thickened overhanging rim (**left**) and narrow rim (**right**). **C:** Placement of the eye in the orbit. Arrow indicates inner canthus.

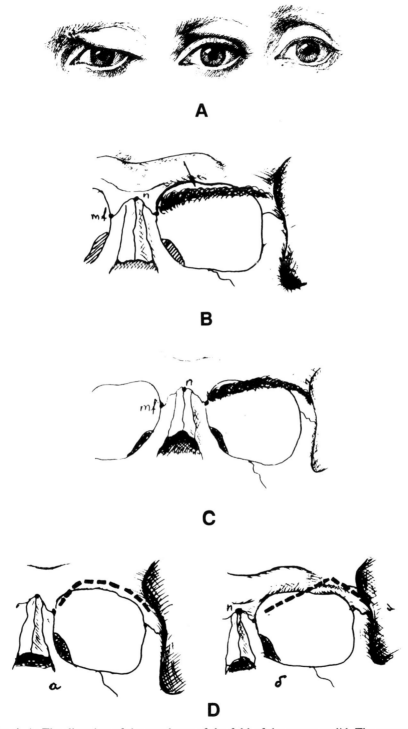

Fig. 4. A: The direction of the overhang of the fold of the upper eyelid. The arrangement of the eyebrow with strongly (**B**) and weakly (**C**) pronounced superior orbital margin. **D**: The form of the upper rim of the eyebrow: arced (**left**) and triangular (**right**).

the structure of the ears. The tragus of the ear corresponds to the upper rim of the external auditory meatus (Fig. 5A).

22. The height of the ear approximates the length of the nose. The protrusion of the ear can be upper, lower, or total. In the case of upper protrusion, the supramastoid crest on the temporal bone is strongly developed and protrudes; with lower protrusion, the outer surface of the mastoid process is rough. When all of these attributes are present, there is total ear protrusion (Fig. 5B,C).

23. The lobe of the ear can be attached (to the cheek) or free. If the mastoid processes are directed downward (with the skull in norma lateralis and set in the Frankfort horizontal), the lobe is attached. If the mastoids point forward, the lobe is free. The features of the ear on the reconstruction cannot be considered absolute except when they are preserved on the body.

24. The cheekbones define the width of the face and its horizontal profile (Fig. 5D). Weak and strong profiling can be approximately differentiated on the frontal surface of the skull, from above and below, depending on the width and height of the curvature of the cheekbones, the depth of the canine fossae, and the value of the nasomalar and zygomaxillary angles.

25. The nose–cheek fold ("smile line") extends from the upper edge of the nostril toward the upper first molar. Its protrusion depends on the depth of the canine fossa, the degree of horizontal face profiling, the projection of the frontal surface of the cheekbones, and the presence or absence of teeth. The depth of the canine fossae—up to 3 mm—is considered shallow. At 4–6 mm it's moderate, and more than 6 mm, deep. Nose–cheek folds are more pronounced when the canine fossae are deep, and profiling of the middle part of the face is strong. This is also the case when teeth are missing and with advancing age.

26. When reconstructing the nose, we can reproduce the nasal ridge (contour, width, root), the tip (shape, width), base, wings (height, shape), the location of the nostrils' axes, and the overall width and the height of the nose. The height of the nose equals the distance from nasion to 1–2 mm below than nasal spine. The width (the greatest distance between the wings of the nose) is defined between the midpoints of the canines or their alveoli (Fig. 6A). The width of the nasal ridge is 1–2 mm greater than the width of the nasal bones.

27. In norma lateralis, the shape of the bony ridge of the nose can be straight, prominent, concave, or wavy. The base of the nose is defined as horizontal, elevated, or prolapsed (Fig. 6B,C). The position of the base of the nose follows the general direction of the central part of the nasal spine.

28. The tip of the nose is formed at the point where imaginary lines, continued from the ridge of the nasal bones and spine, cross. It can be wide (wider than the nose ridge), moderate (equal to the width of the nose ridge), or narrow. A narrow tip of the nose is associated with a long, narrow, pronounced nasal spine and long, narrow nasal (piriform) foramen (Fig. 7A). A wide (fleshy) tip correlates with a short, wide, groovy, nasal spine and low, wide nasal foramen.

29. The wing of the nose begins at the lateral edge of the piriform foramen (nasal sill) at the level of the nasal spine. An exposed nasal septum is characteristic of a crest-shaped base of the nose (Fig. 7B). If the lower edges of the nostrils are positioned at the different levels, this should be reflected on the reconstruction.

31. The closed mouth, under normal conditions, is positioned at the level of the upper edge of the anterior teeth of the mandible. The width of the mouth corresponds to the distance between the mandibular second molars. The height of the lips (when closed) is approximately equal to the height of the enamel of the upper and lower incisors.

32. The width of the philtrum corresponds to the distance between the midpoints of the upper central incisors (Fig. 7C).

33. If prognathism is present, the muzzle area protrudes forward. In case of an overbite or maxillary prognathism, the upper lip projects farther out than the lower one. In the reverse situation, such as an underbite or edge-to-edge occlusion, the lower lip protrudes past the upper one.

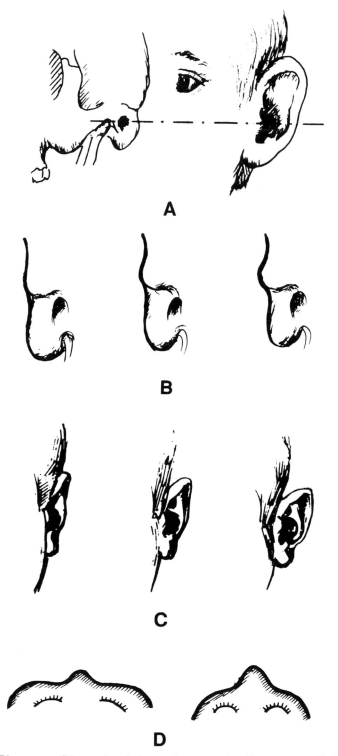

Fig. 5. A: Placement of the ear in relation to the external auditory meatus. **B**: Different degrees of protrusion of the supramastoid crest and the outer surface of the mastoid process: weak (**left**), moderate (**middle**), and strong (**right**). **C**: Protrusion of the ears: weak (**left**), moderate (**middle**), and strong (**right**). **D**: The horizontal profile of the face: weak (**left**) and strong (**right**).

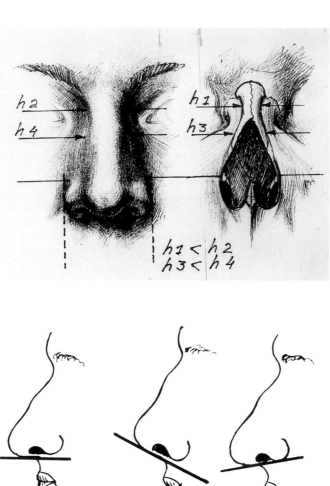

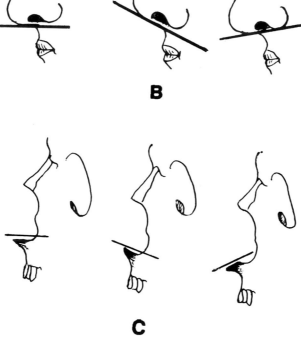

Fig. 6. A: The width of the nose. **B**: Position of the base of the nose: horizontal (**left**), elevated (**middle**), and prolapsed (**right**). **C**: The shapes and direction of the nasal spine: horizontal (**left**), elevated (**middle**), and prolapsed (**right**).

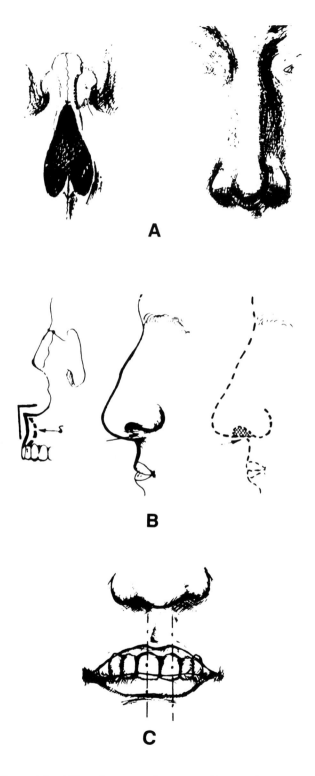

Fig. 7. A: Shape of the piriform foramen and corresponding nose form. **B**: The exposed nasal septum and form of the columella: crest shaped (solid line) and straight (dotted line). **C**: Mouth width, lip height, and the relationship of the philtrum and the central incisors.

34. The line between closed lips can be either straight or arced upward or downward. The direction of this line generally coincides with the line formed when the teeth are closed. In practice, it is difficult to select mouth form corresponding to the majority of examined skull parameters. Therefore, we first consider the width of the mouth and thickness of the lips; the remaining characteristics are derived by "educated guess."

The complex of attributes discussed above is sufficient to draw conclusions from the skull about appearance during life.

DISCUSSION

In the course of scientific and practical work, we have identified some morphological characteristics of the skull and revealed their correlation with appearance as portrayed in photographs of the face. We managed to formulate the concept that individuality can be derived from the skull on this basis.

Individuality is the totality of the variants of the bony structure of every element of the skull. Many of these can be objectively analyzed with our specially developed craniometer, which allows accurate volumetric analysis of the skull with a special computer program (utilizing more than 400 measurements in three-dimensional space). This approach improves the reliability of the method and increases its potential for improvement. The dimensional data were always assessed along with sex, age, and racial or ethnic characteristics. The results were processed both from separately examined elements (areas) and the skull as a whole. Great attention was paid to the objective detection and reproduction of asymmetries of the skull and the face. Our studies have confirmed that this approach can reproduce facial elements and attributes of appearance with three degrees of accuracy: authentically, approximately, and conditionally. Details of the combined graphic method will be published in a subsequent paper.

Authentic reproduction of the total dimen-

sions and shapes of the head, face, mouth, nose, and shape of the eyes is based on their strict correspondence with the bony structure of the skull. The flesh of the face, the lower part of the chin, and the eyes and eyelids can be approximated. Finally, because there is little direct correlation between the skull and features such as the hair, the color of the eyes and skin, the ears, and wrinkles, these can only be conditionally reproduced with less reliability than more anatomically based characteristics. Obviously, the authenticity of reproduced attributes of appearance depends to a considerable degree on the amount of detailed information obtained from the primary examination of the remains by the forensic expert.

Identification is carried out through a comparative examination of objective data collected from the unknown victim, photo superimposition of the images of the skull and photographs, along with other methods generally accepted in forensic medicine and criminalistics. Today, video-based techniques find wider application and make the process of superimposition considerably faster and easier. However, final conclusions are drawn from the examination of the attributes used in the CGM method.

In recent years, the percentage of positive identifications obtained by our method reached 60–70%. In 15–20% of cases, the conclusion was considered probable because of a lack of sufficient objective background data on the missing person, and no match was found for only 10–15% of cases. Thus, the scientific development and successful utilization of this method of facial reconstruction from the skull of contemporary humans has been demonstrated.

In the future, it will be possible to automatically load any metrical data into the computer, execute necessary calculations, and obtain valid recommendations about skulls under investigation. We believe that upon the completion of all planned scientific research (including coupling our craniometer with a computer) and the accumulation of a significant quantity of statistical material on all the dimensional groups, it will be possible to carry out reconstruction on the skull itself automatically, with subsequent correction of individual attributes (if necessary) by the specialist.

ACKNOWLEDGMENTS

The authors express their deep gratitude for the constant consultation and practical assistance during this work to d.m.s. V.N. Zvyagin, S.S. Abramov, and G.V. Lebedinskaya. Particular gratitude goes to the specialists in medical criminalistics, militia officers O.P. Korovansky, L.L. Usatchev, and V.M. Kuzin, who are testing and applying different methods of identification to solve murders for which there is little or no evidence. The editors of this volume are grateful to S.R. Loth for editing this chapter.

REFERENCES

Birkner F (1907) Die Dicke der Gesischtsweichteile bei verschiedenem Alter, Geschlecht und Rasse. Ges Morphol Physiol Munchen 23:140–146.

Djagaryan AD (1984) Facial Morphology and Plastic Reconstruction. Yerevan: Acad Sci Armenian SSR.

Fedosyutkin BA et al. (1984) Investigation of soft tissue thickness by means of ultrasound. In Reports of All-Union Conference on Functional Morphology. Novosibirsk, Siberian Dept AMSc USSR, p 162.

Gerasimov MM (1949) Osnony Vosstanovlieniia Litsa po Cherapu; Gos Izd-vo Sovetskaia (Principles of Reconstruction of the Face on the Skull). Moscow: Nauka (in Russian).

Gerasimov MM (1955) Vosstanovlieniia Litsa po Cherapu; Gos Izd-vo Sovetskaia (Reconstruction of the Face on the Skull). Moscow: Nauka (in Russian).

Gerasimov MM (1971) Face Finder. New York: Lippincott.

Gross H (1899) Die His'sche Regenerastionsmethode. Arch Kriminalanthropol 1:120–121.

Helmer R (1984) Schädelidentifizierung durch elektronische Bildmischung. Zugleich ein Beitrag zur Konstitutionsbiometrie und Dickenmessung der Gesichtsweichteile. Heidelberg: Kriminalstik-Verlag.

His W (1895) Johann Sebastian Bach. Forshungen uber dessen Grabstätte, Gebeine und Antlitz. Bericht an den Rath der Stadt Leipzig. Leipzig: FCW Vogel.

İşcan MY (1988) Rise of forensic anthropology. Yrbk Phys Anthropol 31:203–230.

Kollmann J (1910) Plastische Anatomie des menschlichen Korpers. 3. Absschinitt: Schädel. 3 Aufl. Leipzig: Veith.

Krogman WM, and İşcan, MY (1986) The Human Skeleton in Forensic Medicine. Springfield, Ill: Charles C Thomas.

Kupffer C, and Bessel-Hagen F (1881) Der Schädel Immanuel Kants. Arch Anthropol 13:359–410.

Lebedinskaya GV (1976) Plastic reconstruction of the face on the skull and its developmental trends. Sov Ethnogr 4:63–70 (in Russian).

Lebedinskaya GV, Stepin VS, Surnina TS, Fedosyutkin BA, and Tscherbin LA (1979) The first experience of application of ultrasound for the studies of the thickness of soft facial tissues. Sov Ethnogr 4:121–131 (in Russian).

Leopold D (1978) Personenerkennug durch Superprojektion. In H Hunger and D Leopold (eds): Identification. Leipzig: Johann Absrosius Barth.

Merkel F (1890) Handbuch der Topographischen Anatomie. Braunschweig.

Nainys JV, and Fedosyutkin BA (1988) On skull identification in the Soviet Union. Paper presented at the International Symposium "Advances in Skull Identification via Video Superimposition," 3–5 August, Kiel.

Schaafhausen F (1884) Schädel und Gehirn geisting hervorragen der Männer. Sitzungsber, Niederhein. Ges Natur Heilkunde, Vol 41, Bonn.

Speransky VS (1988) Bases of Medical Craniology. Moscow.

Stieda L (1880) Über die Berechnungen des Schädelindex aus Messungen an lebenden Menschen. Arch Anthropol, Vol 12, Braunschweig.

Tandler Y (1909) Über den Schädel Haydns. Mitt Anthropol Ges 39:260–280.

Virchow H (1912) Die anthropologische untersuchung der nase. Z Ethnol 44:299–337.

Weisbach A (1889) Länge und Breite des Kopfes und Schädels. Mitt Anthropol Ges 7:198–200.

Welcker H (1883) Schiller's Schädel und Todtenmaske, nebst Mittheilungen über Schädel und Todtenmaske Kant's. Braunschweig: Fr Viehweg and Sohn.

Welcker H (1896) Das Profil des menschlichen Schädels mit Röntgenstrahlen am Lebenden dargestellt. Dtch Ges Anthropol 27:38–39.

Yordanov Y (1981) Face Reconstruction from the Skull. Sofia.

Zvyagin VN (1981) Forensic–medical identification of personality from the skull. Autoref dissertation.

Chapter 16

Anatomical and Artistic Guidelines for Forensic Facial Reconstruction

Robert M. George

Universidad Central del Caribe, Hospital Universitario Ramon Ruiz Arnau,
Bayamon, Puerto Rico 00621

Forensic art or medico-legal illustration is a diverse specialty that includes courtroom graphics, evidential and crime scene illustration, composite sketches, and various methods of facial reconstruction and photographic superimposition for purposes of individual identification. Reconstruction techniques were first developed by German anatomists in the late 1800s in attempts to identify historical personages, e.g., Dante, Schiller, Raphael, and Bach (Caldwell, 1981; Krogman and İşcan, 1986). Around the turn of the century and for the next few decades, these methods were primarily used for the museum reconstruction of various species of prehistoric man. It was not until the 1940s that they were first applied to forensic cases of unknown identity. Since the landmark paper of Snow and associates in 1970, the field has rapidly grown in the United States and claims a rather surprising identification rate of nearly 50% (Caldwell, 1981, 1986).

This rate is surprising because, as critics of forensic facial reconstruction are quick to point out: (1) The soft tissue of the face does not fit the skull like a glove (except in cases of extreme emaciation); (2) there are as many facial variations as there are faces (with the negligible exception of identical twins); (3) faces age at different rates and with different intensities; (4) the nutritional status of the face is unpredictable; (5) the subtle details of the eye, nose, and ear cannot possibly be constructed from their gaping cranial apertures; (6) the soft tissues of the lips and chin vary independently from their underlying dental foundations; (7) facial hair patterns are unpredictable, (8) as are dermato-logical and pathological conditions, and so forth. So a 50% identification rate or even a 10% rate is indeed exceptional and calls for an explanation.

Most practitioners of the scientific art of facial reconstruction will readily admit that the ideal of creating a postmortem *portrait* is close to impossible. An *approximation* based on the proper alignment of features that will spark a memory and generate a lead is the best that can be hoped for, and, judging from the statistics, such approximations have been moderately successful. The key words here are "the proper *alignment* of features." It is obviously impossible to precisely predict the intricate details of the eye from the bony orbital outline, the nose from the piriform aperture, the ear from the external auditory meatus, or the lips from the anterior dentition, but it is possible to accurately position these features within and around their bony substrates. Such positioning alone may be sufficient to create the desired approximation. Portrait artists, and especially caricaturists, are well aware of the significance of facial proportions in determining an individual countenance. To quote the distinguished caricaturist Mort Drucker, "We all have the same features, it's the space between them, their proportions and relationships to one another that distinguish one face from another" (Gautier, 1985:99).

Achieving this alignment is the ultimate challenge for the forensic artist and demands a firm grasp of soft–hard tissue correlations, i.e., an exact knowledge of how the soft tissue landmarks of the face relate to the craniometric

Forensic Analysis of the Skull, pages 215–227, ©1993 Wiley-Liss, Inc.

points of the skull. The portrait artist has a subject, the illustrator may rely on the idealized artistic canons of facial proportion in creating characters, but the forensic artist has only the skull. The forensic artist must know what a living face looks and "feels" like, must understand the idealized geometry of the face, and, most importantly, must be an expert in facial anatomy.

These prerequisites lead to natural difficulties resulting from variances in artistic skills. A valid criticism of forensic facial reconstruction is that given the same skull, different artists will create totally different faces. The fact that artists have individual styles is certainly a critical factor, but even so, 10 portraitists drawing or painting Elizabeth Taylor in a variety of media will still produce Ms. Taylor's unmistakable countenance. The more critical problem, the one that clouds the entire field of forensic facial reconstruction, is the current lack of standardization of both methods and measurements. For example, soft tissue thickness data have been obtained in different ways (from embalmed cadavers, autopsy subjects, and X-rays) and are variously lumped and split by sex, race, and nutritional status of the subjects. Thus it is not surprising that the tissue-thickness tables so produced are inconsistent. The goal here is to standardize these tables point by anthropometric point. The most accurate method of obtaining these data is yet to be determined, though the recent application of ultrasound by Helmer (1984) shows great promise. Forensic artists are thus in limbo as to which table to select. Refining these data remains a major and valid area of research in forensic anthropology.

Other inconsistencies arise from the use of contrasting methods. Sculptural methods require different individual techniques from those employed by graphic artists drawing directly over skull photographs or craniographs. Here, I believe the advantage lies initially with the graphic artists, whose techniques are simpler to control. Profile and frontal views worked out by graphic methods can then serve as "blueprints" for more advanced sculptural reconstructions. There is also no reason for this apparent dichotomy, in that any qualified forensic artist should be experienced with both methods. My suggestion is simply that a graphic reconstruction be worked out before attempting a more complex sculpture. To date, unfortunately, graphic and sculptural reconstructions of the same skull have yielded quite different results (İşcan and Charney, 1981).

Photographic superimposition is a more objective method but can only be applied in those cases in which photographs of the decedent(s) have already been retrieved. It is then possible to fit the photographs to the skull (or several skulls to a single photograph) in order to measure anatomical congruence. This comparison effectively eliminates unfit candidates and is the method of choice when leads have already been generated. Even though this is a "nonreconstructive" technique, it still relies on the same craniofacial correlates that are basic to the artistic methods. In the following sections, some basic guidelines are presented for fitting a face to an unidentified skull.

BASIC CAUCASOID FACIAL FEATURES

Before discussing craniofacial landmarks and correlations, it is necessary to identify those features that give the face its unique recognizability. Since the Caucasoid face has received the most attention from artists (with regard to canons of proportion) and orthodontists and maxillo-facial surgeons in the clinical literature, it will serve as the model for this study. In the comprehensive analysis of personal appearance identification by Paley and Zavala (1972:44–54), more than 70 facial attributes were listed that enable one person to recognize another. Those features that are critical to the forensic artist, as opposed to eyewitnesses, may be categorized as follows:

Facial Shape

1. Contours

2. Bilateral asymmetry

Skin

1. Coloring

2. Complexion

3. Blemishes

Hair

1. Head

a. Style (amount, length, hairline)

b. Color

2. Facial

a. Mustache (as above)

b. Beard (as above)

Ear

1. Position

2. Shape

3. Length

4. Angle (to Frankfort plane)

Eye

1. Position

2. Browline—thickness

3. Shape (with lids opened)—width, height

4. Location of medial and lateral canthi

5. Iris color

6. Lid folds

Nose

1. Position

2. Length

3. Width

4. Bridge line

5. Tip angle

6. Tip shape

7. Nostril shape

Lips

1. Position

2. Thickness (upper and lower)

3. Width

4. Shape (including sulci in profile view)

5. Color

Teeth (especially the anterior dentition)

Chin

1. Contour

2. Dimpling

It should be evident that most of these attributes, e.g., hairstyle, ear shape, eye color, and
so on, are beyond the reach of the
reconstructionist working from the bare skull
alone. However, cases do occur in which soft
tissues persist, thus increasing the number of
attributes that can be incorporated in the reconstruction. In a recent forensic case, for example, I had autopsy photographs of a young
woman who had been partially defleshed by
desert scavengers. Though her primary facial
features were largely destroyed, the photographs
clearly revealed her hair (long, blonde, straight),
large patches of skin (pale, taut, blemished), her
brow, an intact ear (uniquely curved), and her
chin and lower lip. Thus, depending on the
condition of the subject, it may be possible in
some cases to accurately reconstruct most of the
above-listed attributes. In the majority of "bare
bones" cases, however, the artist must rely on
the standard methods of reconstruction
(Caldwell, 1981; Gatliff, 1984; Krogman and
İşcan, 1986; George, 1987), concentrating on
the proper alignment of features and developing
common variations where appropriate.

CRANIOFACIAL LANDMARKS

The main task confronting the
reconstructionist or superimpositionist is the
correlation of cranial skeletal landmarks
(craniometric points) with their soft tissue coun-
terparts (cephalometric points). While a great
many of these landmarks are recognized in classical craniometry and cephalometry, only those
that are of critical importance to the forensic
artist have been selected here for definition and
illustration. The following definitions were taken
primarily from Bass (1987) and Rakosi (1982):

Craniometric Points (Figs. 1 and 2)

1. Inion (I): A point at the base of the external
occipital protuberance. It is the intersection of the
midsagittal plane (MSP) with a line drawn tangent to
the uppermost convexity of the superior nuchal line.

2. Lambda (L): The point of intersection of the

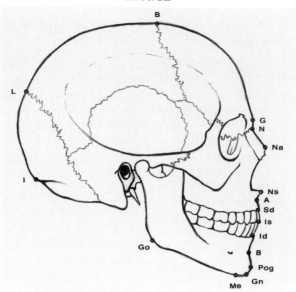

Fig. 1. Craniometric points, lateral view.

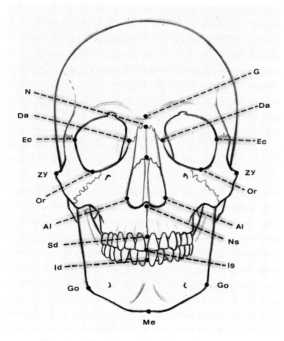

Fig. 2. Craniometric points, frontal view.

sagittal and lambdoidal sutures.

3. Bregma (B): The point of intersection of the sagittal and coronal sutures. The vertex (V) is the highest point of the skull and thus is not fixed.

4. Glabella (G): The most prominent point between the supraorbital ridges in the midsagittal plane (MSP).

5. Nasion (N): The midpoint of the suture between the frontal and the two nasal bones.

6. Nasale (Na): The anterior tip of the nasal bones at their junction with the lateral nasal cartilages.

7. Nasospinale (Ns): The point where a line drawn between the lower margins of the right and left nasal apertures is intersected by the MSP.

8. Alare (Al): The most lateral point on the nasal aperture.

9. Point A (Subspinale in anthropology): The deepest midline point on the indentation between the anterior nasal spine and the supradentale.

10. Supradentale (Sd: alveolare or prosthion in anthropology): The apex of the alveolus in the midline between the maxillary central incisors.

11. Incisor superius (Is): The tip of the crown of the most anterior maxillary central incisor.

12. Infradentale (Id): The apex of the alveolus in the midline between the mandibular central incisors.

13. Point B (Supramentale in anthropology): The deepest midline point on the indentation between the Id and Pog (see below).

14. Pogonion (Pog): The most anterior point in the midline on the mental protuberance.

15. Gnathion (Gn): A constructed point midway between the most anterior (Pog) and most inferior (Me; see below) points on the chin.

16. Menton (Me): The lowest point on the mandible (also considered as the most caudal point in the outline of the mental symphysis in X-rays).

17. Gonion (Go): A constructed point, the intersection of the lines tangent to the posterior margin of the ascending ramus and the mandibular base, or the most lateral point at the mandibular angle.

18. Zygion (Zy): The most lateral point on the zygomatic arch.

19. Dacryon (Da): The point of junction of the frontal, maxillary, and lacrimal bones on the medial wall of the orbit.

20. Ectoconchion (Ec): The most lateral point of the lateral wall of the orbit.

21. Orbitale (Or): The most inferior point on the margin of the orbit.

Cephalometric Points (Figs. 3 and 4)

1. Inion (I'): The soft tissue point directly above I.

2. Lambda (L'): The soft tissue point directly above L.

3. Bregma (B'): The soft tissue point directly above B. The vertex (V') is the highest point of the scalp.

4. Trichion (Tr): The point on the hairline (if present) in the MSP. There is no corresponding definitive craniometric point.

5. Glabella (G'): In the midline, the depression between the eyebrows.

6. Nasion (N'): In the midline, the point of maximum convexity between the nose and forehead. Frontally, this point is located at the midpoint of a tangent between the right and left superior palpebral folds.

7. Nasale (Na'): The soft tissue point directly above Na.

8. Subnasale (Sn): The midpoint of the columella base at the angle where the lower border of the nasal septum meets the upper lip.

9. Alare (Al'): The most lateral point on the alar contour.

10. Superior labial sulcus (Sls): The point of maximum indentation of the upper lip.

11. Labiale superius (Ls): The midpoint on the vermilion line of the upper lip.

12. Stomion (Sto): The point at the intersection of the MSP with the horizontal labial fissure between gently closed lips, with teeth shut in the natural position.

13. Labiale inferius (Li): The midpoint on the vermilion line of the lower lip.

14. Inferior labial sulcus (Ils): The point of maximum indentation of the lower lip, usually at its junction with the soft tissue chin.

15. Cheilion (Ch): The point located at each labial commissure.

16. Pogonion (Pog'): The most anterior point of the soft tissue chin.

17. Gnathion (Gn'): The point on the soft tissue chin midway between Pog' and Me' (see below).

18. Menton (Me'): The lowest point on the MSP of the soft tissue chin.

19. Gonion (Go'): The most lateral point of the jawline at the mandibular angle.

20. Zygion (Zy'): The most lateral point of the cheek (zygomaticomalar) region.

21. Ectocanthion (Ec): The point at the outer commissure (lateral canthus) of the palpebral fissure just medial to the malar tubercle (of Whitnall) to which the lateral palpebral ligaments are attached.

22. Endocanthion (En): The point at the inner commissure (medial canthus) of the palpebral fissure.

CRANIOFACIAL CORRELATIONS

In many illustrations depicting soft tissue thickness data, the overlying cephalometric points are drawn as perpendiculars from their underlying craniometric points. A perusal of Figures 5 and 6 shows that this is not always the case. Thus, in building a face in clay, sculptors should bevel their erasers or cork markers in order to achieve the proper alignment. The points over the scalp are of little consequence but have

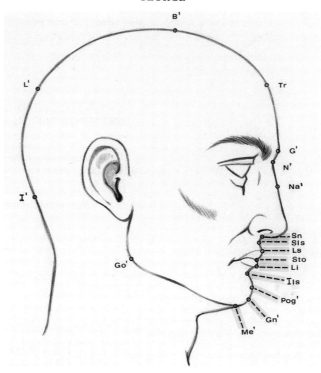

Fig. 3.   Cephalometric points, lateral view.

been included for completeness. For details and depths of the following correlations, see George (1987).

1. I/I': a direct perpendicular

2. L/L': a direct perpendicular

3. B/B': a direct perpendicular

4. G/G': a direct perpendicular

5. N/N': N' is usually 2–3 mm lower than N as determined from lateral craniographs.

6. Na/Na': a direct perpendicular

7. Ns/Sn: Sn is lower than Ns since the medial crus of the greater alar cartilage passes below the anterior nasal spine.

8. Al/Al': On the average, in Caucasoids, Al' is approximately 3 mm lateral to Al (Gatliff and Snow, 1979), but this point is highly variable.

9. Point A/Sls: While point A is fixed, Sls is highly variable. Usually, the upper lip is gently curved, but it may be markedly concave, straight, or convex. The midpoint of the curvature is generally lower

than point A. In some cases the artist must assume "lip strain."

10. Sd/Ls: In Caucasoids, the vermilion border of the upper lip cuts across the upper quarter mark of the maxillary central incisor and thus is lower than Sd.

11. Is/Sto: The stomion is variable and depends upon the state of tension of the lips. Usually, the oral fissure cuts across the lower third or quarter mark of the maxillary central incisor and thus is higher than Is.

12. Id/Li: Li is the most difficult point to assess. In general, the vermilion border of the lower lip cuts across the lower three-quarter mark of the mandibular central incisor and thus is slightly higher than Id.

13. Point B/Ils: Ils is also highly variable. In males this mentolabial contour is more acutely angled than in females and the Ils is usually higher than point B.

14. —/Ch: The cheilion has no direct craniometric counterpoint. In the lateral view, this point usually projects to the maxillary canine tooth, and in the frontal view to a point between the maxillary canine and first premolar. Accuracy in this projection is

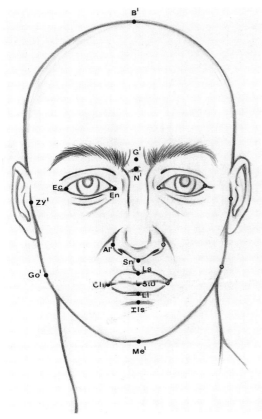

Fig. 4. Cephalometric points, frontal view.

foiled by dental variation.

15. Pog/Pog': Pog' is usually higher (slightly) than Pog, especially in males.

16. Gn/Gn': Gn' is a constructed point and will usually be anterior and inferior to Gn.

17. Me/Me': A direct perpendicular

18. Go/Go': By definition Go' is lateral and inferior to Go.

19. Zy/Zy': A direct lateral perpendicular

20. —/Ec: The ectocanthion has no direct craniometric counterpoint. This is an extremely critical point and projects into the orbit just medial to the malar tubercle (of Whitnall), to which the lateral palpebral ligaments are attached (Stewart, 1983).

21. —/En: The endocanthion has no direct craniometric counterpoint. This point is also extremely critical and projects into the orbit to the midpoint of the posterior (ethmoidal) border of the

lacrimal bone. It is important to note that the medial canthus is usually lower in its orbital projection than the lateral canthus.

ARTISTIC CANONS VERSUS ANTHROPOMETRIC NORMS

The basic observation and wonder that no two people look alike was early recorded by the Roman naturalist Pliny the Elder, who wrote in *Historia Naturalis* (Rackham, 1938:511):

The human features and countenance, although composed of but some ten parts or little more, are so fashioned that among so many thousands of men there are no two in existence who cannot be distinguished from one another.

Pliny, of course, was not the first philosopher to take note of human facial variability. He was easily preceded by the great Greek sculptors, who viewed the phenomenon as an artistic challenge, one of discovering within this seemingly endless range of variation the ideal dimensions of human facial form. Toward this end they constructed the first artistic canons of facial proportion, subjectively guided by their own finely tuned concepts of aesthetics. It must be realized that these so-called canons are not true laws in the scientific sense but merely guidelines for the spacing of facial features in a symmetrical, harmonious, and balanced pattern. And they have changed through time. For example, the Greek ideals of Praxiteles, Phidias, and Polyclitus gave way to the neoclassical Renaissance canons of Francesca and Pacioli, Michelangelo and da Vinci, which in turn were later refined by Dürer, Schadow, and so on (note: Figs. 3 and 4 are tracings of Michelangelo's *David,* sans hair).

Modern anthropometric norms, on the other hand, are scientifically based on statistical means and take into account variations in age, sex, and race. These measurements reveal the actual versus the geometrical ideal, with what is as opposed to what should be. Despite their different objectives, however, both artistic and

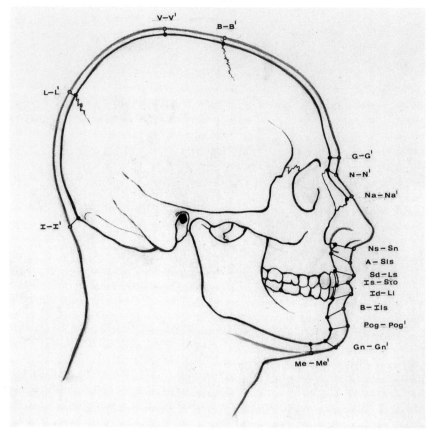

Fig. 5. Craniofacial correlations, lateral view.

anthropometric canons are similar because of the Western artistic view that the ideal face represents a composite of its wide-ranging variants. Da Vinci and Francis Bacon would argue that perfect beauty is never average, but then neither is perfect ugliness. They are the extremes in any given culture.

The exercise of reducing the human facial population to an ideal average is the opposite of that confronting the forensic artist, who must instead proceed from the average to the specific with only the bare skull as a guide. The averages here refer to the average soft tissue thicknesses that have been plotted in various ways for each of the major craniometric points. But tissue thicknesses alone tell little about the critical relations existing between the primary facial features, especially in the frontal view.

In a monumental study of anthropometric facial proportions of normal North American and western European Caucasoid children and young adults, Farkas and Munro (1987) compiled exhaustive tables of facial indices and in a separate chapter analyzed the validity of the neoclassical canons of facial proportion. This work plus the invaluable treatise by Powell and Humphreys (1984) on facial esthetics are the essential references for the following cephalometric descriptions.

1. Facial height canons (Fig. 7): There are several canons for subdividing the face:

a. Two-section division (V'–N' = N'–Me')

b. Three-section division (Tr–N' = N'–Sn = Sn–Me')

c. Four-section division (V'–Tr = Tr–G' = G'–Sn

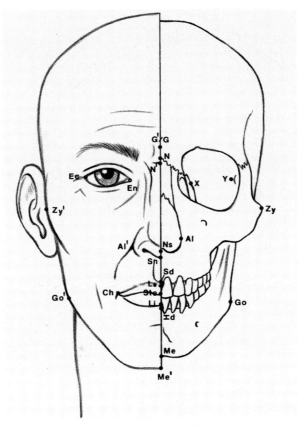

Fig. 6. Craniofacial correlations, frontal view. X, orbital projection of En (to the ethmoidal border of the lacrimal bone); Y, orbital projection of Ec (just medial to the malar tubercle of Whitnall).

= Sn–Me')

In the Farkas-Munro study, the two-section canon was observed in only 10% of the sample and the other idealized proportions were not seen at all. The artistic rule of thumb is that N'–Sn = Sn–Me'; i.e., the distance from the root of the nose to the bottom of the chin is equal to the length of the nose. In reality this makes for a very long nose. In most individuals, N'–Sn < Sn–Me', with a 43% to 57% division representing the norm. This is a vital measurement for reconstruction artists and can be easily taken from the skull.

2. Naso-labio-mental proportions (Fig. 7): There are two artistic canons for subdividing the lower face.

a. Three-section division: (Sn–Sto = Sto–Ils = Ils–Me')

b. Four-section division: (Sn–Sto = Sto–Ils = Ils–Pog' = Pog'–Me')

In a detailed study of these particular canons, Farkas et al. (1984) determined that the average values are closer to 31.2% (Sn–Sto), 26.2% (Sto–Ils), and 42.6% (Ils–Me').

3. Orbital proportion canon (Fig. 8): The distance between the eyes is equal to the width of an eye (En–En = Ec–En).

This canon was true in one-third of the study sample. However, the interocular distance (En–En) was greater than the eye width (Ec–En) in 51.5% of subjects. The ratio 32:36:32 is closer to the norm.

4. Orbitonasal proportion canon (Fig. 8): The distance between the eyes is equal to the width of the nose (En–En = Al'–Al').

This was true in 40.8% of study cases. For comparison, En–En < Al'–Al' in 37.9% and En–En >

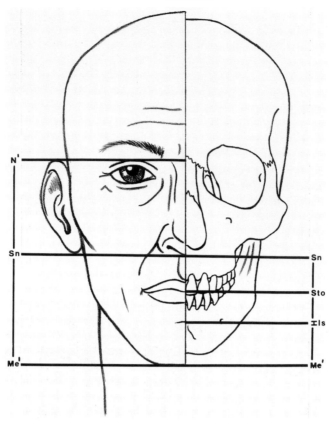

Fig. 7. Facial height proportions (N'–Sn–Me'). Naso-labio-mental proportions (Sn–Sto–Ils–Me').

Al'–Al' in 21.4%. This relationship is measured by drawing the cantho-alar line.

5. Iridio-oral proportion canon (Fig. 8): The width of the mouth is equal to the distance between the medial edges of the irides.

This relationship is measured by drawing the iridio-cheilial line (I–Ch). The interpupillary distance is frequently mentioned in art books, but this gives too wide a mouth. The interiridial distance is illustrated by Powell and Humphreys but without statistics.

6. Facial triangle (Fig. 9): The triangle formed between the lateral canthi (Ec) and the midpoint of the lower lip (Li) is equilateral.

This intriguing relationship is illustrated in an excellent art book by Hamm (1982). In my own studies I have found this canon to be remarkably constant, but here again statistics are lacking. For the reconstruction artist, it is worth noting that the tri-

angle persists in a smiling expression. It is the upper lip that is mobile.

7. Facial "X" (Fig. 10): Lines drawn from the lateral canthi to the corners of the mouth will cross very close to Sn.

This is another intriguing relationship for which there is little statistical data. Still, for the reconstruction artist it is a very handy measurement for cross-checking one's final sketch or sculpture.

By no means does this short list exhaust all known facial relationships. It is possible of course to create facial squares, rectangles, trapezoids, circles, and indices ad infinitum. The seven canons mentioned above, however, are the most critical for the forensic artist, especially for reconstructing the frontal view. The main message from the foregoing is simply that

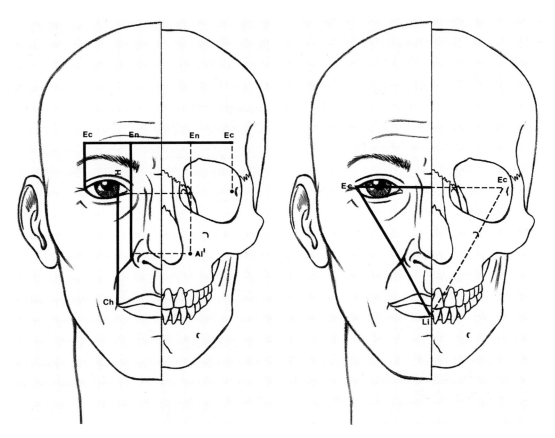

Fig. 8. Orbital proportions (Ec–En–En–Ec). Orbitonasal proportions (En–En = Al'–Al'). Iridiocheilial line (I–Ch).

Fig. 9. The facial triangle (Ec–Li–Ec).

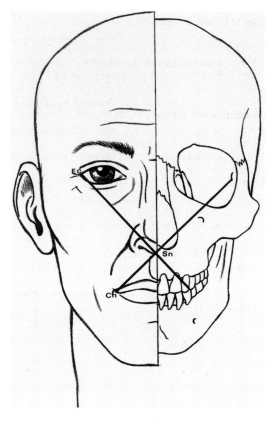

Fig. 10. The facial "X."

the desired lead. Achieving the proper alignment requires a detailed knowledge of craniofacial correlations. In addition to soft tissue thickness data, the artist must also know whether the corresponding points are perpendicular or angled, and, if the latter, by how much. It is also vital to know how best to connect adjacent sets of facial points. To quote Peck and Peck (1970), "the points themselves are meaningless. Ultimate appreciation of the profile depends upon the manner in which these points are connected. Harmonious profile flow may be visualized as a series of waves or reversed 'S, s' on the right profile." Thus, for example, the artist must know: (1) the distance from N–N'; (2) the direction N' takes from N; and (3) how best to connect points G' to N' to Na', and so on. All three of these requisites are valid areas for future research.

The frontal view is even more complex to reconstruct, and some artists lacking the required knowledge of craniofacial landmarks and their relations have been forced to rely on various artistic canons of facial proportion. This is a serious mistake because artistic canons reflect ideals. The forensic artist must always read the skull (or have it translated by a qualified anatomist or physical anthropologist) and not be led astray by artistic generalizations. Otherwise the end result will simply be the reconstruction of "generic" faces, i.e., each new reconstruction will resemble the last. And this should never happen, because to answer Pliny's question, like faces, no two skulls ever look exactly alike.

the neoclassical artistic canons must be treated with extreme caution and never substituted for a careful reading of the skull. The canons are useful rules of thumb, but to correctly position the eyes, nose, and mouth, craniometric landmarks must be followed, not artistic ideals.

SUMMARY

Forensic facial reconstruction is at best a scientific art. In its present state of development, it is not possible for any forensic artist to reconstruct with 100% accuracy the face formerly belonging to a given bare skull (though some intact soft tissues can greatly improve the odds). However, it is possible to accurately position the major facial features, and in some cases this alignment alone is enough to generate

REFERENCES

Bass WM (1987) Human Osteology: A Laboratory and Field Manual. Missouri Archaeological Society.

Caldwell MC (1981) The relationship of the details of the human face to the skull and its application in forensic anthropology. Master's thesis, Arizona State University.

Caldwell PC (1986) New questions (and some answers) on the facial reproduction techniques. In KJ Reichs (ed): Forensic Osteology: Advances in the Identification of Human Remains. Springfield, Ill: Charles C Thomas, pp 229–255.

Farkas LG, Katie MJ, Hreczko TA, Deutsch C, and Munro IR (1984) Anthropometric proportions in the upper lip–lower lip–chin area of the lower face in young white adults. Am J Orthodont 86(1):52–60.

Farkas LG, and Munro IR (1987) Anthropometric Facial Proportions in Medicine. Springfield, Ill: Charles C Thomas, pp 57–66.

Gatliff BP (1984) Facial sculpture on the skull for identification. Am J Forensic Med Pathol 5(4):327–332.

Gatliff BP, and Snow CC (1979) From skull to visage. J Biocommun 6(2):27–30.

Gautier D (1985) The Art of Caricature. New York: Perigee Books.

George RM (1987) The lateral craniographic method of facial reconstruction. J Forensic Sci 32(5):1305–1330.

Hamm J (1982) Drawing the Head and Figure. New York: Perigee Books.

Helmer R (1984) Schadelidentifizierung durch elektronische Bildmischung: Zugl e Beitr zur Konstitutionsbiometrie U Dickermessung d Geshichtsweichteile. Heidelberg: Kriminalistik-Verlag.

İşcan MY, and Charney M (1981) Two-dimensional versus three-dimensional facial reconstruction. AAFS Program 1981, Abstract 173, p 47.

Krogman WM, and İşcan MY (1986) The Human Skeleton in Forensic Medicine. Springfield, Ill: Charles C Thomas.

Paley JJ, and Zavala A (1972) Personal Appearance Identification. Springfield, Ill: Charles C Thomas.

Peck H, and Peck S (1970) A concept of facial esthetics. Angle Orthodontist 40(4):284–318.

Powell N, and Humphreys B (1984) Proportions of the Aesthetic Face. New York: Thieme-Stratton.

Rackham H (1938) Pliny-Historia Naturalis. Vol 2, bk 7. Cambridge, Mass: Harvard University Press.

Rakosi T (1982) An Atlas and Manual of Cephalometric Radiography. London: Wolfe Medical Publications.

Snow CC, Gatliff BP, and McWilliams KR (1970) Reconstruction of facial features from the skull: An evaluation of its usefulness in forensic anthropology. Am J Phys Anthropol 33:221–227.

Stewart TD (1983) The points of attachment of the palpebral ligaments: Their use in facial reconstructions on the skull. J Forensic Sci 28(4):858–863.

Chapter 17

Assessment of the Reliability of Facial Reconstruction

Richard P. Helmer, S. Röhricht, D. Petersen, and F. Möhr

Experimentelle Rechtsmedizin, Institut für Rechtsmedizin der Universität Bonn D-5300 Germany (R.P.H.); Institut für Rechtmedizin, Christian-Albrechts-Universität, Kiel, Germany (S.R., D.P., F.M.)

Attempts to attribute an unknown skull to the photograph of a missing person using the video superimposition technique (VST) represent a direct comparison of the features of the skull with those in the photograph. This generally acknowledged procedure should not be viewed as a mere superimposition of pictures of the skull and face (Helmer, 1980, 1984, 1986; Helmer and Grüner, 1977; Helmer and Beutner, 1988). It must also account for the topographical and anatomical relationships between skull bones and soft tissue, the proportions of the skull and face, as well as all of the other morphological aspects that combine to give the face its individuality.

The identification of a skull via VST requires that the examiner know numerous soft tissue measurements and be familiar with the topography of the skull and face. In the authors' experience, the stated preconditions for this technique enable the expert to assemble a plastic reconstruction of the soft tissue of the head. It is not uncommon to be asked to do a facial reconstruction as a method of last resort in cases where a photograph is not available.

Responses from 33 forensic anthropologists indicated that facial reconstruction is frequently used in the United States (Caldwell, 1981). Forty-two percent said they used this method to identify unknown skulls, 30% used graphic facial reconstruction, and 27% favored photographic superimposition. In the former Soviet Union, Gerassimow (1968) and his team claim to have produced numerous facial reconstructions.

The question of whether a plastic reconstruction of soft tissue on the skull can be regarded as

a serious attempt at identifying an unknown person is closely related to the question of whether a model face with any resemblance to the face of the person in question can be reproduced. Moreover, one must decide what conditions are necessary for this procedure to have validity. Over the years, this question has been examined in many ways by many investigators with highly variable results (Eggeling, 1913; Stadtmüller, 1922; Diedrich, 1926; Gerassimow, 1955, 1968; Snow et al., 1970; Gatliff and Snow, 1979) (Table 1).

It is obvious from the results of these investigations that no consensus has been reached. Von Eggeling and Stadtmüller report slight to no resemblance of the reconstructed face with that of the individual and concluded that a reconstruction provides only an approximation of basic head type. In contrast, Gerassimow concluded that a definite resemblance was established in all of his cases. In between lie the findings of Snow et al. (1970), as well as Gatliff and Snow (1979), who express guarded optimism that reconstruction may produce a face bearing a fundamental resemblance to the unknown individual. The degree of similarity, however, could vary from "relatively little resemblance" to "surprisingly accurate resemblance."

As a measure of the effectiveness of reconstruction, the cases representing successful identification of unknown skulls could be examined. Gerassimow (1968) reported that virtually all of approximately 140 court-ordered reconstructions carried out in his laboratory could be identified. Gatliff and Snow (1979) claim a 70% success rate ($N = 33$). Successful cases

TABLE 1. Overview of Facial Reconstruction Methods Used in Individual Studies

	Eggeling (1913)	Stadtmüller (1922)	Diedrich (1926)	Gerassimow (1955, 1968)	Snow et al. (1970)	Present Study (1989)
No. of cases	1	3	5	12	4	12
No. of facial recon- structions	2	6	5	12	4	24
Investiga- tion concept	Double- blind trial	Double- blind trial	Single- blind trial	Single- blind trial	Single- blind trial	Double- blind trial
Resemblance check based on	Death masks	Corpse photos, death masks	Traced- over corpse photos	Corpse photos	Photos of the living	Photos of the living

were also reported by Krogman (1946), Nagayasu (cited by Furuhata and Yamamoto, 1967), Suzuki (1973), Rathbun (1984), Rhine (1984), and Neave (1988).

Several examples of plastic facial reconstructions from Helmer's personal experience are shown in Figures 1–7.

In the end, however, the successes achieved with this method were not convincing. In many cases it is unclear whether successful identification was based on the quality of the facial reconstruction, or just improved the possibility that others will recognize that individual. Identification also could have stemmed from the particular circumstances and other findings associated with the case.

Consequently, an attempt was made to examine the following questions in a double-blind trial: Can two independent examiners produce similar reconstructions from the original skull, and how good is the resemblance between the reconstructed skull models and the living person?

EXPERIMENTAL ARRANGEMENT AND METHOD

The authors formed a research team and Röhricht and Petersen were assigned the task of

independently reconstructing the soft tissue on 12 identical casts of the original skulls. A preliminary test showed that both co-authors had sufficient and comparable technical and sculpting skill (cf. first reconstruction, Figs. 8 and 10) and neither had artistic training. The details of the procedure were as follows:

1. The molds for the skull and mandible were prepared from silicone and the skulls were cast from polyester resin. The casts were exact duplicates of the original skulls.

2. A specialist produced sets of glass eyes according to measurements from the original skulls.

3. A plan for the reconstruction was drawn up before the test was initiated. Sex, age, and constitutional type of the individual's skull were given as established data for a case investigation. In addition, all important topographic and morphologic details were studied on the original skull. Based on the experience of the team director (Helmer), soft tissue thickness was determined at 34 measuring points on the skull.

4. According to the plans, each member of the reconstruction team independently produced 12 model faces on the respective casts. Problems that arose were discussed individually with the team director, who had no access to antemortem photographs of the individuals in question during this stage of the investigation.

5. Results were discussed jointly only after completion of the respective reconstructions.

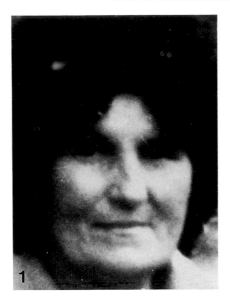
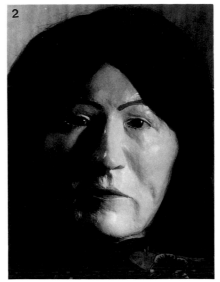
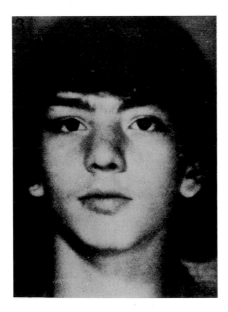
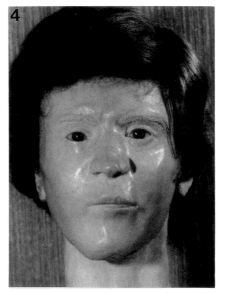

Fig. 1. Photograph of case 1, 1980 murder victim, identified as female, approximately 40 years old (presumed foreigner), height 160 cm, weight 70 kg, obese, dark brown hair up to 45 cm in length, hands and feet free of calluses, fingernails relatively long and manicured, painted red.

Fig. 2. Reconstruction of case 1 in Figure 1.

Fig. 3. Photograph of case 2, 1983 murder victim, identified as young male approximately 20 years old, height about 176 cm, weight approximately 65 kg, boyish build, dark blond hair up to 12 cm in length; exceptional feature: alveolar prognathism of the upper jaw.

Fig. 4. Reconstruction of case 2 in Figure 3.

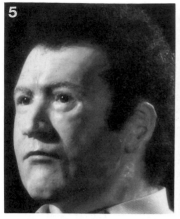 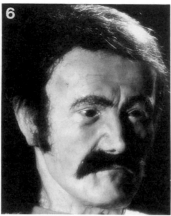 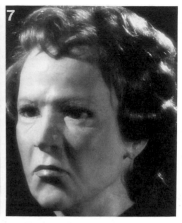

Fig. 5. Reconstruction of case 3, 1984 unidentified, 40–50-year-old male (presumed foreigner, maybe southern European) height 170–175 cm, slender build, short, dark brown hair.

Fig. 6. Reconstruction of case 4, 1985 unidentified murder victim, 40–50-year-old male, height 174 cm, lanky, slim build, dark blond straggly hair combed to the back and up to 10 cm in length, mustache; exceptional features: very poor dental maintenance with partial maxillary denture, mandibular atrophy like that of an extremely old individual.

Fig. 7. Reconstruction of case 5, 1986 unidentified murder victim, 25–35-year-old female, height approximately 160 cm, petite build, short hairstyle, slightly wavy hair dyed a dark reddish blond.

6. A systematic comparison of the reconstructions with each other and with the photographs was made. Finally, the hairstyle was recreated and the finishing touches were applied by a makeup artist (Möhr) corresponding to the photos of the individuals.

With reference to points 2 and 3, it should be noted that the measurements used for soft tissue thickness were established from living persons of all age groups using ultrasound. These values were then "individualized" according to sex, age, and constitutional type (Helmer, 1980, 1984; Helmer and Leopold, 1984).

Compulsory guidelines for the shaping of facial morphology were compiled based on the findings of Merkel (1885–90), Kollmann (1910), Wilder (1912), Stadtmüller (1922), Gerassimow (1955, 1968—the latter results being clearly presented by Ullrich, 1959, 1966), Lebedinskaya (1957), and Krogman (1973), to the extent that they were compatible with each other, as well as with personal experience. We used eyeball prostheses as suggested by Gatliff (1984) because they resulted in a more lifelike appearance.

For the assessment of resemblance between reconstructions, a rating system was chosen that permitted the evaluation of significant details of the model faces as follows:

1—great resemblance
2—close resemblance
3—approximate resemblance
4—slight resemblance
5—no resemblance.

The assessment focused on the following points, whereby the overall impression with regard to the achieved degree of resemblance by no means represents the sum of individual valuations:

1. General impression with regard to age
2. General impression with regard to sex

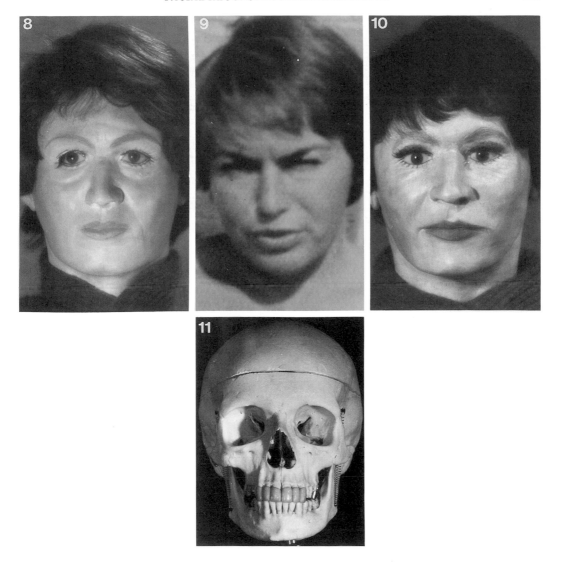

Figs. 8–11. Skull, comparison photograph, and facial reconstruction of a 30–40-year-old female. Constitutional diagnosis from the skull: metromorph, slightly hyperplastic.

3. General impression with regard to body constitution

  4. Profile

  5. Eye region

  6. Nose

  7. Mouth region

  8. Chin region

9. Overall impression of the reconstruction

In the assessment of profile, three regions were distinguished:

  1. Region above the nose

  2. Middle part of the face

  3. Lower part of the face

The following features and regions were examined:

Eye

1. Run of the margin of the eyelid
2. Length of the margin of the eyelid
3. Upper eyelid
4. Lower eyelid
5. Width of palpebral fissure including the position of the canthus
6. Position and run of the eyebrow

Nose

1. Length of the nose
2. Width of the nose
3. Shape of the root of the nose
4. Run of the bridge of the nose
5. Shape of the sides of the nose

Mouth

1. Position of the mouth
2. Width of the mouth
3. Fullness of the lips
4. Curve of the lips
5. Form of the lips
6. Run of the oral fissure

Chin

1. Fullness
2. Form (width, length, point)

The evaluation of the reconstructions was then divided into two steps: (1) Comparison of reconstructions with each other considering the above-mentioned details, and (2) comparison of individual reconstructions with photographs of the individuals.

The evaluation was carried out on a series of photographs of the reconstructed model faces. The assessment of the reconstruction's resemblance with the original was made by three independent and unaffiliated persons whose individual judgments were averaged to maximally exclude subjective factors. Finally, in 3 of the total 12 reconstruction attempts, the video superimposition technique was used to compare the reconstructions with each other, as well as with the original photograph of the individual.

COMPARISON OF THE RECONSTRUCTIONS

As can be seen in Table 2 and Figures 8–59, a comparison of the reconstructions with each other provided the following results in relation to the general impression: 50% of the cases presented approximate resemblance, while 33% showed close resemblance. In two of the cases (17%) only limited resemblance was achieved. The reconstructions showed good to very good agreement with regard to age and sex. The most

TABLE 2. Comparison of the 12 Reconstructed Pairs With Each Other

Frequency in Percent Assessment Rating[a]	1	2	3	4	5
General impression with regard to age	50	33	17		
General impression with regard to sex	75	17		8	
General impression with regard to constitution	25	42	17	17	
Profile	17	42	33	8	
Eye region	8	25	8	59	
Nose	8	50	25	17	
Mouth region		25	8	50	17
Chin region	17	8	50	25	
Overall impression		33	50	17	

[a]Assessment ratings: 1, Great resemblance; 2, close resemblance; 3, approximate resemblance; 4, slight resemblance; 5, no resemblance (see text for further details).

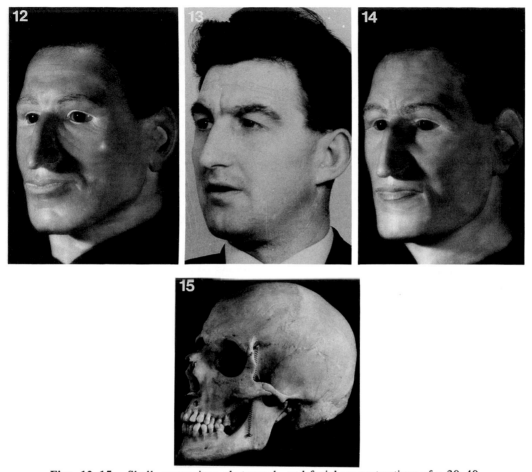

Figs. 12–15. Skull, comparison photograph, and facial reconstructions of a 30–40-year-old man. Constitutional diagnosis from the skull: leptomorph, hyperplastic.

frequent and largest discrepancies were seen in the mouth and eye regions, while in most cases, the nose was reproduced to approximate or close likeness.

It became apparent that each reconstructor developed his own personal style of reconstruction during the course of the experiment. It is important to note, however, that while technical ability greatly improved during the course of 12 reconstructions, this did not influence the results.

In general it was observed that with proper methodological instruction and adherence to the standardized principles of reconstruction,

various reconstructors working on the same skull were able to reproduce a facial model with approximate to close resemblance. Greater discrepancies in detail occurred when the reconstructors deviated from standardized principles. Noncompliance occurred for a number of reasons; for example, due to the vagueness or apparent deficiency of specific standards, or the inexperience of the reconstructor.

Next, the reconstructions were compared with photographs of the individuals, and the following results were obtained for all reconstructions ($N = 24$): 38% showed close resemblance to the original, 17% approximate resemblance, and

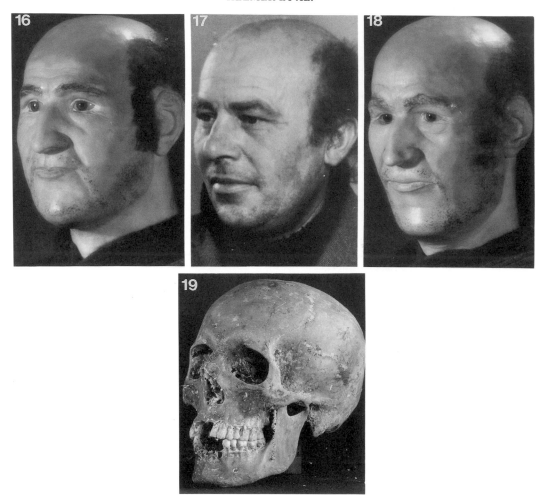

Figs. 16–19. Skull, comparison photograph, and facial reconstructions of a 50–60-year-old man. Constitutional diagnosis from the skull: pyknomorph, slightly hyperplastic. Exceptional features: old fracture of the bridge of the nose, deficiency of front teeth not corrected prosthetically.

42% slight resemblance (Table 3). There was no resemblance in only one case (see Figs. 20–22). More specifically, the reconstructors were able to reproduce the given age and sex of the individual with good to very good accuracy. Greater discrepancy between the original and the reconstructions was found, as anticipated, in the mouth and eye regions, while the nose was reconstructed, for the most part, with approximate to close resemblance.

The most constant agreement in resemblance was produced in relation to the facial profile. Factors related to body constitution also proved to be effectively reproducible characteristics. It was found that skulls with particularly marked characteristics in relation to age, constitution, or illness were the most easily reproduced (see Figs. 12–19). Poorer results were obtained for female and younger individuals (see Figs. 20–22 and 42–44).

In general it can be said that at least a slight and often even a close resemblance was achieved

TABLE 3. Comparison of the 12 Reconstructed Pairs With the Photograph

Assessment Rating[a]	1st Examiner Frequency in Percent					2nd Examiner Frequency in Percent				
	1	2	3	4	5	1	2	3	4	5
General impression with regard to age	42	42	8	8		42	33	17	8	
General impression with regard to sex	84	8		8		92				8
General impression with regard to constitution	33	67				25	33	25	17	
Profile	8	67	25				67	25	8	
Eye region		25	50	17	8		42	42	17	
Nose	25	50	25			8	67	8	17	
Mouth region	8	17	42	33			50	42	8	
Chin region		75	17	8			33	50	8	
Overall impression		42	8	50			33	25	33	8

[a]Assessment ratings: 1, Great resemblance; 2, close resemblance; 3, approximate resemblance; 4, slight resemblance; 5, no resemblance (see text for further details).

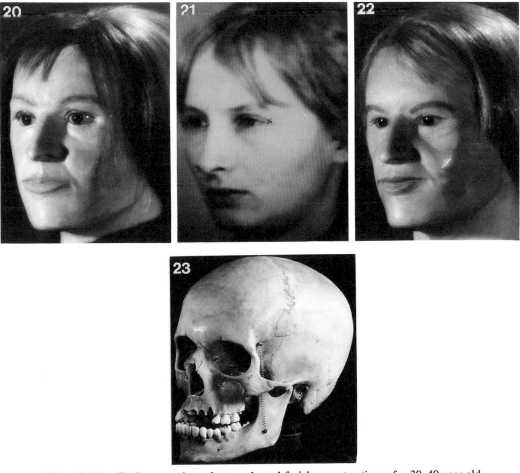

Figs. 20–23. Skull, comparison photograph, and facial reconstructions of a 30–40-year-old woman. Constitutional diagnosis from the skull: metromorph, slightly dysmorph, hypoplastic.

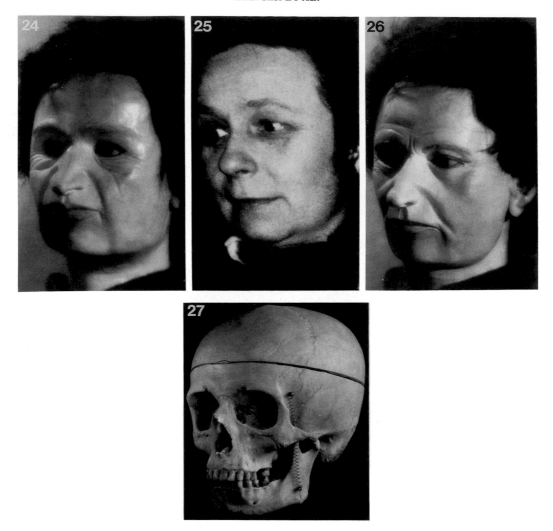

Figs. 24–27. Skull, comparison photograph, and facial reconstructions of a 45–55-year-old woman. Constitutional diagnosis from the skull: pyknomorph to dysmorph, metroplastic.

between the 24 reconstructions and the originals. The extent of similarity was strongly influenced by notable characteristics of the skull. As was found for the comparison of the reconstructions with each other, deviation in terms of the overall impression as well as facial detail occurred most frequently when the reconstructor was unable to follow compulsory guidelines for the reconstruction of morphological details of the soft tissues.

Basic information about the length and color of hair and the hairstyle is essential for every serious attempt at this type of identification. A replica without hair has very limited resemblance to most individuals (see Figs. 36–41 and 46–51). In our experience, a purely intuitive interpretation of hairstyle added to a reconstruction can result in similarity with the individual only by chance and is therefore not dependable.

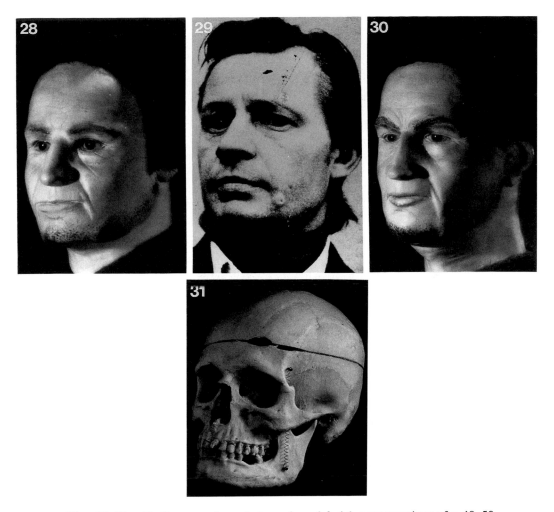

Figs. 28–31. Skull, comparison photograph, and facial reconstructions of a 40–50-year-old man. Constitutional diagnosis from the skull: pyknomorph, slightly hyperplastic.

CONCLUSIONS

The early work of Gerassimow and others concerning the influence of facial bone morphology on the construction and form of soft tissues have made present advances in facial reconstruction possible. Additionally, we have improved our knowledge of facial tissue thickness by studying living persons (Helmer, 1980, 1984; see also Chapter 14, Lebedinskaya et al., this volume). Individual cases and basic demo-graphic research have provided information on age, sex, and constitutional type (see Chapter 6, Novotný et al., and Chapter 14, Leopold et al., this volume). Further advances in reconstruction techniques can be expected when the results of other studies in this field are disseminated (e.g., Rhine and Campbell, 1980; Hodson et al., 1985a,b; Dumont, 1986; Helmer et al., 1986; Macho, 1986; Arries, 1987; Lebedinskaya et al., 1988).

Compulsory guidelines for basic methodology are as essential for every useful attempt at

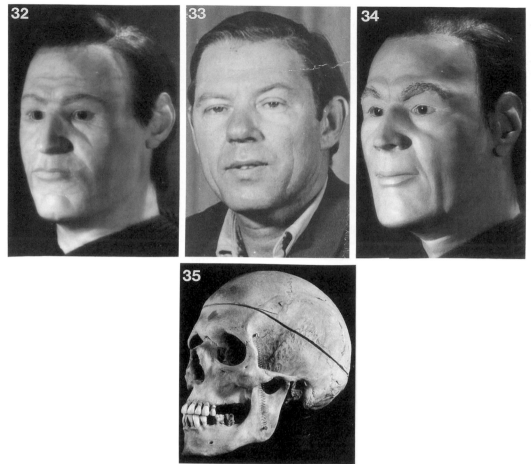

Figs. 32–35. Skull, comparison photograph, and facial reconstructions of a 50–60-year-old man. Constitutional diagnosis from the skull: pyknomorph, hyperplastic.

facial reconstruction. Because the problems involved in the practical application of these techniques are numerous, experience is of primary importance. Our experience has shown, however, that it is not necessary to have a trained artist or sculptor perform the practical work because the result can be negatively influenced by creative intuition. A better approach to test the accuracy of reconstructors would be a series of tests with the participation of several veteran researchers.

What specific expectations can we hold for reconstruction as a means for identifying unknown individuals in relation to our present knowledge? The answer to this question can be found in the following observations by Neave (1980, 1988):

It is, therefore, possible to reconstruct the major features of the human head with some degree of accuracy. However, a reconstruction can only reveal the type of face that may have existed—the position and general shape of the main features can be accurate reconstructions but subtle details such as wrinkles and folds are inevitably speculative as there is no evidence as to their form or even their existence. It appears that facial reconstruction depends as much upon the circumstances pertaining to the subject under investigation as it does upon the accuracy of the technique in order to be successful.

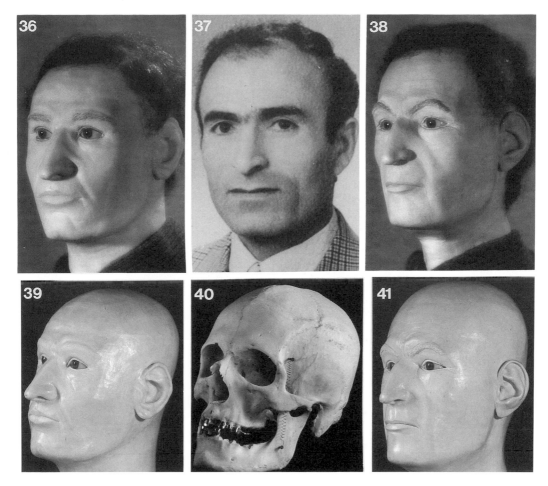

Figs. 36–41. Skull, comparison photograph, and facial reconstructions of a 30–40-year-old man, before and after makeup-artist workover. Constitutional diagnosis from the skull: slightly leptomorph, metroplastic. Exceptional feature: presumably a Turk due to the type of denture.

Gatliff (1984) further states:

Facial sculpture is used as a last-ditch effort when other identifying techniques such as publicizing physical characteristics, describing clothing, and searching missing persons bulletins, etc. have been unsuccessful. The outcome is uncertain in every case, but if the sculpture is done correctly and as accurately as possible within the limitations of the technique, it is usually worth a try.

Our experience has shown that not only the medical professional or forensic anthropologist but also the criminologist plays an important role in the production of a successful facial reconstruction. In addition to the purely physical characteristics of the individual, further clues aid in establishing personal identity. Such factors as hair length and form, the existence of facial hair, signs of illness, or clues to the lifestyle and social standing of the individual are of primary importance and should be included in the reconstruction.

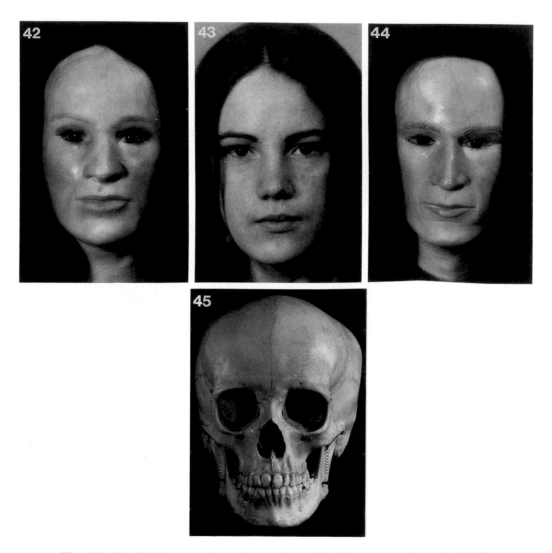

Figs. 42–45. Skull, comparison photograph, and facial reconstructions of a 15–20-year-old woman. Constitutional diagnosis from the skull: metromorph, slightly hypoplastic.

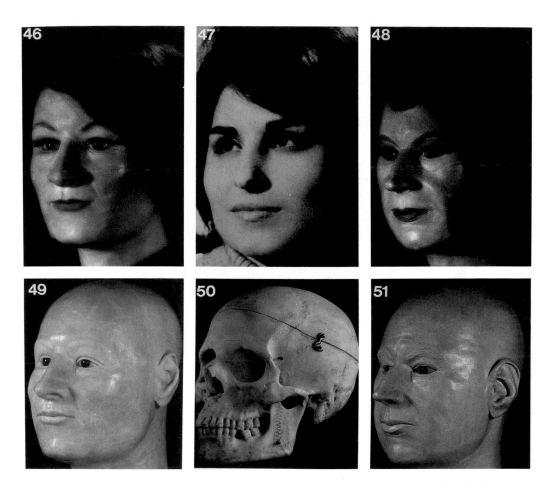

Figs. 46–51. Skull, comparison photograph, and facial reconstructions of a 30–40-year-old woman, before and after makeup-artist workover. Constitutional diagnosis from the skull: metromorph, hyperplastic.

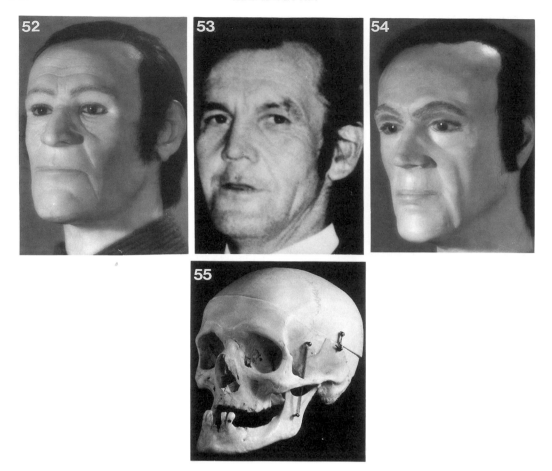

Figs. 52–55. Skull, comparison photograph, and facial reconstructions of a 40–50-year-old man. Constitutional diagnosis from the skull: slightly pyknomorph, dysplastic. Exceptional features: deviation of lower jaw to the right, old mandible condylus fracture to the right, atrophy of the jaw, presumed complete denture-wearer.

REFERENCES

Arries KO (1987) A preliminary study of facial tissue thickness utilizing nuclear magnetic resonance imaging. Paper presented at the 39th Annual Meeting of the American Academy of Forensic Science, February 16–21, San Diego, Calif.

Caldwell MC (1981) The Relationship of the Details of the Human Face to the Skull and Its Application in Forensic Anthropology. MA thesis, Department of Anthropology, Arizona State University.

Caldwell MC (1986) New questions (and some answers) on the facial reproduction techniques. In KJ Reichs (ed): Forensic Osteology: Advances in the Identification of Human Remains. Springfield, Ill: Charles C Thomas, pp 229–255.

Diedrich F (1926) Ein Beitrag zur Prüfung der Leistungsfähigkeit der plastichen Rekonstruktionsmethode der Physiognomie bei der Identifizierung von Schädeln. Dtsch Z Ges Gerichtl Med 8:365–389.

Dumont ER (1986) Mid facial tissue depths of white children: An aid in facial feature reconstruction. J Forensic Sci 31(4):1463–1469.

Eggeling H v (1913) Die Leistungsfähigkeit physiognomischer Rekonstruktionsversuche auf Grundlage des Schädels. Arch Anthropol 12:44–47.

Furuhata T, and Yamamoto K (1967) Superimposition. In: Forensic Odontology. Springfield, Ill: Charles C Thomas, pp. 105–111.

Gatliff BP (1984) Facial sculpture on the skull for identification. Am J Forensic Med Pathol 5(4):327–332.

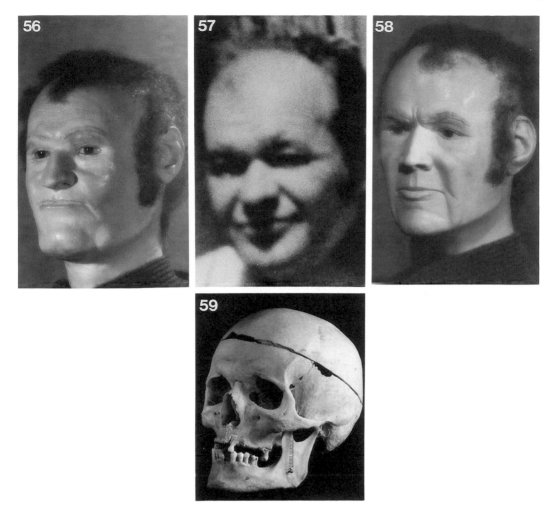

Figs. 56–59. Skull, comparison photograph, and facial reconstructions of a 35–45-year-old man. Constitutional diagnosis from the skull: pyknomorph, hyperplastic. Exceptional feature: questionable denture-wearer.

Gatliff BP, and Snow CC (1979) From skull to visage. J Biocommun 6(2):27–30.

Gerassimow MM (1955) Vosstalovlenie lica po cerepu. (Wiederherstellung des Gesichts aufgrund des Schädels), Izdat. Akad Nauk SSSR, Moscow.

Gerassimow MM (1968) Ich suchte Gesichter: C. Bertelsmann. Gütersloh.

Helmer R (1980) Schädelidentifizierung durch elektronische Bildmischung. Kiel: Habilitationsschrift.

Helmer R (1984) Schädelidentifizierung durch elektronische Bildmischung. Zugleich ein Beitrag zur Konstitutionsbiometrie und Dickenmessung der Gesichtsweichteile. Heidelberg: Kriminalstik-Verlag.

Helmer R (1986) Identifizierung der Leichenüberreste des Josef Mengele. Arch Krim 177:129–144.

Helmer R (1987) Identification of the cadaver remains of Josef Mengele. J Forensic Sci 32(6):1622–1644.

Helmer R, and Beutner KJ (1988) Computer-aided video superimposition applied to skull identification by picture comparison. Paper presented at the International Symposium "Advances in Skull Identification via Video Superimposition," 3–5 August, Kiel.

Helmer R, and Grüner O (1977) Vereinfachte Schädelidentifizierung nach dem Superprojektionsverfahren mit Hilfe einer Video-Anlage. Z Rechtsmed 80:183–187.

Helmer R, and Leopold D (1984) Neuere Aspekte zur Schädelidentifizierung. Kriminal Forens Wiss 55/56:82–88.

Helmer R, Koschorek F, Terwey B, and Frauen T (1986) Dickenmessung der Gesichtsweichteile mit Hilfe der Kernspintomographie zum Zwecke der Identifizierung. Arch Krim 178:139–150.

Helmer R, Schimmler J, and Rieger J (1989) On the conclusiveness of skull identification via the video superimposition technique. Can Soc Forensic Sci J 22(2):177–194.

Helmer R, Schimmler J, and Rieger J (1989) Zum Beweiswert der Schädelidentifizierung mit Hilfe der Video-Bildmischtechnik unter Berücksichtigung der kraniometrischen Individualität menschlicher Schädel. Z Rechtsmed 102:451–459.

Hodson G, Liebermann S, and Wright P (1985a) In vivo measurements of facial tissue thickness in American Caucasoid children. J Forensic Sci 30(4):1100–1112.

Hodson G, Liebermann LS, and Wright P (1985b) In vivo measurements of facial tissue thickness in American black children. Paper presented in the Physical Anthropology Section of the 37th Annual Meeting of the American Academy of Forensic Sciences, February 11–16, Las Vegas, Nevada 1985.

Kollmann J (1910) Plastische Anatomie des menschlichen Körpers. 3. Abschnitt: Schädel, 3rd ed. Leipzig: Veith.

Krogman WM (1946) The reconstruction of the living head from the skull. FBI Law Enforcement Bull 15(7):11–18.

Krogman WM (1973) The Human Skeleton in Forensic Medicine. Springfield, Ill: Charles C Thomas.

Lebedinskaya GV (1957) Kvoprosu ob ob'ektivnom vosproizvedenii razreza glaz pri rekonstrukzii lica po cerepu. Kratkie Soobsc Inst Etnogr 27:55–59.

Lebedinskaya GV, Balueva TS, and Veselovskaya EV (1988) Development of the theoretical principals of the method of reconstruction of the face on the skull (Current Results). Paper presented at the International Symposium "Advances in Skull Identification via Video Superimposition," 3–5 August, Kiel.

Macho GA (1986) An appraisal of plastic reconstruction of the external nose. J Forensic Sci 31(4):1391–1403.

Merkel F (1885–90) Handbuch der topographischen Anatomie. Bd 1, Braunschweig.

Nagayasu S (1962) A case of the restored moulage technique in regio facies. Report Nat Inst Police Sci 15(1) (cited in Furuhata and Yamamoto (1967)).

Neave R (1980) Facial reconstruction of skeletal remains: Three Egyptian examples. MASCA J 1(6):175–177.

Neave R (1988) Facial reconstruction of the unidentified King's cross fire victim and the great Harwood murder victim: An assessment of the problems and results. Paper presented at the International Symposium "Advances in Skull Identification via Video Superimposition," 3–5 August, Kiel.

Petersen D (1992) Die plastische Gesichtsweichteilrekonstruktion als Möglichkeit zur Identifizierung unbekannter Schädel. (I) Med Diss Kiel.

Rathbun TA (1984) Personal identification: Facial reproductions. In TA Rathbun and JE Buikstra (eds): Human Identification: Case Studies in Forensic Anthropology. Springfield, Ill: Charles C Thomas, pp 347–356.

Rhine JS (1984) Facial reproduction in court. In TA Rathbun and JE Buikstra (eds): Human Identification: Case Studies in Forensic Anthropology. Springfield, Ill: Charles C Thomas, pp 357–362.

Rhine JS, and Campbell HR (1980) Thickness of facial tissues in American blacks. J Forensic Sci 25(4):847–858.

Röhricht St (1993) Die plastische Gesichtsweichteilrekonstruktion als Möglichkeit zur Identifizierung unbekannter Schädel. (II) Med Diss Kiel.

Snow CC, Gatliff BP, and McWilliams KR (1970) Reconstruction of facial features from the skull: An evaluation of its usefulness in forensic anthropology. Am J Phys Anthropol 33:221–228.

Stadtmüller F (1922) Zur Beurteilung der plastischen Rekonstruktionsmethode der Physiognomie auf dem Schädel. Z Morphol Anthropol 22:337–372.

Suzuki T (1973) Reconstruction of a skull. Int Crim Pol Rev 28:76–80.

Ullrich H (1959) Die methodischen Grundlagen des plastischen Rekonstruktionsverfahren nach Gerassimow. Z Morphol Anthropol 49:245–258.

Ullrich H (1966) Kritische Bemerkungen zur plastischen Rekonstruktionsmethode nach Gerassimow aufgrund persönlicher Erfahrungen. Ethnogr-Archäol-Z (Berlin) 7:111–123.

Wilder H (1912) The physiognomy of the Indians of southern New England. Am Anthropol 14:415–436.

Index